NAPLEX® Review

THE COMPLETE GUIDE TO LICENSING EXAM CERTIFICATION FOR PHARMACISTS

2013–2014

NAPLEX® Review

THE COMPLETE GUIDE TO LICENSING EXAM CERTIFICATION FOR PHARMACISTS

2013–2014

Steven T. Boyd, PharmD, BCPS, CDE

Amie McCord Brooks, PharmD, FCCP, BCPS

Karen Nagel, BS Pharm, PhD

Cynthia Sanoski, BS, PharmD, FCCP, BCPS

Published by Kaplan Publishing, a division of Kaplan, Inc.
395 Hudson Street, 4th Floor
New York, NY 10014

Printed in the United States of America

10 9 8 7 6 5 4 3 2

ISBN-13: 978-1-60978-736-3

Kaplan Publishing books are available at special quantity discounts to use for sales promotions, employee premiums, or educational purposes. For more information or to purchase books, please call the Simon & Schuster special sales department at 866-506-1949.

About the Authors

Steven T. Boyd, PharmD, BCPS, CDE, is a former associate professor of clinical pharmacy at Xavier University. He received his Doctor of Pharmacy degree from the University of Nebraska and completed a primary care residency at the University of Mississippi. Dr. Boyd's primary and current research endeavors have focused on diabetes, weight loss, student education, medication therapy management, and pharmacoeconomic outcomes at employer worksites. He is a board-certified pharmacotherapy specialist, clinical pharmacist at Causey's Pharmacy, and serves as an instructor with Kaplan Medical, performing multiple NAPLEX reviews across the country.

Amie McCord Brooks, PharmD, FCCP, BCPS, is an associate professor of pharmacy practice at the St. Louis College of Pharmacy and a clinical pharmacy specialist in ambulatory care at St. Louis County Department of Health. Dr. Brooks is the program director for a PGY1 residency program, a board-certified pharmacotherapy specialist, and a fellow of the American College of Clinical Pharmacy. She received her Doctor of Pharmacy degree from the St. Louis College of Pharmacy and completed her pharmacy residency training at the Jefferson Barracks VA Medical Center in St. Louis, Missouri. Her research interests include clinical pharmacy services, diabetes, resistant hypertension, and collaborative practice.

Karen Nagel, BS Pharm, PhD, is an associate professor of pharmaceutical sciences at Midwestern University Chicago College of Pharmacy, where she teaches courses in pharmaceutics, compounding, and biotechnology. She has held national and local offices in pharmacy organizations, including chair of the basic sciences section of the APhA Academy of Pharmaceutical Research and Sciences, chair of the AACP Laboratory Special Interest Group, pharmaceutics section secretary in AACP, and treasurer and chair of the AAPS Chicago discussion group. Her research interests include herbal product analysis and pharmacy education.

Cynthia Sanoski, BS, PharmD, FCCP, BCPS, is the chair of the department of pharmacy practice at the Jefferson School of Pharmacy at Thomas Jefferson University. Dr. Sanoski received her Doctor of Pharmacy degree from Ohio State University, and subsequently completed a 2-year fellowship in cardiovascular pharmacotherapy at the University of Illinois at Chicago. She is also a board-certified pharmacotherapy specialist and a fellow of the American College of Clinical Pharmacy. Dr. Sanoski serves as an instructor with Kaplan Medical, teaching NAPLEX review courses for graduating pharmacy students across the country.

The authors wish to thank the following test item writers: LeAnn C. Boyd, PharmD, BCPS, CDE; Elizabeth Langan, MD; Amy Egras, PharmD, BCPS; Stacey Thacker, PharmD; and Arneka Tillman, PharmD candidate, Xavier University College of Pharmacy.

For Any Test Changes or Late-Breaking Developments

kaptest.com/publishing

The material in this book is up-to-date at the time of publication. However, the NABP® may have instituted changes in the test after this book was published. Be sure to carefully read the materials you receive when you register for the test. If there are any important late-breaking developments—or any changes or corrections to the Kaplan test preparation materials in this book—we will post that information online at kaptest.com/publishing.

Table of Contents

PART ONE

Overview

How to Use This Book

Congratulations! You've taken the first step to prepare yourself for the NAPLEX®. This book contains the information you want and need to do your best.

HIGHLIGHTS OF THE 2013-2014 EDITION

The authors are proud to release the 2013-2014 edition of this NAPLEX® review book. The entire book has been updated with the most current pharmacy information needed to pass the NAPLEX®, focusing on guideline changes and new drug approvals.

The most significant changes to this edition are as follows:

- new sections on antithrombotic drugs (chapter 1, Cardiovascular Disorders), smoking cessation (chapter 3, Pulmonary Disorders), Alzheimer's disease (chapter 8, Psychiatric Disorders), and therapeutic drug levels (chapter 16, Clinical Lab Tests)
- 30 new practice problems with detailed answer explanations (chapter 21, Calculations)
- expanded and enhanced treatment of the following:
  - all aspects of HIV (chapter 2, Infectious Diseases)
  - guidelines for acute uncomplicated cystitis and acute pyelonephritis (chapter 2, Infectious Diseases)
  - storage and administration for gastroesophageal reflux disease/peptic ulcer disease and signs/symptoms for ulcerative colitis and Crohn's disease (chapter 6, Gastrointestinal Disorders)
  - common adverse effects of chemotherapy agents (chapter 7, Oncology)
  - definition of athlete's foot (chapter 17, Over-the-Counter Medications)
- fully revised and updated Practice Test and Practice Test Answers and Explanations, both in the book and online
- updated Top 200 drug lists

REVIEW STRUCTURE

This content of this book is designed to provide a concentrated and concise review of the competency areas tested on the exam. This book is not intended to replace standard textbooks in pharmacy. Rather, it should serve as a primary tool in the weeks and months prior to taking the exam. Since it is not practical to re-read textbooks, you will need a resource that will provide concise, focused review. This book fills that need.

Kaplan suggests that areas in which you feel weakest should be studied first; in this way, you can spend additional review time on difficult concepts.

This book covers all of the areas tested on the NAPLEX® and features an efficient time-management tool to ensure adequate preparation. Each chapter includes a *suggested study time*, prepared by the authors. These are only suggested rates; certainly, the study rate will vary based on your own level of comfort with the subject matter. By gauging yourself, however, you will be able to practice for test day, when your time on the computer will be limited.

The review is arranged by disease states, focusing on the following:

- Definitions of the disease
- Diagnosis
- Signs and Symptoms
- Guidelines
- Guidelines Summary
- Medication Charts
- Storage & Administration Pearls
- Patient Education Pearls

Each chapter also contains a few practice questions, allowing you to apply the information you have just reviewed. The appendix at the end of the book provides tables of the top 200 prescription drugs by units sold, listed by both trade and generic names, which will help you with your memorization skills.

PRACTICE TESTS

The NAPLEX® is a computer-adaptive examination consisting of 185 questions. To assist you in preparing for the test-taking experience, this book offers two complete practice examinations of 185 questions each. One practice exam, along with answer explanations, is included in the text of this book. A second test is available online.

Practice Test 1 should be taken prior to the beginning of your study period. Then, use the results to identify areas of strength and weakness and to tailor an individualized study plan. For example, if you score below average on questions related to oncology therapeutics, plan to spend some additional days studying this subject. Likewise, if cardiovascular therapeutics was the area in which you scored the highest, you may want to leave this section for last.

Both practice tests should be taken in quiet areas—dedicate 4 hours for each test. It is advisable to take the practice exam somewhere with limited distractions, such as a library. The goal is to simulate examlike conditions and to obtain data that will help structure an effective study plan.

As you work through the items, pay particular attention to the explanations. Often, studying the explanations is one of the most valuable study resources. Note that for difficult questions, explanations have been provided that explain the reasoning for not choosing the incorrect answer choices. Use this information to understand the rationale behind eliminating each distracter. The online companion to this book includes animated flashcards to help you with self-assessment on the material prior to the final practice test.

Finally, take Practice Test 2 a week or two prior to your exam date. Test 2 should be taken once the majority of your study has been completed. Test 2 is provided as an online companion to this book and also contains 185 unique questions. Our intention—and our hope—is that this book will be an integral part of your preparation for the NAPLEX®.

ACCESSING THE ONLINE COMPANION:

kaptest.com/booksonline

As owner of this guide, you are entitled to get more practice online. Log on to kaptest.com/booksonline to access:

- 50 animated flashcards
- the second full-length practice test

Just as in the book, the 185-question practice test includes detailed answer explanations. Access to online NAPLEX® practice material is free of charge to purchasers of this book. You'll be asked for a specific password derived from the text in this book, so have your book handy when you log on.

Best of luck to you on your journey toward a successful career as a pharmacist!

Introduction and Test-Taking Strategies

WHAT IS THE NAPLEX®?

NAPLEX stands for North American Pharmacist Licensure Examination. The NAPLEX is issued by the National Association of Boards of Pharmacy (NABP®) and is utilized by the boards of pharmacy as part of their assessment of competence to practice pharmacy. NABP represents each of the 50 states in the United States, the District of Columbia, and the five major U. S. territories. South Africa, New Zealand, Australia, and Canada also utilize the NAPLEX for licensure.

These boards of pharmacy have a mandate to protect the public from unsafe and ineffective pharmacy care, and each board has been given responsibility to regulate the practice of pharmacy in its respective state. In fact, the NAPLEX is often referred to as "The Boards" or "State Boards."

Each state requires applicants to take and pass the NAPLEX in order to obtain a license to practice as a registered pharmacist. The NAPLEX has only one purpose: to determine if it is safe for you to begin practicing as an entry-level pharmacist.

To take the NAPLEX, you must meet the eligibility requirements of the board of pharmacy from which you seek licensure. The board will determine your eligibility in accordance with the jurisdiction's requirements. If you are determined to be eligible, the board will notify NABP of your eligibility. Once that happens, a letter will be issued to you by Pearson VUE, the test administrator, with information about how to schedule your testing appointment.

CONTENT AND STRUCTURE

The NAPLEX is a computer-adaptive test that consists of 185 multiple-choice questions. Of these, 150 questions will be used to calculate your test score. The remaining 35 items serve as experimental questions and do not affect your score.

The NAPLEX is not a test of achievement or intelligence, nor is it designed for pharmacists with years of experience. The questions do not involve high-tech clinical pharmacy or equipment. Note, too, that you will not be tested on all the content you were taught in pharmacy school.

Many of the questions on the NAPLEX are asked in a scenario-based format (i.e., patient profiles with accompanying test questions). To properly analyze and answer the questions, you must refer to the information provided in the patient profile. Other questions are answered solely from the information provided in the question.

There is also a combined-response type question, otherwise called the K question. This type of question includes three Roman-numeral choices. For example:

> Ideally, Lovastatin affects blood lipids by which of the following?
>
> I. Increasing HDLs
> II. Decreasing LDLs
> III. Decreasing triglycerides

The standard response format is typically:

(A) I only
(B) III only
(C) I and II only
(D) II and III only
(E) I, II, and III

K questions can seem confusing if you haven't tackled them before. These are actually a series of true/false questions packaged together. For each question, focus on whether each of the three given statements (I, II, and III) is true or false.

HOW IS THE NAPLEX SCORED, AND WHAT SCORE DO YOU NEED TO PASS?

Your NAPLEX score is a scaled score, not a number-correct score or a percentile score. The scoring scale ranges from 0 to 150. **The minimum passing score is 75.** The algorithms for determining your scaled score are highly confidential and are not released to the public.

Candidates who fail to answer at least 162 of the 185 questions will not receive any score. Since the computer format requires that you answer every question on the screen, the only way you could answer only 162 would be to stop short before the end of the exam. If you complete at least 162 questions but fewer than 185, you will receive a penalty, and your score will be adjusted to reflect the number of questions that remained unanswered. It is certainly in your best interest to answer all questions presented.

NABP will forward your NAPLEX score to the board of pharmacy from which you are seeking licensure. NABP **does not** provide scores to candidates, and score results **are not** released at the test center.

WHAT IF YOU FAIL THE NAPLEX?

First of all, it's unlikely you will fail. Be positive! Currently, the passage rate is approximately 93%. Candidates who receive a failing score on the NAPLEX will automatically be provided with a diagnostic report that indicates their relative performance in each major competency area. The board of pharmacy will notify the candidates of the NAPLEX results and diagnostic report.

THE CAT FORMAT

What Is a CAT?

A computer-adaptive test (CAT) is quite different from a paper-and-pencil test. Each CAT is assembled interactively based on the accuracy of the candidate's response to the questions. This ensures that the questions you are answering are not "too hard" or "too easy" for your skill level. Your first question will be relatively easy; that is, below the level of minimum competency. If you answer that question correctly, the computer selects a slightly more difficult question. If you answer the first question incorrectly, the computer selects a slightly easier question. By continuing to do this as you answer questions, the computer is able to calculate your level of competence.

Because the CAT presents questions on the basis of your responses to previous questions, **you may not change an answer once you have confirmed an answer choice. Likewise, you may not go back to review a question once you have moved on to the next question.** You must answer **all** questions in the order in which they are presented, and you may not skip a question.

In a CAT, the questions are adapted to your ability level. The computer selects questions that represent all areas of pharmacy, as defined by the NAPLEX test plan and by the level of item difficulty. Each question is self-contained, so all of the information you need to answer a question is presented on the computer screen. This difficulty-level determination will then be used to calculate your score.

Strategies for Success with a CAT

1. There is a timer at the top of the computer screen to help you pace yourself. You can hide it if it distracts you—but since the test is timed, you might find it helpful for pacing. You have **4 hours and 15 minutes** to complete all 185 questions.

2. There is a 10-minute break at the 2-hour time point. Make sure to take that break! You need to rest your brain. And while the average candidate takes 2.5 to 3 hours to complete the exam, there are no bonus points for finishing early.

3. It is possible that questions involving mathematical calculations will be weighted more heavily than other questions. Spend extra time solving them, but limit yourself to a maximum of 5 or 6 minutes each.

4. If a question calls for a calculation or a certain mechanism, scratch a rough image. Having a crude diagram to look at, rather than having to imagine it from the computer screen, will help you to see what you're dealing with. Such notes also often stimulate more recall.

5. Look for key words in questions. Words such as "most likely" may help you eliminate some choices even when you don't have comprehensive recall—the most likely choice is probably the one that is most familiar as you review the choices.

6. You cannot cross off an answer choice and banish it from your sight (it's on a computer screen, after all), so you have to be disciplined about not reconsidering choices you've already eliminated.

NAPLEX REGISTRATION

The NAPLEX is administered year-round on business days. There are several steps in registering for the exam. As of this printing, the fee for the exam is $485. (Also, be sure to check with your local board of pharmacy for its fees.)

- **First Step:**
    - Contact the board of pharmacy in the state in which you want to be licensed. The state board will issue paperwork and instructions that determine your eligibility, and will notify the NABP. You will then be issued an authorization to test (ATT), as well as other documents, including:
        - » Test authorization number
        - » Expiration date
        - » Range of dates during which you can take the NAPLEX
- **Second Step:**
    - Once you receive your authorization packet from the NABP, you can call or register online at Pearson VUE to choose your testing center to schedule your test date. You will need your ATT information to schedule a testing date.
    - For more information about registration, go to:
        - » NABP   http://www.nabp.net
        - » Pearson VUE   http://www.pearsonvue.com/

TAKING THE EXAM

There is no time limit for each individual question; however, you have a total of 4 hours and 15 minutes to complete the exam. This does not include the beginning tutorial or the 10-minute break given after the first 2 hours of testing.

Remember, every question counts. There is no warm-up time, so it is important for you to be ready to answer questions correctly from the very beginning. Concentration is also key. You need to give your best thinking to each question.

ON THE DAY OF THE EXAM

1. Arrive at the test center at least 30 minutes before your scheduled testing time to allow for check-in. If you arrive late, you may be required to forfeit your appointment. **If you forfeit your appointment, your testing fee will not be refunded.**

2. Bring two forms of identification: a picture ID that includes your signature and a second form of ID. You will be required to show these IDs for entry. Your thumbprint will also be required when you enter the testing room.

3. You will be provided with laminated note boards, which may be replaced as needed during testing. You will not be allowed to take your own scratch paper or pencil into the testing room.

4. An on-screen, five-function calculator can be activated during the test administration for your use. You may also request a hand-held, five-function calculator from the test administrator.

5. The seating time for the exam is 4 hours and 15 minutes with a 10-minute mandatory break after approximately 2 hours of testing time. Any voluntary breaks will be subtracted from your testing time.

NAPLEX BLUEPRINT

The questions on the NAPLEX involve integrated pharmacy content. The NAPLEX Competency Statements provide a blueprint of the topics covered on the exam. Reviewing these statements will assist you in preparation for the exam.

- **Competence Area 1:** Assess Pharmacotherapy to Assure Safe and Effective Therapeutic Outcomes (about 56% of exam)

- **Competence Area 2:** Assess Safe and Accurate Preparation and Dispensing of Medications (33% of exam)

- **Competence Area 3:** Assess, Recommend, and Provide Healthcare Information that Promotes Public Health (about 11% of exam)

For specific subcategories under each competence areas, go to **www.nabp.net**.

TEST-TAKING STRATEGIES

As you review each chapter in this book, it is important to focus on your own **areas of weakness**. To help you do so, keep the following in mind:

Key Steps toward Preparedness

- **Assess your strengths and weaknesses.** Review your weakest subjects first.
- Focus heavily on the Top 200 drugs by unit. Use the online flashcard component that accompanies this book and spend extra time reviewing the Top 200. These are important.
- Practice calculations to increase your confidence.
- Schedule extra time before your testing date to revisit your weaker areas.
- Complete the practice test under real exam conditions.
- Order and complete the Pre-NAPLEX exam, available from NABP.
- When you review the practice exams, make sure you understand why your incorrect answer choices were incorrect.
- Be sure you understand why you missed a question. Did you simply forget a fact? Choose your answer too quickly? Misunderstand the question? Miss an important clue within the question? Finally, do you keep making the same mistakes over and over? If so, it is important to spend more time on those areas.

Guessing

During the exam, there are sure to be some questions that stump you. For those, just narrow down the choices and take your best guess. You don't want to spend too much time analyzing a question you do not know and then run out of time toward the end of the exam. Remember, you cannot simply leave a question blank, so in some shape or form, you'll have to take your best guess.

Keep in mind that 35 experimental questions are not calculated into your score, so if you answer a few questions incorrectly, it's possible that they won't be scored at all.

When you just don't know the answer: narrow the answer choices to two likely choices, then use the "upper, then lower" decision rule to select one of them. This rule means you alternate your guess, using the upper choice the first time you are stuck, then the lower choice the next time you are stuck. This technique helps keep you moving forward.

Positive Attitude

The most important decision you can make in your studying process is to have a positive attitude, especially on test day. Remember this:

- The odds are on your side; around 93% of pharmacy graduates pass the NAPLEX.
- This is a minimal competency exam.
- You spent a minimum of 6 years in school to become a pharmacist. If you did that, you can conquer this exam!

You **are** prepared, and this book is a tool to increase your confidence.

Part Two

Review of Therapeutics

Cardiovascular Disorders

1

This chapter covers the following diseases:

- **Hypertension**
- **Dyslipidemia**
- **Heart failure**
- **Ischemic heart disease**

The text also provides an overview of the antiarrhythmic drugs and antithrombotic drugs commonly used in clinical practice.

 Suggested Study Time: **2.5 hours**

HYPERTENSION

Definitions

Hypertension (HTN) is defined as a systolic blood pressure (SBP) >140 mmHg, a diastolic blood pressure (DBP) >90 mmHg, or any patient requiring antihypertensive therapy. Most patients with HTN have primary (essential) HTN (due to an unknown cause, likely genetic), while less than 10% have secondary HTN (due to chronic kidney disease [CKD], pheochromocytoma, Cushing's syndrome, or medications [nonsteroidal anti-inflammatory drugs (NSAIDs), corticosteroids, cyclosporine, tacrolimus, sibutramine, estrogens, erythropoietin, venlafaxine, sympathomimetics, cocaine]).

Diagnosis

- Normal blood pressure (BP): SBP <120 mmHg and DBP <80 mmHg
- Prehypertension: SBP 120–139 mmHg or DBP 80–89 mmHg

- Hypertension is categorized into two stages:
  - Stage 1 HTN: SBP 140–159 mmHg or DBP 90–99 mmHg
  - Stage 2 HTN: SBP ≥160 mmHg or DBP ≥100 mmHg

Signs and Symptoms

- Can develop target organ damage with chronic, uncontrolled HTN:
  - Cardiac
    - » Angina, myocardial infarction (MI), history of coronary revascularization (e.g., percutaneous coronary intervention [PCI], coronary artery bypass graft [CABG] surgery), left ventricular hypertrophy (LVH), left ventricular (LV) dysfunction (i.e., heart failure [HF])
  - Cerebrovascular
    - » Stroke, transient ischemic attack (TIA)
  - Renal
    - » CKD
  - Ophthalmologic
    - » Retinopathy, blindness
  - Vascular
    - » Peripheral arterial disease (PAD)

Guidelines

Seventh Joint National Committee on the Detection, Evaluation, and Treatment of High Blood Pressure (JNC 7), *JAMA*, no. 289 (2003): 2560–71. www.nhlbi.nih.gov/guidelines/hypertension.

American Heart Association (Treatment of HTN in the Prevention and Management of Ischemic Heart Disease guidelines). *Circulation*, no. 15 (2007): 2761–88.

Guidelines Summary

- BP goals:
  - Uncomplicated HTN: <140/90 mmHg
  - Diabetes mellitus (DM), CKD, known coronary artery disease (CAD) or CAD equivalent (e.g., carotidartery disease, peripheral arterial disease, abdominal aortic aneurysm), 10-year Framingham risk score (FRS) ≥10%, stable/unstable angina (UA), or MI: <130/80 mmHg
  - HF: <120/80 mmHg
- Lifestyle modifications: weight loss (goal body mass index [BMI] 18.5–24.9 kg/m^2), diet rich in fruits, vegetables, and low-fat dairy products with ↓ saturated and total

fat, ↓ sodium (Na+) intake (≤2.4 g/day), ↑ physical activity (30 minutes most days of the week), moderation of alcohol use (≤1 ounce of ethanol/day), smoking cessation

- Pharmacologic therapy:
  - Initial antihypertensive drug selection: Based upon degree of BP elevation and whether compelling indications are present
  - Compelling indications for specific antihypertensive drug therapy:
    » HF: Diuretic, angiotensin-converting enzyme inhibitor (ACEI), β-blocker (carvedilol, metoprolol, or bisoprolol), angiotensin II receptor blocker (ARB), aldosterone receptor antagonist (ARA), hydralazine/isosorbide dinitrate (for African-Americans)
    » Post-MI: β-blocker, ACEI (or ARB), ARA
    » High coronary disease risk: β-blocker, ACEI, diuretic, calcium channel blocker (CCB)
    » DM: ACEI, ARB, diuretic, β-blocker, CCB
    » CKD: ACEI, ARB
    » Recurrent stroke prevention: ACEI, diuretic
  - Management of pre-HTN:
    » No compelling indication present → Lifestyle modifications only
    » If patient has CKD or DM → Treat with drugs listed for these compelling indications (see above)
  - Management of HTN:
    » No compelling indication present:
      - Stage 1 HTN → Initiate thiazide diuretic (may also consider ACEI, ARB, β-blocker, CCB, or combination of these drugs)
      - Stage 2 HTN → Initiate two antihypertensive drugs (one of the drugs should be a thiazide diuretic)
    » Compelling indication present:
      - Use drugs indicated for these specific conditions (see above)

Diuretics

Thiazide Diuretics – inhibit Na$^+$ reabsorption in the distal convoluted tubule

Generic	Brand	Dose	Contra-indications	Primary Side Effects	Key Monitoring	Pertinent Drug Interactions	Med Pearl	Top 200
Chlorothiazide	Diuril	500–2,000 mg/day	Sulfa allergy	• Hypokalemia • Hypomagnesemia • Hyponatremia • Hypercalcemia • Hyperglycemia • Hyperuricemia • Photosensitivity	• BP • Electrolytes • Blood urea nitrogen (BUN)/serum creatinine (SCr) • Blood glucose • Uric acid	• May ↑ risk of lithium toxicity • May ↓ effect of antidiabetic agents • NSAIDs ↓ antihypertensive effects	• Often used as 1st-line therapy for HTN • Synergistic effect with other antihypertensives • Not effective (except metolazone) when creatinine clearance (CrCl) <30 mL/min; use loop diuretics • Have ceiling dose (unlike loop diuretics)	No
Chlorthalidone	Thalitone	12.5–100 mg/day						No
Hydrochlorothiazide	Microzide	12.5–50 mg/day						Yes
Indapamide	Only available generically	1.25–5 mg/day						Yes
Metolazone	Zaroxolyn	2.5–5 mg/day						Yes

Loop Diuretics – inhibit Na$^+$ reabsorption in the ascending limb of loop of Henle (should only be used for HTN in patients with renal insufficiency [maintain efficacy when CrCl <30 mL/min], severe edema, or HF) (see HF section for further details)

Potassium-Sparing Diuretics – inhibit Na$^+$ reabsorption in the collecting ducts

Generic	Brand	Dose	Contra-indications	Primary Side Effects	Key Monitoring	Pertinent Drug Interactions	Med Pearl	Top 200
Amiloride	Only available generically	5–10 mg/day	• Hyperkalemia • CKD	Hyperkalemia	• BP • Potassium (K$^+$) • BUN/SCr	Use with K$^+$ supplements, ACEIs, ARBs, ARAs, or NSAIDs may ↑ risk of hyperkalemia	• Not used often as monotherapy (weak antihypertensives) • Often used with hydrochlorothiazide to ↓ K$^+$ loss	No
Triamterene	Dyrenium	50–100 mg/day						No

Combination products:
Triamterene/hydrochlorothiazide (Dyazide, Maxzide)
Amiloride/hydrochlorothiazide (Moduretic)

Aldosterone Receptor Antagonists – have similar mechanism of action to K$^+$-sparing diuretics (also block the effects of aldosterone) (not used often for HTN) (see HF section for further details)

Combination products:
Spironolactone/hydrochlorothiazide (Aldactazide)

β-Blockers

Mechanism of action — ↓ cardiac output (CO) by negative inotropic (↓ contractility) and negative chronotropic (↓ heart rate [HR]) effects

- Cardioselective — bind more to β_1 than β_2 receptors (at low doses); less likely to cause bronchoconstriction or vasoconstriction at low doses (safer to use in patients with asthma, chronic obstructive pulmonary disease [COPD], PAD, or DM); cardioselectivity may be lost at higher doses
  - Bisoprolol, atenolol, metoprolol, betaxolol, acebutolol (BAMBA)
- Intrinsic sympathomimetic activity (ISA) — have partial β-receptor agonist activity
  - Carteolol, acebutolol, pindolol, penbutolol (CAPP)
- Lipophilic vs. hydrophilic — lipophilic (propranolol, metoprolol, carvedilol, labetalol, pindolol) more likely to cause central nervous system (CNS) side effects (e.g., depression, fatigue) than hydrophilic (atenolol)

Generic	Brand	Dose	Contraindications	Primary Side Effects	Key Monitoring	Pertinent Drug Interactions	Med Pearl	Top 200
Cardioselective:								
Acebutolol	Sectral	200–1,200 mg/day	• ≥2nd degree heart block (in absence of pacemaker) • HF (except metoprolol succinate or bisoprolol)	• Bradycardia/heart block • HF exacerbation • Bronchospasm • Cold extremities • Fatigue • ↓ exercise tolerance • Depression • Glucose intolerance • Mask hypoglycemia (in patients with DM)	• BP • HR • S/S HF • Blood glucose (in patients with DM)	Use with other negative chronotropes (e.g., digoxin, verapamil, diltiazem, or clonidine) may ↑ risk of bradycardia	Abrupt discontinuation may cause angina, MI, or hypertensive emergency; need to taper over 2 wks	No
Atenolol	Tenormin	25–100 mg/day						Yes
Betaxolol	Kerlone	5–20 mg/day						No
Bisoprolol	Zebeta	2.5–20 mg/day						No
Metoprolol	• Tartrate: Lopressor (2x daily) • Succinate: Toprol XL (1x daily)	25–400 mg/day						Yes
Nonselective:								
Carvedilol	Coreg, Coreg CR	Immediate-release (IR): 12.5–50 mg/day (in two divided doses) Controlled-release (CR): 20–80 mg/day (1x daily)	• ≥2nd degree heart block (in absence of pacemaker) • HF (except carvedilol)	Same as with selective β-blockers	Same as with selective β-blockers	Same as with selective β-blockers	• Same as with selective β-blockers • Labetalol and carvedilol also have α_1-blocking properties	Yes
Labetalol	Trandate	200–2,400 mg/day						Yes
Nadolol	Corgard	20–320 mg/day						No
Pindolol	Only available generically	5–60 mg/day						No
Propranolol	Inderal, Inderal LA, InnoPran XL	80–640 mg/day (IR given 2–3x daily; extended-release [ER] given 1x daily)						Yes
Timolol	Blocadren	20–60 mg/day						No

Combination products:

Atenolol/chlorthalidone (Tenoretic)

Bisoprolol/hydrochlorothiazide (Ziac)

Nadolol/bendroflumethiazide (Corzide)

Propranolol/hydrochlorothiazide (Inderide)

Metoprolol/hydrochlorothiazide (Lopressor HCT)

Angiotensin-Converting Enzyme Inhibitors

Mechanism of action – inhibit angiotensin-converting enzyme and prevent the conversion of angiotensin I to angiotensin II → vasodilation, ↓ aldosterone production; also inhibit degradation of bradykinin

Generic	Brand	Dose	Contraindications	Primary Side Effects	Key Monitoring	Pertinent Drug Interactions	Med Pearl	Top 200
Benazepril	Lotensin	5–40 mg/day	• Pregnancy • History of angioedema or renal failure with prior use • Hyperkalemia • Bilateral renal artery stenosis	• Hyperkalemia • Renal insufficiency • Cough (dry) • Angioedema	• BP • BUN/SCr • K+	• Use with ARBs, K+ supplements, K+-sparing diuretics, ARAs, or NSAIDs may ↑ risk of hyperkalemia • May ↑ risk of lithium toxicity	• Captopril has shortest duration of action • If patient has intolerable dry cough, may switch to ARB • Hyperkalemia and renal insufficiency also likely to occur with ARBs (risk of angioedema cross-sensitivity with ARBs controversial)	Yes
Captopril	Capoten	12.5–450 mg/day						No
Enalapril	Vasotec	2.5–40 mg/day						Yes
Fosinopril	Monopril	5–80 mg/day						No
Lisinopril	Prinivil, Zestril	2.5–40 mg/day						Yes
Moexipril	Univasc	3.75–30 mg/day						No
Perindopril	Aceon	4–16 mg/day						No
Quinapril	Accupril	10–80 mg/day						Yes
Ramipril	Altace	1.25–20 mg/day						Yes
Trandolapril	Mavik	0.5–4 mg/day						No

Combination products:

Benazepril/amlodipine (Lotrel)
Benazepril/hydrochlorothiazide (Lotensin HCT)
Captopril/hydrochlorothiazide (Capozide)
Enalapril/hydrochlorothiazide (Vaseretic)
Fosinopril/hydrochlorothiazide (Monopril-HCT)
Lisinopril/hydrochlorothiazide (Prinzide, Zestoretic)
Moexipril/hydrochlorothiazide (Uniretic)
Quinapril/hydrochlorothiazide (Accuretic)
Trandolapril/verapamil (Tarka)

Angiotensin II Receptor Blockers

Generic	Brand	Dose	Contraindications	Primary Side Effects	Key Monitoring	Pertinent Drug Interactions	Med Pearl	Top 200
Mechanism of action — inhibit the binding of angiotensin II to the angiotensin type 1 (AT$_1$) receptor → ▼vasodilation, ↓ aldosterone production; no effect on bradykinin								
Azilsartan	Edarbi	40–80 mg/day	Same as for ACEIs	Same as for ACEIs (except no cough)	Same as for ACEIs	• Use with ACEIs, K$^+$ supplements, K$^+$-sparing diuretics, ARAs, or NSAIDs may ↑ risk of hyperkalemia • May ↑ risk of lithium toxicity	Hyperkalemia and renal insufficiency also likely to occur with ACEIs (risk of angioedema cross-sensitivity with ACEIs is controversial)	No
Candesartan	Atacand	4–32 mg/day						Yes
Eprosartan	Teveten	400–800 mg/day						No
Irbesartan	Avapro	75–300 mg/day						Yes
Losartan	Cozaar	25–100 mg/day						Yes
Olmesartan	Benicar	20–40 mg/day						Yes
Telmisartan	Micardis	20–80 mg/day						Yes
Valsartan	Diovan	80–320 mg/day						Yes

Combination products:

Azilsartan/chlorthalidone (Edarbyclor)
Candesartan/hydrochlorothiazide (Atacand HCT)
Eprosartan/hydrochlorothiazide (Teveten HCT)
Irbesartan/hydrochlorothiazide (Avalide)
Losartan/hydrochlorothiazide (Hyzaar)
Olmesartan/amlodipine (Azor)
Olmesartan/amlodipine/hydrochlorothiazide (Tribenzor)
Olmesartan/hydrochlorothiazide (Benicar HCT)
Telmisartan/amlodipine (Twynsta)
Telmisartan/hydrochlorothiazide (Micardis HCT)
Valsartan/amlodipine (Exforge)
Valsartan/hydrochlorothiazide (Diovan HCT)
Valsartan/amlodipine/hydrochlorothiazide (Exforge HCT)

Renin Inhibitor

Generic	Brand	Dose	Contraindications	Primary Side Effects	Key Monitoring	Pertinent Drug Interactions	Med Pearl	Top 200
Mechanism of action — inhibits renin and prevents the conversion of angiotensinogen to angiotensin I, which then ↓ production of angiotensin II								
Aliskiren	Tekturna	150–300 mg/day	• Pregnancy • History of ACEI- or ARB-induced angioedema • Hyperkalemia • Bilateral renal artery stenosis	• Headache • Dizziness • Diarrhea • May also cause hyperkalemia and renal insufficiency	• BP • BUN/SCr • K$^+$	• Use with ACEIs, ARBs, K$^+$ supplements, K$^+$-sparing diuretics, ARAs, or NSAIDs may ↑ risk of hyperkalemia • Atorvastatin, ketoconazole, or cyclosporine may ↑ effects	• Use with caution in patients with CrCl <30 mL/min • Avoid taking with high-fat meals • Should not use with cyclosporine	Yes

Combination products:

Aliskiren/amlodipine (Tekamlo)
Aliskiren/hydrochlorothiazide (Tekturna HCT)
Aliskiren/amlodipine/hydrochlorothizide (Amturnide)
Aliskiren/valsartan (Valturna)

Calcium Channel Blockers

Mechanism of action – bind to L-type channels in heart and coronary/peripheral arteries to block inward movement of calcium (Ca^{2+}) → vascular smooth-muscle relaxation (vasodilation); all (except for amlodipine and felodipine) have negative inotropic effects (↓ contractility)
- Dihydropyridines (DHPs) – more selective to vasculature; more potent vasodilators; have no effect on cardiac conduction
- Non-DHPs – cause less peripheral vasodilation than DHPs; have negative chronotropic properties (↓ HR)

Generic	Brand	Dose	Contra-indications	Primary Side Effects	Key Monitoring	Pertinent Drug Interactions	Med Pearl	Top 200
DHPs:								
Amlodipine	Norvasc	2.5–10 mg/day	None	• Reflex tachycardia • Headache • Flushing • Peripheral edema • Gingival hyperplasia • HF exacerbation (except amlodipine and felodipine)	• BP • HR • S/S HF	• CYP3A4 inhibitors may ↑ effects • CYP3A4 inducers may ↓ effects	• Sublingual nifedipine should not be used → may ↑ risk of MI, death • Do not use grapefruit juice	Yes
Felodipine	Plendil	2.5–20 mg/day						Yes
Isradipine	DynaCirc CR	5–10 mg/day						No
Nicardipine	Cardene, Cardene SR	60–120 mg/day (IR given 3x daily; sustained-release [SR] given 2x daily)						No
Nifedipine	Adalat CC, Afeditab CR, Nifediac CC, Nifedical XL, Procardia XL	30–180 mg/day						Yes
Nisoldipine	Sular	ER: 10–40 mg/day Geomatrix: 17–34 mg/day						No
Non-DHPs:								
Diltiazem	Cardizem CD, Cardizem LA, Cartia XT, Dilacor XR, Taztia XT, Tiazac	120–540 mg/day	• ≥2nd degree heart block (in absence of pacemaker) • Systolic HF	• Bradycardia/heart block • Constipation • Peripheral edema • Gingival hyperplasia • HF exacerbation	Same as for DHPs	• Same as for DHPs • Use with other negative chronotropes (e.g., digoxin, β-blockers, or clonidine) may ↑ risk of bradycardia • May ↑ effect/toxicity of CYP3A4 substrates • May ↑ risk of digoxin toxicity	Do not use grapefruit juice	Yes
Verapamil	Calan, Calan SR, Covera-HS, Isoptin SR, Verelan, Verelan PM	120–360 mg/day (IR given 2–3x daily, SR given 1–2x daily)						Yes

α₁-Receptor Antagonists

Generic	Brand	Dose	Contraindications	Primary Side Effects	Key Monitoring	Pertinent Drug Interactions	Med Pearl	Top 200
Mechanism of action – block the α₁ receptor on peripheral blood vessels → arterial and venous vasodilation								
Doxazosin	Cardura	1–16 mg/day	Should not be used with phosphodiesterase (PDE)-5 inhibitors (e.g., sildenafil, tadalafil, vardenafil) → ↑ risk of hypotension	• Orthostatic hypotension • Reflex tachycardia • Peripheral edema • Headache • Drowsiness	• BP • HR	↑ risk of hypotension with PDE-5 inhibitors (avoid concurrent use)	• Take dose at bedtime to minimize risk of orthostatic hypotension • ALLHAT trial → 25% ↑ in cardiovascular events with doxazosin • Also available as epidural injection	No
Prazosin	Minipress	1–20 mg/day						No
Terazosin	Hytrin	1–20 mg/day						Yes

Central α₂-Receptor Agonists

Generic	Brand	Dose	Contra-indications	Primary Side Effects	Key Monitoring	Pertinent Drug Interactions	Med Pearl	Top 200
Mechanism of action – stimulate α₂ receptors in brain → ↓ sympathetic outflow (release of norepinephrine) → ↓ BP and HR								
Clonidine	Catapres, Catapres-TTS	Oral: 0.2–2.4 mg/day Transdermal: 0.1–0.3 mg weekly	Methyldopa: Liver disease	• Sedation • Orthostatic hypotension • Depression • Peripheral edema • Dry mouth • Bradycardia • Hepatitis (methyldopa)	• BP • HR • Liver function tests (LFTs) (methyldopa)	Use with other negative chronotropes (e.g., digoxin, verapamil, diltiazem, or β-blockers) may ↑ risk of bradycardia	• Clonidine patch should be applied once weekly • Abrupt discontinuation (especially in presence of β-blockers) may cause angina, MI, or hypertensive emergency; need to taper over 2 wks • When starting clonidine patch, overlap with oral for 2–3 days, then discontinue oral • Should not be used as first-line therapy • Also available as epidural injection	Yes
Methyldopa	Aldomet	250–1,000 mg/day						No

Direct Vasodilators

Generic	Brand	Dose	Contra-indications	Primary Side Effects	Key Monitoring	Pertinent Drug Interactions	Med Pearl	Top 200
Mechanism of action – ↑ cyclic GMP → arterial vasodilation								
Hydralazine	Apresoline	25–300 mg/day	• Acute MI • Aortic dissection	• Reflex tachycardia • Orthostatic hypotension • Peripheral edema • Lupus-like syndrome (hydralazine) • Hirsutism (minoxidil)	• BP • HR • S/S lupus (e.g., stabbing chest pain, joint pain, fever, rash)	None	• Should not be used as 1st-line therapy	Yes
Minoxidil	Loniten	2.5–100 mg/day					• Minoxidil is usually absolutely last-line therapy (because of side effects)	No

Storage and Administration Pearls

- When initiating antihypertensive drug therapy in the elderly, initiate at a low dose and slowly titrate to achieve goal BP ("start low and go slow").

Patient Education Pearls

- Diuretics should be taken in the morning to avoid nocturia. Patients receiving diuretics should wear sunscreen and protective clothing. Also, they should report any episodes of muscle cramps, as this may be a symptom of hypokalemia or hypomagnesemia.
- Patients receiving K^+-sparing diuretics, ARAs, ACEIs, or ARBs should avoid excessive intake of foods high in K^+ (e.g., green leafy vegetables, potatoes, apricots, bananas, dates, oranges, avocados) and K^+-containing salt substitutes.
- α_1-receptor antagonists should be taken at bedtime to minimize the risk of developing orthostatic hypotension.
- Patients receiving α_1-receptor antagonists, α_2-receptor agonists, or direct vasodilators should rise slowly from a sitting position.
- Patients receiving ACEIs or ARBs should call 911 immediately if he/she experiences lip, tongue, or facial swelling or has difficulty breathing.
- ACEIs, ARBs, and renin inhibitors should be avoided in pregnant patients. Antihypertensive drugs that can be safely used in pregnancy include methyldopa, labetalol, or CCBs.

DYSLIPIDEMIA

Definitions

Dyslipidemia can refer to any lipid disorder including ↑ total cholesterol (TC), low-density lipoprotein cholesterol (LDL-C), and triglycerides (TGs), and ↓ high-density lipoprotein cholesterol (HDL-C). Dyslipidemia can predispose patients to the development of cardiovascular disease, cerebrovascular disease, or PAD. While most forms of dyslipidemia are due to genetic factors, certain drugs may also cause elevated lipid concentrations, including β-blockers, diuretics, corticosteroids, isotretinoin, protease inhibitors, cyclosporine, and estrogens.

Diagnosis

Classification of TC, LDL-C, HDL-C, and TGs

TC	HDL-C
• <200 mg/dL → Desirable • 200–239 mg/dL → Borderline high • ≥240 mg/dL → High	• <40 mg/dL → Low • ≥60 mg/dL → High
LDL-C	**TGs**
• <100 mg/dL → Optimal • 100–129 mg/dL → Near/above optimal • 130–159 mg/dL → Borderline high • 160–189 mg/dL → High • ≥190 mg/dL → Very high	• <150 mg/dL → Normal • 150–199 mg/dL → Borderline high • 200–499 mg/dL → High • ≥500 mg/dL → Very high (↑ risk for pancreatitis)

- Fasting lipid profile should be obtained in adults ≥20 years every 5 years.

- The Friedewald LDL equation (applies if TG <400 mg/dL) is LDL = TC − (HDL-C + TG/5).

- To determine LDL-C goal and appropriate lipid-lowering therapy, a risk factor assessment should be performed.

  - Major risk factors for coronary heart disease (CHD) are:

    » Age ≥45 years (males), ≥55 years (females)

    » Cigarette smoking

    » HTN (BP >140/90 mmHg or on antihypertensive therapy)

    » HDL-C <40 mg/dL

    » Family history of premature CHD (male first-degree relative <55 years, female first-degree relative <65 years)

  - A negative risk factor (if present, subtract one risk factor from total count above) is:

    » HDL-C ≥60 mg/dL

  - Patient's risk factors should be counted up. If ≥2 risk factors, FRS should be calculated. You do not need to calculate FRS in patients with 0–1 risk factors, or those with CHD or CHD-risk equivalent (see below).

  - You will not need to calculate FRS for exam!

  - CHD-risk equivalents (confer the same degree of risk for developing a CHD event as an individual who has established CHD) are:

    » PAD

    » Abdominal aortic aneurysm

    » Symptomatic carotid artery disease (i.e., stroke, TIA)

    » DM

    » Stage 5 CKD

    » Multiple (≥2) risk factors that confer ≥20% risk of CHD at 10 years (as determined by FRS)

Signs and Symptoms

- Most patients with dyslipidemias are asymptomatic until a significant degree of atherosclerosis occurs.
- Complications of dyslipidemias may include MI, stroke, PAD, erectile dysfuction, and sudden cardiac death.

Guidelines

National Cholesterol Education Program (NCEP) Adult Treatment Panel III. *Circulation*, no. 110 (2004): 227–39. http://nhlbi.nih.gov/guidelines/cholesterol/index.htm.

Guidelines Summary

Risk Category	LDL-C Goal
CHD or CHD-risk equivalent	<100 mg/dL (<70 mg/dL reasonable for patients with CHD, PAD, atherosclerotic aortic disease, stroke/TIA, or DM)
Multiple (≥2) risk factors	<130 mg/dL (<100 mg/dL optional goal for patients with FRS of 10–20%)
0–1 risk factors	<160 mg/dL

- Lifestyle modifications (to be initiated in all patients): Therapeutic lifestyle changes, weight loss, ↑ physical activity, use of plant stanols/sterols (may help ↓ LDL-C)
- Pharmacologic therapy
  - Selection of drug therapy should be based on lipid abnormality.
  - Achieving LDL-C goal should be the primary goal for all patients, except for when TG >500 mg/dL (↓ TG to <500 mg/dL then becomes the primary goal).
  - For 3-hydroxyl-3-methylglutaryl-coenzyme A (HMG-CcA) reductase inhibitors (statins), select dose that will achieve % LDL-C reduction that will get patient to their LDL-C goal.
    - » % LDL-C reduction: [(Baseline LDL-C – Goal LDL-C)/Baseline LDL-C] × 100

Lipid-Lowering Effects of Various Drug Classes

Drug Class	Effect on LDL-C	Effect on HDL-C	Effect on TGs
Bile acid resins	↓ 15–30%	↑ 3–5%	↑ 1–10%
Niacin	↓ 5–25%	↑ 15–35%	↓ 20–50%
Fibric acid derivatives	↓/↑ 5–20%	↑ 10–20%	↓ 20–50%
Statins	↓ 18–55%	↑ 5–15%	↓ 7–30%
Cholesterol absorption inhibitors	↓ 15–20%	↑ 1%	↓ 8%

Bile Acid Resins

Mechanism of action – bind bile acids in intestines, forming insoluble complex that is excreted in feces → ↓ in bile acids causes liver to convert cholesterol into bile acids, which then ↓ cholesterol stores → ↑ demand for cholesterol in liver → upregulation of LDL receptors → ↑ LDL-C clearance from bloodstream

Generic	Brand	Dose	Contra-indications	Primary Side Effects	Key Monitoring	Pertinent Drug Interactions	Med Pearl	Top 200
Cholestyramine	Prevalite, Questran	4–24 g/day	Complete biliary obstruction	• Constipation • Bloating • Abdominal pain • Nausea/vomiting (N/V) • Flatulence • ↑ TGs	Lipid panel	Bind to and ↓ absorption of many drugs (e.g., warfarin, digoxin, thiazides, levothyroxine)	• Used to ↓ LDL-C • Can be used in patients with liver disease • Do not use in patients with ↑ TGs • Colesevelam has fewer gastro-intestinal (GI) side effects and drug interactions	No
Colesevelam	Welchol	3.75 g/day						No
Colestipol	Colestid	• Granules: 5–30 g/day • Tablets: 2–16 g/day						No

Niacin

Mechanism of action – ↓ production of very low density lipoproteins (VLDL) in liver → ↓ synthesis of LDL-C

Generic	Brand	Dose	Contra-indications	Primary Side Effects	Key Monitoring	Pertinent Drug Interactions	Med Pearl	Top 200
Niacin	Niaspan; also available as over-the-counter (OTC) product	500–3,000 mg/day	• Hepatic dysfunction • Active gout • Active peptic ulcer disease	• Flushing/itching • Nausea • Orthostatic hypotension • ↑ LFTs • Myopathy • Hyperuricemia • Hyperglycemia	• Lipid panel • LFTs • Creatine kinase (CK) (if muscle aches) • Uric acid • Blood glucose (if patient has DM)	None significant	• Used to ↓ LDL-C, ↓ TGs, and ↑ HDL-C • Most effective drug for ↑ HDL-C • Do not ↑ dose by >500 mg in 4-week period • Avoid use of OTC SR products (↑ risk of hepatotoxicity)	Yes

Combination products: Niacin/lovastatin (Advicor)   Niacin/simvastatin (Simcor)

Fibric Acid Derivatives

Mechanism of action – ↑ activity of lipoprotein lipase → ↑ catabolism of VLDL → ↓ TGs

Generic	Brand	Dose	Contra-indications	Primary Side Effects	Key Monitoring	Pertinent Drug Interactions	Med Pearl	Top 200
Fenofibrate	Antara, Fenoglide, Lipofen, Lofibra, TriCor, Triglide	43–200 mg/day (depending on brand)	• Hepatic dysfunction • Severe renal dysfunction • Gallbladder disease	• Nausea/vomiting/diarrhea (N/V/D) • Abdominal pain • ↑ LFTs • Myopathy	• Lipid panel • LFTs • CK (if muscle aches)	• Avoid using gemfibrozil with statins (↑ risk of myopathy) • ↑ effects of warfarin and sulfonylureas • ↑ cyclosporine level	• Used to ↓ TGs and/or ↑ HDL-C • Gemfibrozil should not be used with statins →↑ risk of myopathy • Fenofibrate preferred with statins • Adjust dose in renal insufficiency	Yes
Gemfibrozil	Lopid	1,200 mg/day						Yes

Omega-3 Polyunsaturated Fatty Acids (Fish Oil)

Mechanism of action — ↓ production of TGs in the liver

Generic	Brand	Dose	Contraindications	Primary Side Effects	Key Monitoring	Pertinent Drug Interactions	Med Pearl	Top 200
Omega-3-Acid Ethyl Esters	Lovaza; also available as OTC product	2–4 g/day	Fish allergy	• Belching ("fishy taste") • Dyspepsia	Lipid panel	May ↑ risk of bleeding with antiplatelets or warfarin	• Used to ↓ TGs • May ↑ LDL-C	Yes

HMG-CoA Reductase Inhibitors (Statins)

Mechanism of action — inhibit HMG-CoA reductase → prevent the conversion of HMG-CoA to mevalonate (rate-limiting step in cholesterol synthesis)

Generic	Brand	Dose	Contraindications	Primary Side Effects	Key Monitoring	Pertinent Drug Interactions	Med Pearl	Top 200
Atorvastatin	Lipitor	10–80 mg/day	• Hepatic dysfunction • Pregnancy (Pregnancy Category X) • Concomitant use with cyclosporine (pitavastatin) • CrCl <30 mL/min (pitavastatin) • Concomitant use with strong CYP3A4 inhibitors (simvastatin and lovastatin) • Concomitant use with gemfibrozil, cyclosporine or danazol (simvastatin)	• ↑ LFTs • Myopathy • N/V • Constipation	• Lipid panel • LFTs • CK (if muscle aches)	• Atorvastatin, lovastatin, rosuvastatin, and simvastatin are CYP3A4 substrates; CYP3A4 inhibitors may ↑ risk of side effects; may ↑ effects of warfarin • Fluvastatin and pitavastatin metabolized by CYP2C9; may ↑ effects of warfarin • Pravastatin not metabolized by CYP enzymes • Cyclosporine, erythromycin, rifampin, and atazanavir may ↑ risk of side effects	• Most effective drugs for ↓ LDL-C • Lower maximum dosage of simvastatin and lovastatin when used with amiodarone, verapamil, amlodipine, diltiazem, ranolazine, or niacin • Adjust rosuvastatin dose if CrCl <30 mL/min • Lower maximum dosage of rosuvastatin when used with cyclosporine, lopinavir/ritonavir, or atazanavir/ritonavir • Lower maximum dosage of pitavastatin when used with erythromycin or rifampin • Adjust pitavastatin dose if CrCl 15–59 mL/min	Yes
Fluvastatin	Lescol, Lescol XL	20–80 mg/day						No
Lovastatin	Altoprev, Mevacor	20–80 mg/day						Yes
Pitavastatin	Livalo	1–4 mg/day						No
Pravastatin	Pravachol	10–80 mg/day						Yes
Simvastatin	Zocor	10–80 mg/day						Yes
Rosuvastatin	Crestor	5–40 mg/day						Yes

Combination products: Atorvastatin/amlodipine (Caduet)   Simvastatin/ezetimibe (Vytorin)   Simvastatin/sitagliptin (Juvisync)

Cholesterol Absorption Inhibitor

Mechanism of action – prevents absorption of cholesterol from small intestine

Generic	Brand	Dose	Contraindications	Primary Side Effects	Key Monitoring	Pertinent Drug Interactions	Med Pearl	Top 200
Ezetimibe	Zetia	10 mg/day	None	• Headache • Diarrhea	Lipid panel	• Cyclosporine and fibrates may ↑ effects • ↑ cyclosporine levels • ↑ effects of warfarin	• Used to ↓ LDL-C • Can add to statin to further ↓ LDL-C or if dose-limiting side effects occur with statin	Yes

KAPLAN) MEDICAL

Storage and Administration Pearls

- Bile acid resins
  - Cholestyramine available as powder; colestipol available as granules and tablets; colesevelam available as tablets
  - Should be administered with meals
  - Powder can be mixed in applesauce, pudding, oatmeal, Jell-O, etc. to improve its palatability (do not mix in carbonated beverages)
  - Give other medications 1 hour *before* or 4 hours *after* cholestyramine or colestipol
- Niacin: Give at bedtime (so flushing reaction can occur while patient is sleeping)
- Fibric acid derivatives: Can be administered with meals to ↓ GI effects
- Statins: IR lovastatin administered with meals; ER lovastatin administered at bedtime
- Most statins administered in the evening (at bedtime)—most hepatic cholesterol production occurs during the night (~2 A.M.); atorvastatin, rosuvastatin, and pitavastatin administered in the morning or evening
- After initiating lipid-lowering therapy, lipid profile reassessed in 6 weeks to determine if any changes in therapy are needed.
- LDL-lowering potential of statins: Rosuvastatin >atorvastatin >simvastatin >pravastatin = lovastatin = pitavastatin >fluvastatin

Patient Education Pearls

- Fiber/fiber supplements may help minimize GI side effects associated with bile acid resins.
- Any episodes of muscle pain/aches or dark urine should be reported.
- Flushing reaction associated with niacin may be minimized by taking aspirin (325 mg) or an NSAID at least 30 minutes before dose, taking with food, slowly titrating the dose, and avoiding alcohol or hot beverages. Tolerance usually develops.
- Statins should be avoided if the patient is pregnant (Category X).

HEART FAILURE

Definition

HF is a condition in which the heart is unable to pump out enough blood (CO) to meet the metabolic demands of the body. The decrease in CO leads to the activation of numerous compensatory mechanisms, which attempt to improve CO. There are two types of HF: systolic (pumping function/contractility impaired; left ventricular ejection fraction [LVEF] ≤40%) or diastolic (impaired ability to relax, which leads to underfilling; normal LVEF [>40%]). The majority of HF cases are due to either CAD or HTN. A number of drugs can also precipitate or worsen HF by causing negative inotropic effects (e.g., β-blockers, CCBs [except amlodipine and felodipine], antiarrhythmics [except amiodarone and dofetilide], itraconazole, terbinafine), causing Na+ and water retention (e.g., corticosteroids, NSAIDs, thiazolidinediones), causing vasoconstriction (e.g., sympathomimetics), or acting as a direct cardiotoxin (e.g., anthracyclines, cyclophosphamide, trastuzumab).

Diagnosis

- Diagnosis is primarily based on the patient's physical exam findings in conjunction with the past medical history and results from laboratory and diagnostic tests.

- Echocardiogram provides information regarding LV function and can reflect whether the patient has systolic or diastolic dysfunction.

- B-type natriuretic peptide (BNP) concentration can also be obtained to help differentiate between acute HF and other causes of dyspnea (e.g., pneumonia, bronchitis, COPD, pulmonary embolus) (>500 pg/mL in patients with acute decompensated HF [ADHF]).

Signs and Symptoms

- Signs and symptoms of left-sided HF (reflect pulmonary congestion)
  - Symptoms: Dyspnea, orthopnea, paroxysmal nocturnal dyspnea, cough
  - Signs: Rales (usually bibasilar), pulmonary edema, pleural effusion, S_3 gallop
- Signs and symptoms of right-sided HF (reflect systemic congestion)
  - Symptoms: Anorexia, N/V, constipation, abdominal pain, bloating
  - Signs: Jugular venous distention, (+) hepatojugular reflux, ascites, peripheral edema, hepatomegaly, splenomegaly

Classification of HF

New York Heart Association (NYHA) Functional Classification	American College of Cardiology/ American Heart Association Staging System
• Functional class I = Patients have LV dysfunction but no physical limitations; lack symptoms with ordinary physical activity ("well compensated") • Functional class II = Slight limitation of physical activity; symptoms with ordinary physical activity (e.g., walking two blocks) • Functional class III = Marked limitation of physical activity; minimal activity (e.g., activities of daily living) causes symptoms • Functional class IV = Unable to carry on physical activity without discomfort; symptoms at rest	• Stage A = At high risk for development of HF but have no structural heart disease or symptoms of HF. Includes patients with HTN, DM, and CAD • Stage B = Structural heart disease (e.g., LVH, previous MI, LV systolic dysfunction, or valvular heart disease) but no symptoms of HF (NYHA class I symptoms) • Stage C = Structural heart disease with current or previous symptoms of HF (NYHA class I, II, III, or IV symptoms) • Stage D = Refractory symptoms of HF at rest despite maximal medical therapy (often hospitalized) (end-stage HF) (NYHA class IV symptoms)

Guidelines

Heart Failure Society of America. *J Card Fail*, no. 16 (2010): e1-194. www.heartfailureguidelines.com.

American College of Cardiology American Heart Association. *J Am Coll Cardiol*, no. 53 (2009): el-90.

Guidelines Summary

The goals of therapy are to relieve symptoms, improve quality of life, improve survival, reduce hospitalizations, and slow the progression of disease.

■ Nonpharmacologic therapy: Regular low-intensity physical activity, ↓ Na$^+$ (≤3 g/day), ↓ fluid intake (<2 L/day), weight loss (if obese), alcohol restriction, and smoking cessation

■ Pharmacologic therapy:

• Stage A: Modify risk factors and control HTN, DM, CAD, and dyslipidemia; ACEI or ARB in patients with risk factors for vascular disease

• Stage B: ACEI + β-blocker

• Stage C: ACEI + β-blocker + diuretic

» Other drugs to be considered:

– ARA: Current or recent NYHA class IV symptoms who are already receiving ACEI (or ARB), β-blocker, and diuretic (± digoxin)

- ARBs: Patients who cannot tolerate an ACEI due to intractable cough; patients who remain symptomatic despite optimal therapy with ACEI and β-blocker

- Digoxin: Patients who remain symptomatic despite optimal therapy with ACEI (or ARB), β-blocker, and diuretic

- Hydralazine/isosorbide dinitrate: Patients with intolerance or contraindications (renal insufficiency, hyperkalemia) to ACEI or ARB; African-American patients with NYHA class III or IV symptoms who remain symptomatic despite optimal therapy with ACEI (or ARB) and β-blocker

- Stage D: Chronic positive inotrope therapy (e.g., dobutamine, milrinone), mechanical circulatory support (e.g., LV assist device), heart transplant, end-of-life care/hospice

Medication Charts

Loop Diuretics

Mechanism of action – inhibit Na^+ reabsorption in the ascending limb of loop of Henle; ↓ preload

Generic	Brand	Dose	Contra-indications	Primary Side Effects	Key Monitoring	Pertinent Drug Interactions	Med Pearl	Top 200
Bumetanide	Bumex	0.5–10 mg/day	Sulfa allergy	• Hypocalcemia • Hypokalemia • Hypomagnesemia • Hyponatremia • Hyperglycemia • Hyperuricemia • Metabolic alkalosis • Azotemia	• BP • Electrolytes • BUN/SCr • Blood glucose • Uric acid • Jugular venous pressure • Urine output • Weight (↓ by 0.5–1 kg/day initially)	• May ↑ risk of lithium toxicity • May ↑ risk of ototoxicity with aminoglycosides • May ↓ effect of antidiabetic agents • NSAIDs ↓ effects	• ↓ symptoms; effect on mortality unknown • If initial dose inadequate, double dose, dose 2x daily, add metolazone, or use IV • Similar side effects as thiazides (except ocps cause hypocalcemia) • BUN/SCr ratio >20:1 → dehydration (prerenal azotemia) • Furosemide PO dose = 2x IV dose	No
Furosemide	Lasix	20–600 mg/day						Yes
Torsemide	Demadex	10–200 mg/day						No

ACE Inhibitors

- See HTN monograph for further details
- Medication pearls specific to their use in HF:
  - ↓ mortality; ↓ preload and afterload
  - Strive to achieve target dose, if possible (titrate dose to symptoms, not BP)

Drug	Initial Dose	Target Dose
Captopril	6.25 mg TID	50 mg TID
Enalapril	2.5 mg BID	10 mg BID
Lisinopril	2.5 mg daily	40 mg daily
Ramipril	1.25 mg daily	10 mg daily
Trandolapril	1 mg daily	4 mg daily
Fosinopril	5 mg daily	40 mg daily
Quinapril	5 mg BID	20 mg BID
Perindopril	2 mg daily	16 mg daily

β-Blockers

Mechanism of action – ↓ activation of the sympathetic nervous system; slows and potentially reverses detrimental effects (e.g., ventricular remodeling) of catecholamines

Generic	Brand	Dose	Contraindications	Primary Side Effects	Key Monitoring	Pertinent Drug Interactions	Med Pearl	Top 200
Bisoprolol	Zebeta	1.25–10 mg/day Target dose: 10 mg daily	• Symptomatic bradycardia • ≥2nd-degree heart block (in absence of pacemaker) • SBP <85 mmHg • Severe asthma • Decompensated HF	See HTN section	• BP • HR • S/S HF • Weight		• ↓ mortality • Metoprolol succinate (not tartrate) approved for HF	No
Carvedilol	Coreg, Coreg CR	IR: 6.25–100 mg/day (in two divided doses) Target dose: <85 kg = 25 mg BID; >85 kg = 50 mg BID CR: 10–80 mg/day (1x daily) Target dose: 80 mg daily				Carvedilol may ↑ digoxin levels	• Patient should be fairly euvolemic before starting • Strive to achieve target dose, if possible • Dose can be doubled every 2–4 wks to achieve target dose (unless side effects) • Manage worsening HF by ↑ diuretic dose • If hypotension occurs, may ↓ dose of ACEI, ARB, or other vasodilator (more common with carvedilol) • If bradycardia occurs, ↓ dose • Abrupt discontinuation may cause worsening HF	Yes
Metoprolol succinate	Toprol XL	12.5–200 mg/day Target dose: 200 mg daily						Yes

Digoxin

Mechanism of action – inhibits Na⁺/K⁺ ATPase pump → ↑ intracellular Ca²⁺ → ↑ myocardial contractility; also ↓ neurohormonal activation

Generic	Brand	Dose	Contra-indications	Primary Side Effects	Key Monitoring	Pertinent Drug Interactions	Med Pearl	Top 200
Digoxin	Digitek, Lanoxin	0.125–0.25 mg/day (loading doses not necessary in HF)	≥2nd-degree heart block (in absence of pacemaker)	• Bradycardia/heart block • S/S digoxin toxicity (visual disturbances, N/V, confusion, anorexia, arrhythmias)	• HR • Electrolytes (predisposed to toxicity if hypokalemia, hypomagnesemia, or hypercalcemia) • BUN/SCr • Digoxin concentrations	• Amiodarone, dronedarone, quinidine, verapamil, and clarithromycin may ↑ levels • Antacids may ↓ levels (separate by 1–2 hours) • Use with other negative chronotropes (e.g., β-blockers, verapamil, diltiazem, or clonidine) may ↑ risk of bradycardia	• Improves symptoms, ↓ hospitalizations; no effect on mortality • Used to ↑ contractility in systolic HF and to ↓ HR in atrial fibrillation (AF) • Abrupt discontinuation may cause worsening HF • ↓ dose by 50% when starting amiodarone or dronedarone • Adjust dose in patients with renal dysfunction • Target level: 0.5–1 ng/mL (↑ mortality if >1 ng/mL)	Yes

Aldosterone Receptor Antagonists

Mechanism of action – inhibit the effects of aldosterone → ↓ remodeling and Na$^+$/water retention
- Spironolactone is nonselective ARA (also blocks androgen and progesterone receptors → associated with endocrine side effects)
- Eplerenone is selective ARA (not associated with endocrinologic side effects)

Generic	Brand	Dose	Contraindications	Primary Side Effects	Key Monitoring	Pertinent Drug Interactions	Med Pearl	Top 200
Eplerenone	Inspra	25–50 mg/day	• K$^+$ >5 mEq/L • SCr >2.5 mg/dL (or CrCl ≤30 mL/min) • Concomitant ACEI and ARB use • Also for eplerenone: Use of strong CYP3A4 inhibitors (e.g., ritonavir, ketoconazole, itraconazole, nefazodone, clarithromycin, nelfinavir)	• Hyperkalemia • Also for spironolactone: Gynecomastia, breast tenderness, menstrual changes, hirsutism	• BP • K$^+$ • BUN/SCr	Use with ACEIs, ARBs, K$^+$ supplements, or NSAIDs may ↑ risk of hyperkalemia	• ↓ mortality • Should consider discontinuing or ↓ dose of K$^+$ supplements • Eplerenone tends to be used in patients who develop endocrine side effects (≥, gynecomastia) with spironolactone	No
Spironolactone	Aldactone	12.5–25 mg/day						Yes

Angiotensin II Receptor Blockers

- See HTN monograph for further details
- Medication pearls specific to their use in HF:
  - Only candesartan, losartan, or valsartan recommended for the management of HF (only candesartan and valsartan approved for HF)
  - Should not be considered equivalent or superior to ACEIs

Hydralazine/Isosorbide Dinitrate

Mechanism of action:
- Hydralazine – causes arterial vasodilation (↓ afterload)
- Isosorbide dinitrate – causes venous vasodilation (↓ preload)

Generic	Brand	Dose	Contra-indications	Primary Side Effects	Key Monitoring	Pertinent Drug Interactions	Med Pearl	Top 200
Hydralazine	Apresoline	40–300 mg/day	None	• Headache • Dizziness • Reflex tachycardia • Peripheral edema (hydralazine) • Lupus-like syndrome (hydralazine)	• BP • HR	None	• ↓ mortality (when used together) • Often used in patients who cannot tolerate ACEIs or ARBs due to renal insufficiency, hyperkalemia, or angioedema • Do not use hydralazine alone (↑ mortality)	Yes
Isosorbide dinitrate	Isordil	30–120 mg/day						No

Combination product:

Hydralazine/isosorbide dinitrate (BiDil) – approved for African-American patients with NYHA class III or IV HF due to LV systolic dysfunction (LVEF ≤40%) who are receiving an ACEI (or ARB) and a β-blocker (can also use individual products together if there are financial concerns)

Intravenous Drugs for Treatment of ADHF

Drug	Mechanism of Action	Primary Side Effects	Med Pearl
Vasodilators			
Nitroglycerin (NTG)	• Venous vasodilation → ↓ preload • Can cause arterial vasodilation at higher doses	Hypotension, tachycardia, headache, tolerance	• Especially useful in patients with myocardial ischemia • Tolerance can develop (overcome by ↑ infusion rate)
Nitroprusside	Arterial and venous vasodilation → ↓ preload and afterload	Hypotension, N/V, cyanide/thiocyanate toxicity (risk ↑ if infusion >24 hours)	Avoid in patients with renal dysfunction
Nesiritide (Natrecor)	• BNP • Arterial and venous vasodilation → ↓ preload and afterload	Hypotension, headache	Infusion should not be titrated more frequently than every 3 hours
Positive Inotropes			
Dopamine	• 0.5–3 mcg/kg/min → Stimulates dopamine receptors → ↑ urine output • 3–10 mcg/kg/min → Stimulates β_1 receptors → ↑ CO, ↑ HR • >10 mcg/kg/min → Stimulates α_1 receptors → ↑ BP	Arrhythmias, tachycardia, myocardial ischemia, N/V	Avoid in patients with myocardial ischemia
Dobutamine	β_1 and β_2 receptor agonist and weak α_1 receptor agonist → ↑ CO and vasodilation	Arrhythmias, tachycardia, myocardial ischemia, hypokalemia, tremor	• Avoid in patients with myocardial ischemia • Should not be used in patients receiving chronic β-blocker therapy • Tolerance can develop
Milrinone	PDE III inhibitor → ↑ CO and vasodilation	Hypotension, arrhythmias	• Can be used in patients receiving chronic β-blocker therapy, or in those not responding to or tolerating dobutamine • Tolerance does not develop • Use lower initial dose in patients with renal dysfunction

Storage and Administration Pearls

- Captopril should be administered at least 1 hour *before* or 2 hours *after* meals.
- Carvedilol should be administered with food to minimize the risk of orthostatic hypotension.
- Nitroprusside infusions should be protected from light.

Patient Education Pearls

- If a patient is taking >1 dose of diuretic each day, the last dose should be taken before 5 P.M. to minimize nocturia.
- Patients should weigh themselves daily (first thing in the morning after urinating) and should contact their healthcare provider if they gain more than 3–5 lb in a week.
- Patients receiving diuretics should wear sunscreen and protective clothing. Also, they should report any episodes of muscle cramps, as this may be a symptom of hypokalemia or hypomagnesemia.
- A patient who is receiving ARAs, ACEIs, or ARBs should avoid excessive intake of foods high in K^+ (e.g., green leafy vegetables, potatoes, apricots, bananas, dates, oranges, avocados) and K^+-containing salt substitutes.
- A patient who is receiving ACEIs or ARBs should call 911 immediately if he/she experiences lip, tongue, or facial swelling or is having difficulty breathing.
- ACEIs and ARBs should be avoided in patients who are pregnant.
- Patients should not stop their β-blocker or digoxin therapy abruptly, as this may cause a sudden worsening of HF symptoms.

ANTIARRHYTHMIC DRUGS

Class IA

Generic	Brand	Dose	Contra-indications	Primary Side Effects	Key Monitoring	Pertinent Drug Interactions	Med Pearl	Top 200
Mechanism of action – Na$^+$ channel blockers; slow conduction velocity, prolong refractoriness, ↓ automaticity								
Disopyramide	Norpace, Norpace CR	400–1,600 mg/day	• HF • ≥2nd-degree heart block (in absence of pacemaker) • Long QT syndrome	• Dry mouth • Urinary retention • Blurred vision • Constipation • HF exacerbation • Hypotension • Torsades de pointes (TdP)	• Electrocardiogram (ECG) (QTc interval, QRS duration) • BP • S/S HF • Electrolytes • Disopyramide concentrations	• CYP3A4 inhibitors and anticholinergics may ↑ risk of side effects • CYP3A4 inducers may ↓ effects • ↑ risk of TdP with other drugs that prolong QT interval	• Used for atrial and ventricular arrhythmias • Therapeutic range: 2–5 mcg/mL • Adjust dose in renal dysfunction	No
Procainamide	Pronestyl	IV: *Loading dose:* 15–17 mg/kg over 25–60 min *Maintenance dose:* 1–4 mg/min continuous infusion	• ≥2nd-degree heart block (in absence of pacemaker) • Long QT syndrome	• Lupus-like syndrome • TdP • Hypotension • Agranulocytosis	• ECG (QTc interval, QRS duration) • BP • S/S lupus (e.g., stabbing chest pain, joint pain, rash) • Procainamide/N-acetylprocainamide (NAPA) concentrations • Complete blood count (CBC) with differential • Electrolytes	↑ risk of TdP with other drugs that prolong QT interval	• Used for atrial and ventricular arrhythmias • Therapeutic range: 4–10 mcg/mL (procainamide); 15–25 mcg/mL (NAPA); 10–30 mcg/mL (total) • Use with caution, if at all, in renal insufficiency	No
Quinidine	Quinaglute, Quinidex	• Sulfate: 800–2,400 mg/day • Gluconate: 648–2,916 mg/day	• ≥2nd-degree heart block (in absence of pacemaker) • Long QT syndrome • Use of ritonavir	• Diarrhea • Stomach cramps • TdP • Hypotension • Cinchonism (tinnitus, blurred vision, headache) • Thrombocytopenia	• ECG (QTc interval, QRS duration) • BP • Quinidine concentrations • CBC with differential • LFTs • Electrolytes	• CYP3A4 inhibitors may ↑ risk of side effects • CYP3A4 inducers may ↓ effects • ↑ risk of digoxin toxicity • May ↑ toxicity of CYP3A4 and CYP2D6 substrates • ↑ risk of TdP with other drugs that prolong QT interval	• Used for atrial and ventricular arrhythmias • Therapeutic range: 2–5 mcg/mL • Administer with food to minimize GI effects	No

- Avoid all Class IA antiarrhythmics in patients with structural heart disease (i.e., HF, CAD, left ventricular hypertrophy, valvular disease)

Class IB

Mechanism of action – Na⁺ channel blockers; little effect on conduction velocity, shorten refractoriness, ↓ automaticity

Generic	Brand	Dose	Contraindications	Primary Side Effects	Key Monitoring	Pertinent Drug Interactions	Med Pearl	Top 200
Lidocaine	Xylocaine	*Loading dose:* 1–1.5 mg/kg, up to 3 mg/kg (total) *Maintenance dose:* 1–4 mg/min	≥2nd-degree heart block (in absence of pacemaker)	CNS toxicity (dizziness, blurred vision, slurred speech, confusion, paresthesias, seizures)	• ECG (QRS duration) • BP • Neurologic exam • Lidocaine concentrations (if duration of therapy >24 hours)	Amiodarone may ↑ risk of toxicity	• Used only for ventricular arrhythmias • Therapeutic range: 1.5–5 mcg/mL • Use lower infusion rate in elderly, HF or hepatic dysfunction	No
Mexiletine	Mexitil	600–1,200 mg/day	Same as for lidocaine	• CNS toxicity (same as lidocaine) • N/V	• ECG (QRS duration) • BP • LFTs • Neurologic exam	• ↑ risk of theophylline toxicity • CYP1A2 and CYP2D6 inhibitors may ↑ risk of toxicity	• Used only for ventricular arrhythmias • Take with food to minimize GI effects • ↓ dose in HF or hepatic dysfunction	No

- Class 1B antiarrhythmics do not cause TdP

Class IC

Class II

(See medication chart in HTN section for discussion on β-blockers)

Generic	Brand	Dose	Contraindications	Primary Side Effects	Key Monitoring	Pertinent Drug Interactions	Med Pearl	Top 200
Mechanism of action – Na$^+$ channel blockers (most potent); markedly slow conduction velocity, no effect on refractoriness, ↓ automaticity; propafenone also has nonselective β-blocking properties								
Flecainide	Tambocor	*Loading dose (for conversion of AF):* 200–300 mg x 1 dose *Maintenance dose:* 100–400 mg/day	• ≥2nd-degree heart block (in absence of pacemaker) • History of MI • HF	• Dizziness • Tremor • HF exacerbation • Ventricular tachycardia (VT)	• ECG (QRS duration) • Echocardiogram (at baseline to evaluation LV function) • Electrolytes	↑ risk of digoxin toxicity	• Used for atrial and ventricular arrhythmias • Adjust dose in renal dysfunction	No
Propafenone	Rythmol, Rythmol SR	IR: *Loading dose (for AF conversion):* 450–600 mg x 1 *Maintenance dose:* 450–900 mg/day (in three divided doses) SR: *Maintenance dose:* 450–950 mg/day (in two divided doses)	• ≥2nd-degree heart block (in absence of pacemaker) • Bradycardia • Bronchospastic disorders • HF • History of MI	• Bradycardia/ heart block • HF exacerbation • Bronchospasm • Taste disturbances • VT	• ECG (QRS duration, PR interval) • BP • HR • Echocardiogram (at baseline to evaluation LV function) • Electrolytes	• ↑ risk of digoxin toxicity • ↑ effects of warfarin • Use with other negative chronotropes (e.g., β-blockers, digoxin, verapamil, diltiazem, or clonidine) may ↑ risk of bradycardia	• Used for atrial and ventricular arrhythmias	No

- Avoid Class IC antiarrhythmics in patients with structural heart disease
- Class IC antiarrhythmics do not cause TdP

Class III

Mechanism of action – K+ channel blockers; no effect on conduction velocity or automaticity; amiodarone and dronedarone also have Na+-channel blocking, β-blocking, and CCB properties; sotalol also has nonselective β-blocking properties

Generic	Brand	Dose	Contraindications	Primary Side Effects	Key Monitoring	Pertinent Drug Interactions	Med Pearl	Top 200
Amiodarone	Cordarone, Pacerone	Loading dose (IV): *Stable VT / ventricular fibrillation:* 150 mg over 10 min *Pulseless VT / ventricular fibrillation:* 300 mg IV push AF: 5 mg/kg over 30–60 min Loading dose (PO): *Ventricular arrhythmias:* 1,200–1,600 mg/day *Atrial arrhythmias:* 800–1200 mg/day until 10 g total Maintenance dose: IV: 1 mg/min x 6 hrs, then 0.5 mg/min PO: 100–400 mg/day	≥2nd-degree heart block (in absence of pacemaker)	IV: • Hypotension • Bradycardia/ heart block • Phlebitis PO: • Hypo-/ hyper- thyroidism • Pulmonary fibrosis • Bradycardia/ heart block • Corneal microdeposits • Optic neuritis • N/V • ↑ LFTs • Ataxia • Paresthesias • Photosensitivity • Blue-gray skin discoloration	• ECG (QTc interval, QRS duration, PR interval) • BP • HR • Chest x-ray (baseline; then every 12 months) • Pulmonary function tests (if symptoms) • Thyroid function tests (TFTs) (baseline; then every 6 months) • LFTs (baseline; then every 6 months) • Ophthalmologic exam (baseline if significant visual abnormalities; then if symptoms develop)	• Inhibits CYP1A2, CYP2C9, CYP2D6, and CYP3A4 • CYP3A4 substrate • ↑ risk of digoxin toxicity (↓ digoxin dose by 50%) • ↑ effects of warfarin (↓ warfarin dose by 30%) • Use with other negative chronotropes (e.g. β-blockers, digoxin, verapamil, diltiazem, or clonidine) may ↑ risk of bradycardia • May ↑ cyclosporine or phenytoin levels • May ↑ risk of side effects of simvastatin and lovastatin	• Used for atrial and ventricular arrhythmias • Safe to use in HF • Half-life = 40–60 days • If pulmonary fibrosis or blurred vision occur, discontinue therapy • If TFTs abnormal, treat thyroid disorder • If ↑ LFTs occur, ↓ amiodarone dose • Take with food to minimize GI effects	No

Class III *(cont'd)*

Generic	Brand	Dose	Contraindications	Primary Side Effects	Key Monitoring	Pertinent Drug Interactions	Med Pearl	Top 200
Dronedarone	Multaq	400 mg 2x daily with meals	• Permanent AF • NYHA class IV HF or NYHA class II–III HF with recent decompensation requiring hospitalization or referral to specialized HF clinic • ≥2nd-degree heart block (in absence of pacemaker) • Bradycardia • Concurrent use of strong CYP3A4 inhibitors (e.g., ketoconazole, itraconazole, voriconazole, cyclosporine, telithromycin, clarithromycin, nefazodone, ritonavir) or strong CYP3A4 inducers (e.g., rifampin, phenobarbital, phenytoin, carbamazepine, St. John's wort) • Concurrent use of other drugs that prolong QT interval • QTc interval ≥500 msec • PR interval >280 msec • Severe hepatic impairment • Liver toxicity related to previous amiodarone use • Pregnancy	• N/V/D • ↑ SCr • Bradycardia • ↑ LFTs • New-onset or worsening HF	• ECG (QTc interval, PR interval) • HR • SCr • S/S HF • LFTs	• Inhibits CYP2D6 and CYP3A4 • CYP3A4 substrate • May ↑ toxicity of CYP3A4 and CYP2D6 substrates • CYP3A4 inhibitors may ↑ risk of side effects • CYP3A4 inducers may ↓ effects • ↑ risk of digoxin toxicity (↓ digoxin dose by 50% or consider discontinuing) • Use with other negative chronotropes (e.g. β-blockers, digoxin, verapamil, diltiazem, or clonidine) may ↑ risk of bradycardia • ↑ effects of dabigatran (↓ dose of dabigatran to 75 mg BID if CrCL 30–50 mL/min) • May ↑ risk of side effects of simvastatin and lovastatin	• Used only for atrial arrhythmias • Structurally related to amiodarone (does not have iodine component); less likely to cause organ toxicities; also has shorter half-life	No

Class III *(cont'd)*

Generic	Brand	Dose	Contraindications	Primary Side Effects	Key Monitoring	Pertinent Drug Interactions	Med Pearl	Top 200
Dofetilide	Tikosyn	• 500 mcg 2x daily (if CrCl >60 mL/min) • Adjust dose if CrCl ≤60 mL/min	• CrCl <20 mL/min • QTc interval >440 msec • Hypokalemia/hypomagnesemia • Use of verapamil, ketoconazole, cimetidine, trimethoprim, prochlorperazine, hydrochlorothiazide, megestrol, or other drugs that prolong QT interval	TdP	• ECG (QTc interval) • SCr • Electrolytes	↑ risk of TdP with other drugs that prolong QT interval	• Used only for atrial arrhythmias • Adjust dose based on renal function and QT interval • Must be initiated in hospital • Safe to use in HF	No
Ibutilide	Corvert	1 mg over 10 min; repeat x 1, if needed	• QTc interval >440 msec • Hypokalemia/hypomagnesemia • Concurrent use of other drugs that prolong QT interval	TdP	• ECG (QTc interval) • Electrolytes	↑ risk of TdP with other drugs that prolong QT interval	Used only for atrial arrhythmias	No
Sotalol	Betapace, Betapace AF, Sorine	• 160–640 mg/day (in 2 divided doses) • Extend dosing interval if CrCl ≤60 mL/min	• ≥2nd-degree heart block (in absence of pacemaker) • Concurrent use of other drugs that prolong QT interval • CrCl <40 mL/min (for AF) • Long QT syndrome • HF	• TdP • Bradycardia/heart block • Bronchospasm • HF exacerbation	• ECG (QTc interval, PR interval) • HR • SCr • Electrolytes	• ↑ risk of TdP with other drugs that prolong QT interval • Use with other negative chronotropes (e.g. β-blockers, digoxin, verapamil, diltiazem, or clonidine) may ↑ risk of bradycardia	• Used for atrial and ventricular arrhythmias • Adjust dosing interval in renal dysfunction	No

Class IV Antiarrhythmics

(See medication chart in HTN section for discussion on CCBs)

ANTITHROMBOTIC DRUGS

Warfarin (Coumadin)

- Commonly prescribed for patients with a variety of conditions where clotting is a risk, such as AF, to prevent the formation of thrombi.
- Mechanism of action: Interferes with the synthesis of the vitamin K-dependent clotting factors of the liver (II, VII, IX, and X) as well as protein C and S
  - Regular monitoring of the PT/INR is necessary.
- Contraindications: Pregnancy (Category X), recent surgery
- Side effects: Bleeding, skin necrosis (especially with Protein C deficiency), purple toe syndrome
- Drug interactions:

Increased Anticoagulant Effect	Decreased Anticoagulant Effect
Alcohol (acute ingestion), amiodarone, azole antifungals, cephalosporins, cimetidine, corticosteroids, dronedarone, fluoroquinolones, lovastatin, macrolides, omeprazole, penicillins, simvastatin, sulfonamides, thyroid hormones	Alcohol (chronic ingestion), barbiturates, carbamazepine, cholestyramine, phenytoin, rifampin, St. John's wort, vitamin K

- Antidote: Vitamin K
- Dosing:
  - Must be individualized
  - The full effect of a specific warfarin dose (or dosage change) is not seen for 72–96 hours (3–4 days). A good rule to follow is that 50% of warfarin's effect will be evident after 1 day, 25% more (75% total) on day 2 and 25% more (100% total effect) on days 3–4.
  - The INR obtained "today" is a reflection of the last 3 doses.
  - Continually monitor for trends related to changes in the INR.
  - Review all medications (new and existing) that may have been added or changed.
  - Consider the possibility of drug-drug interactions with warfarin.
  - Monitor for signs/symptoms of bleeding (labs and physical).

Dabigatran (Pradaxa)

- Indicated for prevention of stroke and systemic embolism in patients with AF
- Considered as an alternative to warfarin
- Mechanism of action: Direct thrombin inhibitor (oral)

- Contraindications: Active bleeding
- Side effects: Bleeding, dyspepsia
- Drug interactions:
  - Dronedarone and ketoconazole →↑ anticoagulant effects
    » ↓ dabigatran dose to 75 mg BID if CrCl 30–50 mL/min
  - Rifampin →↓ anticoagulant effects (avoid concomitant use)
- Antidote: None available
- Recommended dose:
  - CrCl >30 mL/min: 150 mg BID
  - CrCl 15–30 mL/min: 75 mg BID
  - CrCl <15 mL/min: NOT recommended

Rivaroxaban (Xarelto)

- Indicated for prevention of stroke and systemic embolism in patients with AF and for venous thromboembolism prophylaxis in patients undergoing hip or knee replacement surgery
- Mechanism of action: Factor Xa inhibitor (oral)
- Contraindications: Active bleeding
- Side effects: Bleeding
- Drug interactions:
  - Avoid concomitant use with COMBINED P-gp and strong CYP3A4 inhibitors (e.g., ketoconazole, itraconazole, ritonavir)
  - Avoid concomitant use with COMBINED P-gp and strong CYP3A4 inducers (e.g., carbamazepine, phenytoin, rifampin, St. John's wort)
- Antidote: None available
- Recommended dose:
  - VTE prophylaxis: 10 mg daily
  - AF
    » CrCl >50 mL/min: 20 mg daily
    » CrCl 15–50 mL/min: 15 mg daily
    » CrCl <15 mL/min: NOT recommended

ISCHEMIC HEART DISEASE

Definitions

Ischemic heart disease (IHD) is characterized by a lack of oxygen resulting from inadequate perfusion of the myocardium, which is often due to narrowing or blockage in a coronary artery. Patients with IHD may present with chronic stable angina, vasospastic angina (variant or Prinzmetal's angina), or an acute coronary syndrome (ACS). ACS can include UA, non–ST-segment-elevation MI (NSTEMI), or ST-segment–elevation MI (STEMI). An ACS is precipitated by rupture of an atherosclerotic plaque, followed by formation of a thrombus at the site of plaque rupture. In NSTEMI, the thrombus tends to contain more platelets than fibrin ("white clot") and does not completely occlude the vessel. In STEMI, the thrombus contains more fibrin and red blood cells than platelets ("red clot") and completely occludes the vessel.

This section reviews the management of NSTEMI and STEMI.

Diagnosis

- If ischemic-like chest pain persists for at least 20 minutes, ACS should be suspected.
  - An ECG should be performed and serial cardiac enzymes (troponin, CK-MB) should be obtained.

Findings	UA	NSTEMI	STEMI
Cardiac enzymes (troponin, CK-MB)	Negative	Positive	Positive
ECG changes	ST-segment depression, T-wave inversion, or no ECG changes (any changes are usually transient)	ST-segment depression, T-wave inversion, or no ECG changes	ST-segment elevation

Signs and Symptoms

- Chest pain/pressure (substernal, crushing) that may radiate to the left arm, jaw, shoulders, and back are common symptoms.
- Other symptoms include dyspnea, diaphoresis, N/V.
- When compared to chronic stable angina, pain in ACS may be more severe, occur at rest, occur more frequently, be precipitated by less exertion, and be refractory to sublingual NTG.
- Patients may also present with signs/symptoms of HF or with arrhythmias.

Guidelines

American College of Cardiology/American Heart Association (NSTEMI guidelines). *J Am Coll Cardiol*, no. 57 (2011): e215-e367.

American College of Cardiology/American Heart Association (STEMI guidelines, 2009 Focused Update). *J Am Coll Cardiol*, no. 54 (2009): 2205–41.

Guidelines Summary

ACUTE PHARMACOLOGIC MANAGEMENT OF UA/NSTEMI

Anti-Ischemic and Analgesic Therapy

Morphine

- Can be given to patients who continue to have chest discomfort despite the use of NTG or have recurrence of chest pain despite the use of other anti-ischemic therapies
- Dose: 1–5 mg IV every 5–30 minutes as needed for pain

NTG

- Can be given to patients with ongoing chest discomfort (0.4 mg sublingually every 5 min × 3 doses); following these doses, give IV NTG within the initial 48 hours if patients continue to have ischemia, or if they present with HF or are hypertensive
- Dose: 5–10 mcg/min continuous infusion; can be titrated up to 100 mcg/min for relief of symptoms
- Adverse effects: Reflex tachycardia, hypotension, headache

β-Blockers

- Oral β-blockers: Given within the first 24 hours to patients who **do not** have signs/symptoms of HF, risk factors for developing cardiogenic shock (age >70 years, SBP <120 mmHg, HR >110 beats per minute (bpm) or <60 bpm, or prolonged duration since presenting with UA/NSTEMI), PR interval >0.24 sec, ≥2nd-degree heart block, or severe reactive airway disease
- IV β-blockers can be used as an alternative

CCBs

- A non-DHP CCB (verapamil or diltiazem) can be used alternatively if the patient has a contraindication to β-blocker therapy and does not have evidence of LV dysfunction
- A long-acting non-DHP CCB can be used in patients who have recurrent ischemia despite being on a β-blocker and nitrate therapy

ACEIs

- Should be given within the first 24 hours to patients with pulmonary congestion or LVEF ≤40%, provided they are not hypotensive (SBP <100 mmHg) or have contraindications
- Can also be useful if given within the first 24 hours to patients without pulmonary congestion or LVEF ≤40%, provided they are not hypotensive (SBP <100 mmHg) or have contraindications
- An ARB can be used alternatively in patients who cannot tolerate ACEIs

Antiplatelet Therapy

Aspirin

- All patients should receive 162–325 mg (non–enteric-coated) at the onset of chest pain (should be chewed and swallowed).
- Patients experiencing UA/NSTEMI should continue to receive the following aspirin regimens (based on whether or not they received a stent):

Procedure	Initial Therapy	Indefinite Therapy
No stent		75–162 mg daily
Bare-metal stent (BMS)	162–325 mg daily for ≥1 month	75–162 mg daily
Drug-eluting stent (DES)—Sirolimus-eluting	162–325 mg daily for ≥3 months	75–162 mg daily
DES—Paclitaxel-eluting	162–325 mg daily for ≥6 months	75–162 mg daily

Clopidogrel (Plavix)

- Prodrug; must be converted via CYP2C19 to active drug
- This is an alternative to aspirin in patients who are allergic or have a major GI intolerance to aspirin.
- A loading dose of 300–600 mg, followed by a maintenance dose of 75 mg daily, should be given to all patients regardless of whether an invasive (PCI) or conservative treatment strategy is planned (should be given **with** aspirin).
- Clopidogrel should be continued (**with** aspirin) for the following durations of time:
  - BMS or DES (sirolimus or paclitaxel): At least 12 months
  - No stent: At least 1 month, ideally up to 1 year
- Discontinue ≥5 days before CABG

Prasugrel (Effient)

- Prodrug
- Alternative to clopidogrel in patients with ACS managed with PCI
- Achieves faster inhibition of platelet aggregation than clopidogrel
- Administered as a loading dose of 60 mg prior to PCI, followed by maintenance dose of 10 mg daily (↓ dose to 5 mg daily in patients <60 kg)
- Not recommended for patients ≥75 years (↑ risk of bleeding) or in patients with prior history of stroke or TIA
- Prasugrel should be continued (**with** aspirin) for the following duration of time:
  - BMS or DES: At least 12 months
- Discontinue ≥7 days before CABG

Ticagrelor (Brilinta)

- NOT a thienopyridine
  - Reversibly binds the P2Y12 receptor
  - Does not require conversion to an active metabolite (NOT a prodrug)
- Alternative antiplatelet in patients with ACS managed medically or with PCI
- Administered as a loading dose of 180 mg prior to PCI, followed by maintenance dose of 90 mg BID (dose of aspirin during maintenance therapy should not exceed 100 mg/day)
- Should be continued (**with** aspirin) for the following duration of time:
  - BMS or DES: At least 12 months
- Discontinue ≥5 days before CABG

Glycoprotein IIb/IIIa Receptor Blockers (GPBs)

- PCI planned: Clopidogrel and/or GPB (eptifibatide or tirofiban) can be initiated prior to angiography. Do not need GPB if bivalirudin + 300 mg loading dose of clopidogrel (given ≥6 hours before angiography) are used.
- Conservative strategy: Adding eptifibatide or tirofiban to clopidogrel can be considered (especially if patient has recurrent ischemia and requires angiography).

Anticoagulant Therapy

- PCI planned: Either unfractionated heparin (UFH) or enoxaparin should be added to antiplatelet therapy; fondaparinux or bivalirudin can be used alternatively.
- Conservative strategy: Either enoxaparin or fondaparinux should be added to antiplatelet therapy; UFH can be used alternatively.

ACUTE PHARMACOLOGIC MANAGEMENT OF STEMI

Anti-Ischemic and Analgesic Therapy

Morphine, NTG, β-Blockers, ACEIs

- Same recommendations as for UA/NSTEMI

Antiplatelet Therapy

Aspirin

- Same recommendations as for UA/NSTEMI

Clopidogrel

- This is an alternative to aspirin in patients who are allergic or have a major GI intolerance to aspirin.
- Clopidogrel 75 mg daily should be added to aspirin therapy in all patients regardless of whether or not they undergo reperfusion with a fibrinolytic. A loading dose of 300–600 mg can be considered in patients age <75 years.
- Clopidogrel should be continued (**with** aspirin) for the following durations of time:
  - BMS or DES: At least 12 months (and up to 15 months)
  - No stent: At least 14 days (can be considered for up to 1 year)
- Discontinue ≥ 5 days before CABG

Prasugrel

- Same recommendations as for UA/NSTEMI

Ticagrelor

- Same recommendations as for UA/NSTEMI

GPBs

- Can be used if patient undergoing primary PCI

Fibrinolytic Therapy

- Should be used in patients presenting to a hospital without the capability to perform PCI or cannot perform PCI within 90 minutes of first medical contact ("door-to-balloon" time)
- Should be initiated within 30 minutes of presenting to the hospital ("door-to-needle" time)

Anticoagulant Therapy

- Fibrinolytic administered: UFH, enoxaparin, or fondaparinux can be used; should be continued for up to 8 days; UFH should only be used if the treatment duration is <48 hours because of risk for heparin-induced thrombocytopenia (HIT) with prolonged therapy.
- Primary PCI: UFH, bivalirudin, or enoxaparin can be used.

SECONDARY PREVENTION OF MI

- **Aspirin:** See recommendation above regarding dosing and duration of therapy.
- **Clopidogrel, prasugrel, or ticagrelor:** See recommendations above in respective NSTEMI and STEMI sections regarding dosing and duration of therapy.
- **β-blockers:** Continue indefinitely.
- **ACEIs:** Should be given and continued indefinitely in all patients; ARB can be used in patients intolerant of ACEIs.
- **ARAs:** Should be given to patients with LVEF ≤40% receiving optimal ACEI and β-blocker therapy who have DM or HF.
- **Statins:** Should be given and continued indefinitely in all patients (LDL-C goal <100 mg/dL; <70 mg/dL is considered reasonable).

Glycoprotein IIb/IIIa Receptor Blockers

Mechanism of action – block the glycoprotein IIb/IIIa receptor on platelets to prevent the binding of fibrinogen → Inhibit platelet aggregation

Generic	Brand	Dose	Contra-indications	Primary Side Effects	Key Monitoring	Pertinent Drug Interactions	Med Pearl
Abciximab	ReoPro	*Loading dose:* 0.25 mg/kg IV bolus *Maintenance dose:* 0.125 mcg/kg/min (max of 10 mg/min); continue for 12 hr after PCI	• Active bleeding • Prior stroke within past 30 days or any hemorrhagic stroke • History of intracranial neoplasms or aneurysm • Thrombocytopenia • BP >180/110 mmHg • Dialysis-dependent (for eptifibatide)	• Bleeding • Thrombocytopenia	• CBC • Prothrombin time (PT)/activated partial thromboplastin time (aPTT) • Activated clotting time (ACT) (with PCI) • S/S bleeding • SC (baseline)	Anticoagulants and other antiplatelets may ↑ risk of bleeding	• Abciximab preferred over others in NSTEMI only if there is no significant delay to PCI (otherwise, eptifibatide or tirofiban preferred) • Adjust maintenance dose infusion of tirofiban and eptifibatide in renal dysfunction
Eptifibatide	Integrilin	*Loading dose:* 180 mcg/kg IV bolus x 2 (given 10 min apart) *Maintenance dose:* 2 mcg/kg/min; continue for 18–24 hr after PCI					
Tirofiban	Aggrastat	NSTEMI: *Loading dose:* 0.4 mcg/kg/min x 30 min *Maintenance dose:* 0.1 mcg/kg/min; continue for 18–24 hr after PCI STEMI (with PCI): *Loading dose:* 25 mcg/kg IV bolus *Maintenance dose:* 0.1 mcg/kg/min; continue for up to 18 hr after PCI					

Anticoagulants

Mechanism of action:
- UFH: Potentiates the action of antithrombin III, which inactivates the clotting factors, IIa (thrombin), IXa, Xa, XIa, and XIIa, and ultimately prevents the conversion of fibrinogen to fibrin
- Low molecular-weight heparins (LMWHs): Similar mechanism as UFH, but primarily inhibit factor Xa
- Fondparinux: Selective inhibitor of factor Xa
- Bivalirudin: Direct thrombin inhibitor

Generic	Brand	Dose	Contra-indications	Primary Side Effects	Key Monitoring	Pertinent Drug Interactions	Med Pearl
UFH	None	*Loading dose:* 60 units/kg IV bolus (max = 4,000 units) *Maintenance dose:* 12 units/kg/hr (max = 1,000 units/hr)	• Active bleeding • History of HIT • Recent stroke	• Bleeding • Thrombocytopenia (UFH and LMWH)	• PT/aPTT (only for UFH) • CBC • Anti-Xa levels (for LMWHs) (consider in obese or renal dysfunction) • S/S bleeding	Antiplatelets and other anticoagulants may ↑ risk of bleeding	• If platelets <100,000 or ↓ by >50% from baseline, test for HIT; discontinue UFH and start direct thrombin inhibitor (eg., lepirudin, argatroban) • Protamine can be used to reverse effects
Enoxaparin	Lovenox	*Loading dose:* 30 mg IV x 1 *Maintenance dose:* 1 mg/kg SC every 12 hr					• ↓ enoxaparin dose to 1 mg/kg every 24 hr if CrCl <30 mL/min • Avoid using dalteparin in renal dysfunction • Should not use in patients with suspected HIT • Protamine only partially reverses effects
Dalteparin	Fragmin	120 units/kg (max = 10,000 units) SC every 12 hr					
Fondaparinux	Arixtra	2.5 mg SC daily	• Active bleeding • CrCl <30 mL/min				For STEMI, can give initial dose IV
Bivalirudin	Angiomax	*Loading dose:* 0.1 mg/kg IV bolus *Maintenance dose:* 0.25 mg/kg/hr	Active bleeding		• PT/aPTT • ACT		Can also be used during PCI in patients with HIT

Fibrinolytic Agents

Generic	Brand	Dose	Contra-indications	Primary Side Effects	Key Monitoring	Pertinent Drug Interactions	Med Pearl
Mechanism of action – activate and convert plasminogen into plasmin, which then degrades fibrin (lyses the clot) to form fibrin degradation products							
Reteplase (rPA)	Retavase	10 units IV x 2 doses (separated by 30 min)	• Active bleeding • Any history of intracranial hemorrhage • Known intracranial neoplasm or arteriovenous malformation • Suspected aortic dissection • Significant closed head or facial trauma within 3 months	Bleeding	• CBC • ECG (for signs of reperfusion) • S/S bleeding	Antiplatelets and other anticoagulants may ↑ risk of bleeding	tPA also approved for treatment of acute ischemic stroke and pulmonary embolism
Tenecteplase (TNK)	TNKase	All doses given as IV bolus: • <60 kg: 30 mg • 60–69.9 kg: 35 mg • 70–79.9 kg: 40 mg • 80–89.9 kg: 45 mg • ≥90 kg: 50 mg					
Tissue plasminogen activator (tPA)	Alteplase	15 mg IV bolus, then 0.75 mg/kg (max = 50 mg) over 30 min, then 0.5 mg/kg (max = 35 mg) over 60 min					

LEARNING POINTS

- **HTN**
  - For patients with stage 1 HTN who do not have a compelling indication, a thiazide diuretic should be considered 1st-line therapy. If these patients have stage 2 HTN, two antihypertensives should be started initially, one of which should be a thiazide diuretic. If patients have a compelling indication, antihypertensive agent(s) that can also be used to treat this disease state should be initiated.

- **Dyslipidemia**
  - For all patients (except for those with TG >500 mg/dL), the primary objective of therapy is achieving their individualized LDL-C goal.
  - Statins are the most effective drugs for ↓ LDL-C.
  - Niacin is the most effective drug for ↑ HDL-C.
  - Myopathy and ↑ LFTs are potential side effects of niacin, fibric acid derivatives, and statins.

- **Heart Failure**
  - ACEIs, β-blockers, ARAs, and hydralazine/isosorbide dinitrate have been shown to ↓ mortality in patients with systolic HF.
  - β-blockers should not be initiated in patients who have evidence of fluid overload (peripheral or pulmonary); patients should be relatively euvolemic before starting β-blocker therapy.
  - ARBs can be used in patients who develop intolerable cough from ACEI therapy. Hyperkalemia and renal insufficiency can be associated with both ACEIs and ARBs. If patients are unable to tolerate ACEIs or ARBs because of hyperkalemia or renal insufficiency, hydralazine/isosorbide dinitrate can be used as an alternative.

- **Antiarrhythmic Drugs**
  - Know which antiarrhythmic drugs belong in which class and their basic mechanism of action (e.g., Na^+-channel blocker)
  - Dosages of disopyramide, procainamide, flecainide, sotalol, and dofetilide must be adjusted in patients with renal dysfunction.
  - Amiodarone and dofetilide are the antiarrhythmics of choice in patients with AF who have HF.
  - Dronedarone should not be used in patients with severe HF.
  - Class IA and IC antiarrythmics should be avoided in patients with structural heart disease.
  - Lidocaine and mexiletine are only effective for ventricular arrhythmias.

- Amiodarone has a large volume of distribution and a very long half-life. It can be associated with toxicities that affect just about every organ system in the body. Chest x-ray should be performed annually while TFTs and LFTs should be evaluated every 6 months. Pulmonary function tests can be performed if patient complains of symptoms, such as shortness of breath or cough. An ophthalmologic exam can be performed if patient complains of visual changes.

- **Ischemic Heart Disease**
  - Fibrinolytic drugs should only be used for STEMI.
  - For patients undergoing PCI and receiving a BMS or a DES, clopidogrel, prasugrel, or ticagrelor should be administered for at least 12 months.
  - Know examples of GPBs, LMWHs, factor Xa inhibitors, direct-thrombin inhibitors, and fibrinolytic drugs.
  - Drugs used for the secondary prevention of MI include aspirin, statins, β-blockers, ACEIs, clopidogrel/prasugrel/ticagrelor, and ARAs.

PRACTICE QUESTIONS

1. Which of the following drugs may be associated with bradycardia?

    I. Bisoprolol
    II. Clonidine
    III. Amlodipine

    (A) I only
    (B) III only
    (C) I and II only
    (D) II and III only
    (E) I, II, and III

2. A patient has been on simvastatin 80 mg PO at bedtime for 3 weeks and is now complaining of muscle pain. Which of the following laboratory tests should be obtained?

    (A) Blood glucose
    (B) Creatine kinase
    (C) Complete blood count
    (D) Simvastatin blood concentration
    (E) Thyroid function tests

3. Which of the following are potential side effects of nitroglycerin?

    I. Arrhythmias
    II. Headache
    III. Tachycardia

    (A) I only
    (B) III only
    (C) I and II only
    (D) II and III only
    (E) I, II, and III

4. Which of following drugs are considered positive inotropes?

    I. Nesiritide
    II. Hydralazine
    III. Dobutamine

    (A) I only
    (B) III only
    (C) I and II only
    (D) II and III only
    (E) I, II, and III

ANSWERS

1. C

Both bisoprolol and clonidine decrease atrioventricular (AV) nodal conduction, and therefore may cause bradycardia and/or heart block. Thus, choice (C) is correct. The non-DHP CCBs (i.e., verapamil, diltiazem) also decrease AV nodal conduction and can cause bradycardia. However, the DHP CCBs, including amlodipine, have no effect on AV nodal conduction. Instead, these drugs can actually cause reflex tachycardia.

2. B

For a patient on a statin who complains of muscle pain, a creatine kinase should be obtained. Therefore, choice (B) is correct.

3. D

Nitroglycerin could potentially cause headaches and tachycardia, so choice (D) is correct. Nitroglycerin does not cause cardiac arrhythmias.

4. B

Dobutamine stimulates β_1 receptors in the heart and increases myocardial contractility and is therefore considered a positive inotrope. Nesiritide is an arterial and venous vasodilator, while hydralazine is a direct arterial vasodilator. While these drugs may increase CO, they do so by decreasing afterload and not by increasing myocardial contractility. Therefore, choice (B) is correct.

Infectious Diseases

2

This chapter reviews various antibiotic agents, including antibacterial, antifungal, and antiviral agents. A brief overview of the recommended pharmacologic treatments of the following infections is also provided:

- **Urinary tract infections (UTIs)**
- **Pneumonia**
- **Meningitis**
- **Sexually transmitted diseases (STDs) (chlamydia, gonorrhea, syphilis)**
- **Human immunodeficiency virus (HIV)**
- **Tuberculosis (TB)**

 Suggested Study Time: **3 hours**

PRINCIPLES OF ANTIBIOTIC THERAPY

Factors to Consider When Selecting Antibiotic Therapy

- Identity/susceptibility of bacteria
  - Important to know which bacteria may be causing the infection
    - » Can begin empiric antibiotic therapy without knowing the actual identity (or sensitivities) of the organism; select antibiotic(s) (usually broad-spectrum) based on the organism(s) *most* likely to cause a particular infection
    - » Once organism (and sensitivities) are identified, can adjust/narrow antibiotic therapy, as needed, to cover this organism
- Site of infection
  - Especially important for meningitis, UTIs, prostatitis, and osteomyelitis

» Only certain antibiotics can penetrate into these areas to target the infection; these drugs may need to be used at higher doses, especially for meningitis, prostatitis, and osteomyelitis

- Patient allergies
- Concomitant medications
  - May need to be concerned with potential drug interactions when selecting an antibiotic
- Hepatic and renal function
  - May need to adjust antibiotic dosages if hepatic or renal dysfunction present
- Past medical history
  - Certain antibiotics may need to be avoided in particular disease states (e.g., seizure disorders)
- Patient age
  - Some antibiotics are contraindicated in pediatric patients
- Pregnancy/breastfeeding
  - Some antibiotics are contraindicated in these patients

URINARY TRACT INFECTIONS

Common Organisms

Community-Acquired	Nosocomial (Hospital-Acquired)
• *E. coli* • *Staphylococcus saprophyticus* • *Klebsiella pneumoniae* • *Proteus mirabilis*	• *E. coli* • *Pseudomonas aeruginosa* • *Klebsiella pneumoniae* • *Proteus mirabilis* • *Enterobacter* spp. • *Staphylococcus aureus* • Fungus (e.g., *Candida*)

Diagnosis

- Confirmed by urinalysis
  - Bacteruria: $>10^2$ cfu/mL
  - Pyuria: >5–10 white blood cells (WBCs)/mm^3
  - Nitrite-positive
  - Leukocyte esterase–positive
  - Casts (may be present in pyelonephritis)

Signs and Symptoms

- Lower UTI (cystitis)
  - Dysuria
  - Urgency
  - Frequency
  - Nocturia
  - Suprapubic pressure/pain
- Upper UTI (pyelonephritis)
  - All of the above symptoms, *plus*
  - Flank pain
  - Fever
  - Nausea/vomiting (N/V)
- Complicated UTI factors
  - Male
  - Elderly
  - Pregnancy
  - Children
  - Nosocomial
  - Recent use of antibiotics
  - Diabetes
  - Immunosuppressed
  - Catheterized

Guidelines

Infectious Disease Society of America and European Society for Microbiology and Infectious Diseases. *Clin Infect Dis*, no. 52 (2011): e103–20.

Guidelines Summary

Acute Uncomplicated Cystitis

- First-line therapy: Nitrofurantoin x 5 days
- Second-line therapy: Trimethoprim/sulfamethoxazole (TMP/SMX) double strength (DS) x 3 days
- Third-line therapy: Fosfomycin x 1 dose

- *Alternative agents:*
  - Fluoroquinolone (FQ) x 3 days
    - » Only use when other agents cannot be used
  - β-lactams (i.e., amoxicillin-clavulanate, cefdinir, cefaclor, cefpodoxime) x 3–7 days
    - » Avoid unless other agents are not appropriate

Acute Pyelonephritis (outpatient therapy)

- First-line therapy:
  - Ciprofloxacin 500 mg PO BID x 7 days
  - Cipro XR 1 g PO daily x 7 days
  - Levofloxacin 750 mg PO daily x 5 days

  +/–
  | Ceftriaxone 1 g IV x 1 |
  | OR |
  | Gentamicin 5–7 mg/kg IV x 1 |

- Second-line therapy: TMP/SMX DS PO BID x 14 days
- Third-line therapy: Oral β-lactam (i.e., amoxicillin-clavulanate) x 10–14 days AND one-time dose of ceftriaxone 1 g IV or gentamicin 5–7 mg/kg IV

Acute Pyelonephritis (inpatient therapy)

- IV FQ
- Aminoglycoside +/- IV ampicillin
- IV extended-spectrum cephalosporin or penicillin +/- aminoglycoside
- IV carbapenem (e.g., imipenem/cilastatin)

Complicated UTIs

- Duration of therapy: 10–14 days

PNEUMONIA

Common Organisms

Community-Acquired	Hospital-Acquired (occurs ≥48 hours after admission)
• Mycoplasma pneumoniae	• Staphylococcus aureus
• Streptococcus pneumoniae	• Pseudomonas aeruginosa
• Haemophilus influenzae	• Klebsiella pneumoniae
• Chlamydia pneumoniae	• Enterobacter
• Legionella pneumophila	• E. coli
• Moraxella catarrhalis	• Acinetobacter spp.
• Viruses	• Serratia spp.
	• Anaerobes

Diagnosis

- Symptoms and ausculatory findings consistent with pneumonia, plus an infiltrate on chest x-ray
- Diagnosis can often be made on history and physical exam findings

Signs and Symptoms

- Fever, chills, dyspnea, cough (may or may not be productive), rigors, pleuritic pain
- Physical examination:
  - Tachypnea
  - Tachycardia
  - Dullness to percussion
  - Inspiratory crackles
  - ↓ breath sounds over affected area
- Laboratory findings
  - ↑ WBCs
- Infiltrate on chest x-ray

Guidelines

Community-acquired pneumonia, Infectious Disease Society of America/American Thoracic Society. *Clin Infect Dis*, no. 44 (Suppl 2) (2007): S27–72.

Hospital-acquired, ventilator-associated, and healthcare-associated pneumonia, American Thoracic Society/Infectious Disease Society of America. *Am J Respir Crit Care Med*, no. 171 (2005): 388–416.

Guidelines Summary

Diagnosis	Treatment	Duration
Community-acquired (ambulatory)	*Previously healthy and no antibiotic therapy in past 3 months:* Macrolide (clarithromycin or azithromycin) **OR** Doxycycline	≥5 days
	With comorbidities (see below)[1] risk for drug-resistant Streptococcus pneumoniae or antibiotic use in past 3 months: FQ (moxifloxacin, gemifloxacin, or levofloxacin) **OR** Macrolide (or doxycycline) *plus* one of the following: • High-dose amoxicillin • Amoxicillin/clavulanate • Cephalosporin (ceftriaxone, cefuroxime, or cefpodoxime)	
Community-acquired (hospitalized)	*Moderate:* FQ (moxifloxacin, gemifloxacin, or levofloxacin) **OR** Macrolide (or doxycycline) *plus* one of the following: • Ampicillin • Ceftriaxone • Cefotaxime	
	Severe: FQ (moxifloxacin, gemifloxacin, or levofloxacin) **OR** azithromycin *plus* one of the following: • Ampicillin/sulbactam • Ceftriaxone • Cefotaxime	
Hospital-acquired	*Hospitalized <5 days and no risk factors for multidrug-resistant (MDR) organisms (see below) (select one of the following drugs):* [2] • 3rd-generation cephalosporin (ceftriaxone or cefotaxime) • FQ (ciprofloxacin, moxifloxacin, or levofloxacin) • Ampicillin/sulbactam • Ertapenem	8 days (14 days if due to *Pseudomonas*)
	Hospitalized ≥5 days or risk factors for MDR organisms (see below) [2]: FQ (ciprofloxacin or levofloxacin) **OR** aminoglycoside *plus* one of the following: • Ceftazidime or cefepime • Imipenem/cilastatin or meropenem • Piperacillin/tazobactam	

[1] *Comorbidities: Chronic obstructive pulmonary disease (COPD), diabetes, chronic renal failure, chronic liver failure, heart failure (HF), cancer, asplenia, immunosuppressed*

[2] *Risk factors for MDR organisms: Recent antibiotic therapy (in last 90 days), hospitalized ≥5 days, ↑ resistance in environment, nursing home resident, chronic dialysis, home infusion therapy, immunosuppressed*

MENINGITIS

Common Organisms

Age Group	Most Common Organisms
<1 mo	• *Streptococcus agalactiae* (Group B Strep) • *E. coli* • *Listeria monocytogenes* • *Klebsiella* spp.
1–23 mo	• *Streptococcus pneumoniae* • *Neisseria meningitidis* • Group B Strep • *Haemophilus influenzae* • *E. coli*
2–50 yr	• *Neisseria meningitidis* • *Streptococcus pneumoniae*
>50 yr	• *Streptococcus pneumoniae* • *Neisseria meningitidis* • Group B Strep

Diagnosis

- Confirmed by analysis of cerebrospinal fluid (CSF)
  - Bacterial meningitis: $\downarrow$ glucose, $\uparrow$ protein, $\uparrow$ WBCs
  - Gram stain can help identify organism

Signs and Symptoms

- Symptoms
  - Fever, chills
  - Headache, photophobia
  - Nuchal rigidity
  - N/V
  - Altered mental status
  - Petechiae/purpura (*Neisseria meningitidis*)
- Signs
  - Brudzinski's sign (flexion of hips and knees upon flexing the neck)
  - Kernig's sign (pain develops when the knee is extended after flexing the hip to 90 degrees)
  - Bulging fontanelle (children)

Guidelines

Infectious Disease Society of America. *Clin Infect Dis*, no. 39 (2004): 1267–84.

Guidelines Summary

Empiric Treatment

Age Group	Treatment
<1 mo	Ampicillin + aminoglycoside **OR** Ampicillin + cefotaxime
1–23 mo	Third-generation cephalosporin (cefotaxime or ceftriaxone) + vancomycin
2–50 yr	Third-generation cephalosporin (cefotaxime or ceftriaxone) + vancomycin
>50 yr	Third-generation cephalosporin (cefotaxime or ceftriaxone) + vancomycin + ampicillin

- Dexamethasone may considered as adjunctive therapy
- Infants and Children: *H. influenzae* meningitis
- Adults: *Streptococcus pneumonia* meningitis

SEXUALLY TRANSMITTED DISEASES

Causative Organisms

Disease	Organisms
Chlamydia	*Chlamydia trachomatis*
Gonorrhea	*Neisseria gonorrhoeae*
Syphilis	*Treponema pallidum*

Diagnosis

- Chlamydia: Test performed on urine swab or endocervical/vaginal/male urethral swab
- Gonorrhea: Gram-stained smears or culture (endocervical/vaginal/male urethral/urine specimen)
- Syphilis: Dark field examination and direct fluorescent antibody stains of exudates
  - Serologic testing
    » Nontreponemal: Venereal Disease Research Laboratory (VDRL) slide test, rapid plasma regain (RPR) test; can be used for screening
    » Treponemal: Fluorescent treponemal antibody absorbed (FTA-ABS), *T. pallidum* particle agglutination (TP-PA); can be used to confirm diagnosis

Signs and Symptoms

- Chlamydia
  - Penile/vaginal discharge, dysuria
  - May also be asymptomatic
- Gonorrhea
  - Penile/vaginal discharge, dysuria, urinary frequency
  - May also be asymptomatic
- Syphilis
  - Primary (10–90 days after exposure): Presence of chancre
  - Secondary (2–8 wk after development of primary stage): Variety of rashes/lesions, flu-like symptoms, and lymphadenopathy
  - Latent (positive serologic test but no clinical manifestations)
  - Tertiary: Cardiovascular (e.g., aortic insufficiency) and neurologic abnormalities (e.g., deafness, blindness, dementia, paresis)

Guidelines

Department of Health and Human Services, Centers for Disease Control and Prevention. *MMWR Recomm Rep*, no. 59 (RR-12) (2010): 1–110.

Guidelines Summary

Disease	Treatment
Chlamydia	Azithromycin 1 g PO x 1 dose **OR** Doxycycline 100 mg PO q12h x 7 days
Gonorrhea	Ceftriaxone 250 mg IM x 1 dose **OR** Cefixime 400 mg PO x 1 dose **PLUS** Treatment for chlamydia (if not ruled out)
Syphilis	*Primary, secondary, or early latent syphilis (<1 yr in duration):* • Benzathine penicillin G 2.4 million units IM x 1 dose *Late latent syphilis (>1 yr in duration), latent syphilis of unknown duration, or tertiary syphilis (not neurosyphilis):* • Benzathine penicillin G 2.4 million units IM once weekly x 3 weeks *Neurosyphilis:* • Aqueous penicillin G 3–4 million units IV or as continuous infusion q4h x 10–14 days

HUMAN IMMUNODEFICIENCY VIRUS

Definitions

Human immunodeficiency virus (HIV) is a human retrovirus that infects lymphocytes and other cells that bear the CD4 surface protein. Infection leads to CD4 T-cell depletion, impaired cell-mediated immunity, and polyclonal B-cell activation. Over time, this immune system dysfunction leads to acquired immune deficiency syndrome (AIDS) and illnesses such as opportunistic infections and malignancies.

Diagnosis

- The Centers for Disease Control and Prevention (CDC) recommends routine HIV screening for adults, adolescents and pregnant women in healthcare settings in the United States.
- Persons at a high risk for HIV infection should be screened for HIV at least annually:
  - Healthcare workers, intravenous drug users, men who have sex with men, hemophiliacs, sexual partners of persons living with HIV, commercial sex workers and their partners, persons with a history of sexually transmitted infections, and persons with multiple sex partners or those with a history of unprotected sexual encounters
- Pregnant women should receive HIV testing during the routine panel of prenatal screening tests.
- Laws requiring informed consent for HIV testing vary depending upon the state. Most states have adopted the "opt-out" testing strategy recommended by the CDC. This strategy notifies a patient that HIV screening will be taking place unless the patient declines.
- Screening for HIV is performed with an enzyme-linked immunosorbent assay (ELISA) test. Positive results must always be confirmed with a Western blot.

Signs and Symptoms

Acute HIV infection most commonly presents with a "flu-like" illness that resolves within 2-4 weeks. After acute infection, patients may remain symptom-free for 8–9 years or more. As the virus continues to multiply and destroy immune cells, the patient may develop chronic symptoms such as:

- Swollen lymph nodes, diarrhea, weight loss, rash, fever, cough, and shortness of breath

When a patient's CD4 cell count declines to <200 cells/mm3, the immune system is significantly compromised and the patient is at an increased risk for opportunistic infections such as:

- Oropharyngeal candidiasis, *Pneumocystis jirovecii* pneumonia, *Toxoplasma gondii*, *Cryptococcus neoformans*, and *Mycobacterium avium intracellulare*

Guidelines

Panel on Antiretroviral Guidelines for Adults and Adolescents. Guidelines for the use of antiretroviral agents in HIV-1-infected adults and adolescents. Department of Health and Human Services. January 10, 2011; 1–166. Available at http://www.aidsinfo.nih.gov/ContentFiles/AdultandAdolescentGL.pdf.

Guidelines Summary

For the NAPLEX®, you should make learning the names of the medications and their respective classes a priority. Below are some helpful learning tips:

- Memorize the non-nucleoside reverse transcriptase inhibitors (NNRTIs)
  - Efavirenz, nevirapine, etravirine, rilpivirine
- All protease inhibitors (PIs) end in "-navir"
  - Examples: Darunavir, atazanavir, ritonavir
- There is only one integrase inhibitor: Raltegravir
- There is only one fusion inhibitor: Enfuvirtide
- There is only one CCR5 inhibitor: Maraviroc
- The remaining agents are nucleoside reverse transcriptase inhibitors (NRTIs)
  - Examples: Tenofovir, emtricitabine, abacavir, lamivudine, zidovudine

For the NAPLEX®, know the indications for initiating an antiretroviral regimen in treatment-naïve patients:

- CD4 cell count <500 cells/mm^3
- An AIDS-defining illness or history of an opportunistic infection
- HIV-associated nephropathy
- Hepatitis B co-infection that requires treatment
- Pregnancy

For the NAPLEX®, know the signature side effects for the major drug classes (NNRTIs, NRTI, and PIs) and know the four antiviral regimens that are preferred for starting therapy in treatment-naïve patients:

- Tenofovir/emtricitabine/efavirenz
- Tenofovir/emtricitabine/raltegravir
- Tenofovir/emtricitabine/darunavir/ritonavir
- Tenofovir/emtricitabine/atazanavir/ritonavir

Below is a summary of acceptable initial combination regimens for antiretroviral naïve patients:

- NNRTI-based regimen: 1 NNRTI + 2 NRTIs
- PI-based regimen: PI (preferably boosted with ritonavir) + 2 NRTIs
- Integrase inhibitor-based regimen: Integrase inhibitor + 2 NRTIs
- CCR5 antagonist-based regimen: CCR5 inhibitor + 2 NRTIs

Non-Nucleoside Reverse Transcriptase Inhibitors (NNRTIs)

Generic	Brand	Dose	Contra-indications	Primary Side Effects	Key Monitoring	Pertinent Drug Interactions	Med Pearl	Top 200
Mechanism of action – binds to an allosteric site on reverse transcriptase that results in a conformational change to the enzyme's active site								
Nevirapine	Viramune	200 mg PO daily x 2 weeks, then 200 mg BID or 400 mg (XR) daily thereafter	None	• Rash • ↑ LFTs	LFTs	• 3A4, 2B6 substrate • Inhibits: 3A4, 2D6, 1A2 • Induces: 3A4, 2B6	• Risk of hepatotoxicity in men and women with CD4 count > 400 and 250 cells/mm³, respectively • Hepatotoxicity often associated with a rash	No
Efavirenz	Sustiva	600 mg PO QHS on an empty stomach	None	• Rash • ↑ LFTs • Drowsiness • Dizziness • Insomnia • Abnormal vivid dreaming • Agitation	LFTs	• 3A4, 2B6 substrate • Inhibits: 3A4, 2C9 • Induces: 3A4, 2B6	Can cause a false positive cannabinoid or benzodiazepine screening test	No
Etravirine	Intelence	200 mg PO BID with food	None	• Rash • ↑ LFTs	LFTs	• 3A4, 2C9, 2C19 substrate • Inhibits: 2C9, 2C19 • Induces: 3A4	May disperse tabs in water	No
Rilpivirine	Edurant	25 mg PO daily with food	None	• Rash • ↑ LFTs	LFTs	• 3A4 substrate • Not expected to induce or inhibit CYP enzymes	• Requires at least a 500-calorie meal • ↑ virologic failure with high baseline HIV RNA (>100,000 copies/mL)	No

Nucleoside Reverse Transcriptase Inhibitors (NRTIs)

Mechanism of action – triphosphate moiety competes with natural substrates for incorporation into proviral DNA that is developed by reverse transcriptase

Generic	Brand	Dose	Contra-indications	Primary Side Effects	Key Monitoring	Pertinent Drug Interactions	Med Pearl	Top 200
Abacavir	Ziagen	300 mg PO BID or 600 mg PO daily	Discontinue drug promptly and do not rechallenge in patients with hypersensitivity	Hypersensitivity reaction	Hypersensitivity symptoms: fever, rash, N/V/D, malaise, fatigue, cough	None	Perform HLA-B*5701 test prior; only use if negative	No
Didanosine	Videx EC	≥60 kg: 400 mg PO daily <60 kg: 250 mg PO daily	None	• Peripheral neuropathy • Pancreatitis • Diarrhea • Nausea	None	Tenofovir ↑ levels (avoid combination)	• Administer on an empty stomach • Do not crush or open	No
Emtricitabine	Emtriva	200 mg PO daily	None	• N/V • Hyperpigmentation of palms/soles	None	None	Also active against hepatitis B	No
Lamivudine	Epivir	300 mg PO daily	None	• N/V/D	None	None	Also active against hepatitis B	No
Stavudine	Zerit	≥60 kg: 40 mg PO BID <60 kg: 30 mg PO BID	None	• Peripheral neuropathy • Pancreatitis • Lipoatrophy	None	Additive risk of pancreatitis with concurrent didanosine	None	No
Tenofovir	Viread	300 mg PO daily	None	• Renal insufficiency • Fanconi syndrome	SCr	↓ atazanavir levels	Also active against hepatitis B	No
Zidovudine	Retrovir	300 mg PO BID	Concurrent ribavirin due to additive toxicity	• Anemia • Neutropenia • Headache • Nausea	CBC with differential	None	First antiretroviral for HIV	No

Protease Inhibitors (PIs)

Mechanism of action – inhibits HIV protease enzyme from processing the gag-pol polyprotein precursor, thereby preventing development and maturation of new HIV particles

Generic	Brand	Dose	Contra-indications	Primary Side Effects	Key Monitoring	Pertinent Drug Interactions	Med Pearl	Top 200
Atazanavir	Reyataz	400 mg PO daily OR 300 mg PO daily + ritonavir 100 mg PO daily	None	• Indirect hyperbilirubinemia • PR prolongation • Dyslipidemia (greater with ritonavir) • Hepatotoxicity • GI upset	• LFTs • Bilirubin • Lipids	• 3A4 inhibitor and substrate • Tenofovir ↓ levels; atazanavir must be boosted by ritonavir	• Acid dependent absorption; follow guidelines for using in combination or with PIs, H_2 blockers and antacids	No
Darunavir	Prezista	• Therapy naïve: 800 mg PO daily • Therapy experienced: 600 mg PO BID	None	• Dyslipidemia • Rash • Hepatotoxicity • GI upset	• LFTs • Lipids	• 3A4 inhibitor and substrate • ↑ atorvastatin and rosuvastatin levels	• Must be taken with food • Always boosted by ritonavir	No
Fosamprenavir	Lexiva	• Therapy naïve: 1,400 mg PO BID OR 1,400 mg PO daily + ritonavir 100 mg PO daily OR 700 mg PO BID + ritonavir 100 mg PO BID • Therapy experienced: 700 mg PO BID + ritonavir 100 mg PO BID	None	• Dyslipidemia • Rash • Hepatotoxicity • GI upset	• LFTs • Lipids	• 3A4 inhibitor and substrate • Separate administration from H_2 blockers	Available as a suspension	No
Indinavir	Crixivan	800 mg PO BID + ritonavir 100–200 mg PO BID	None	• Dyslipidemia • Hepatotoxicity • GI upset • Nephrolithiasis • Indirect hyperbilirubinemia	• LFTs • Lipids	3A4 inhibitor and substrate	Patients are advised to drink six 8 oz glasses of water per day	No

Protease Inhibitors (PIs) *(cont'd)*

Generic	Brand	Dose	Contra-indications	Primary Side Effects	Key Monitoring	Pertinent Drug Interactions	Med Pearl	Top 200
Lopinavir/ Ritonavir	Kaletra	Lopinavir 400 mg/ritonavir 100 mg PO BID OR Lopinavir 800 mg/ritonavir 200 mg PO daily	None	• Dyslipidemia • Hepatotoxicity • GI upset	• LFTs • Lipids	3A4 substrate and inhibitor	• Available in solution • Recommended PI for pregnant women (BID dosing only)	No
Nelfinavir	Viracept	1250 mg PO BID	Concurrent use of PPIs	• Diarrhea • Dyslipidemia • Hepatotoxicity	• LFTs • Lipids	• 3A4 and 2C19 substrate • 3A4 inhibitor	• Administer with food • May disperse in water	No
Ritonavir	Norvir	100 mg–200 mg to boost other PIs	None	• Dyslipidemia • Hepatotoxicity • GI upset	• LFTs • Lipids	• 3A4, 2D6 substrate and inhibitor • 2C9, 2C19 and UGT inducer	• Only used for boosting • Administer with food • Available in solution (43% alcohol)	No
Saquinavir	Invirase	1000 mg PO BID + ritonavir 100 mg PO BID	Concurrent use of class IA or class III antiarrhythmics	• PR prolongation • QT prolongation • Dyslipidemia • Hepatotoxicity • GI upset	• LFTs • Lipids	3A4 substrate and inhibitor	Administer with food	No
Tipranavir	Aptivus	500 mg PO BID + ritonavir 200 mg PO BID	None	• Hepatotoxicity • Rash • Dyslipidemia	• LFTs • Lipids	• 3A4 substrate • 3A4 and 2D6 inhibitor • Separate dosing from antacids	Available in solution	No

Integrase Inhibitor

Generic	Brand	Dose	Contra-indications	Primary Side Effects	Key Monitoring	Pertinent Drug Interactions	Med Pearl	Top 200
Mechanism of action – inhibits integration of proviral DNA into host CD4 T-cell genome								
Raltegravir	Isentress	400 mg PO BID	None	• Nausea • Headache • Diarrhea • ↑ CPK • Muscle weakness • Rhabdomyolysis	None	Rifampin ↓ levels (↑ dose to 800 mg PO BID)	No CYP450 metabolism; only UGT1A1 glucuronidation	No

CCR5 Inhibitor

Generic	Brand	Dose	Contra-indications	Primary Side Effects	Key Monitoring	Pertinent Drug Interactions	Med Pearl	Top 200
Mechanism of action – acts as an antagonist for the CCR5 receptor, a chemokine coreceptor that can facilitate HIV entry into CD4 ⁺-cells								
Maraviroc	Selzentry	300 mg PO BID	None	• Abdominal pain • Cough • Dizziness • Musculoskeletal symptoms • Rash • Hepatotoxicity • Orthostatic hypotension	LFTs	• 3A4 substrate • ↑ dose to 600 mg PO BID with strong 3A4 inducers • ↓ dose to 150 mg PO BID with strong 3A4 inhibitors	Hepatotoxicity may be preceded by systemic hypersensitivity reaction (rash, eosinophilia)	No

Fusion Inhibitor

Generic	Brand	Dose	Contra-indications	Primary Side Effects	Key Monitoring	Pertinent Drug Interactions	Med Pearl	Top 200
Mechanism of action – blocks conformational changes in gp41 on the surface of HIV that are required for HIV fusion with CD4 cell membranes								
Enfuvirtide	Fuzeon	90 mg SC BID	None	Local injection site reactions (pain, erythema, induration, nodules and cysts, pruritus, ecchymosis)	Injection sites	None	Only HIV medication available as SC injection	No

Combination Products: See individual drug components for important points

Brand	Components	Dosing
Atripla	Efavirenz, tenofovir, emtricitabine	1 tablet PO daily
Combivir	Lamivudine, zidovudine	1 tablet PO BID
Complera	Rilpivirine, tenofovir, emtricitabine	1 tablet PO daily
Epzicom	Abacavir, lamivudine	1 tablet PO daily
Trizivir	Abacavir, lamivudine, zidovudine	1 tablet PO BID

TUBERCULOSIS

Definitions

Tuberculosis (TB) is a communicable infection disease caused by *Mycobacterium tuberculosis*. It can produce a silent, latent infection, as well as an active disease state. Although TB is far less common today in the United States, it remains the most prevalent infection on the planet. Effective therapy for *Mycobacterium tuberculosis* infections require combination chemotherapy designed to prevent the emergence of resistant organisms. Increased resistance to the conventional antituberculous agents has led to the use of more complex regimens.

Diagnosis

- Diagnosis relies on skin testing with the tuberculin purified protein derivative (PPD).
- PPD should be performed on high-risk patients.
  - High-risk patients include HIV-infected, hospital employees, nursing home staff and residents, workers in prisons, immigrants, and healthcare students.
- The intracutaneous PPD injection should produce a small, raised, blanched wheal. This test should be read by an experienced professional in 48 to 72 hours.
  - Measured area >5 mm is considered positive for HIV-infected persons, recent contact of a person with TB disease, persons with fibrotic changes on chest radiograph consistent with prior TB, patients with organ transplants, and persons who are immunosuppressed for other reasons.
  - Measured area >10 mm is considered positive for recent immigrants from high-prevalence countries, injection drug users, residents and employees of high-risk congregate settings, mycobacteriology laboratory personnel, persons with clinical conditions that place them at high risk, children <4 years of age, and infants, children, and adolescents exposed to adults in high-risk categories.
  - Measured area >15 mm is considered positive for any person, including persons with no known risk factors for TB.
- After a positive PPD skin test, a diagnostic test must be performed to rule out active disease.
  - Confirmatory diagnosis is performed with chest radiographs and microbiologic examination or sputum.
  - A total of three sputum samples should be collected and sent for acid-fast bacillus testing.

Signs and Symptoms

TB can present with generalized symptoms of weight loss, malaise, fever, and night sweats. As the disease progresses, the patient may develop a persistent cough, which is often productive of sputum. Frequently, the onset of TB is insidious and the diagnosis may not be considered until a chest radiograph is performed.

Guidelines

Currently, there are two sets of guidelines from two national associations. Overall, there are minor differences and the information has been combined for clarity.

American College of Chest Physicians, Medical Specialty Society. (January 2006). NGC:004834. http://guidelines.gov/browse/browsemode.aspx?node=27945&type=1.

American Thoracic Society, Medical Specialty Society Centers for Disease Control and Prevention–Federal Government Agency [U.S.] Infectious Diseases Society of America–Medical Specialty Society. (June 20, 2003). http://guidelines.gov/browse/browsemode.aspx?node=27945&type=1.

Centers for Disease Control and Prevention. Tuberculosis. http://www.cdc.gov/tb.

Department of Health and Human Services Centers for Disease Control and Prevention. American Thoracic Society, CDC, and Infectious Diseases Society of America. Treatment of Tuberculosis. MMWR. 2003;52(11).

Guidelines Summary

The overall goals for treatment of TB are: (*1*) To cure the individual patient, and (*2*) to minimize the transmission of *Mycobacterium tuberculosis* to other persons.

- Risk factors
  - Location of birth (New York, New Jersey, California, Florida, and Texas account for 92% of cases)
  - Close contact (>40 hours per week) with TB patients
  - Increase in age
  - Race and ethnicity: Hispanics, African Americans, and Asian Pacific Islanders
- Successful treatment of TB has benefits for both the individual patient and the community in which the patient resides.
- Prescribing physician responsibility for treatment completion is a fundamental principle in TB control.
- Treatment of patients with TB is most successful within a comprehensive framework that addresses both clinical and social issues of relevance to the patient.

- It is strongly recommended that patient-centered care be the initial management strategy, regardless of the source of supervision. This strategy should always include an adherence plan that emphasizes directly observed therapy (DOT).
- There are four recommended regimens for treating patients with TB caused by drug-susceptible organisms following a continuation phase:

Drug	Duration	Interval	Minimum doses
Isoniazid	9 months	Daily	270
		Twice weekly	76
Isoniazid	6 months	Daily	180
		Twice weekly	52
Isoniazid and Rifapentine	3 months	Once weekly	12
Rifampin	4 months	Daily	120

Tuberculosis

Generic	Brand	Dose	Contra-indications	Primary Side Effects	Key Monitoring	Pertinent Drug Interactions	Med Pearl	Top 200
Mechanism of action – inhibition of mycolic acid synthesis resulting in disruption of the bacterial cell wall								
Isoniazid (INH)	Isotamine	• Latent: 300 mg/day for 9 months • Active: multiple scenarios	• Acute liver disease • Previous severe reactions (drug fever, chills, arthritis)	• Hypertension • Depression • Flushing • Jaundice, increased LFTs	• Baseline LFTs • Sputum cultures, until two consecutive negatives • Hepatitis	• CYP3A4 inhibitor: CYP1A2, CYP2A6, CYP2C19, CYP2D6, CYP2E1, CYP3A4 • inducers: CYP2E1	• Severe and sometimes fatal hepatitis may occur within 3 months of treatment • Drinking alcohol is not recommended during treatment • Empty stomach • Pyridoxine should be administered to prevent peripheral neuropathy	No
Mechanism of action – inhibits bacterial RNA synthesis by binding to the beta subunit of DNA-dependent RNA polymerase, blocking RNA transcription								
Rifampin (RIF)	Rifadin	• Oral/IV: 10 mg/kg/day • Max: 600 mg/day	Concurrent use of amprenavir, saquinivir/ritonivir	• Numbness • Flu-like syndrome • Rash • Discoloration of urine • Neutropenia/leukopenia	• Baseline LFT • CBC • Sputum cultures • Chest x-ray 23 months into treatment	CYP450 inducers: CYP A2, CYP2A6, CYP2B6, CYP2C8, CYP2C9, CYP2C19, CYP3A4	Rifabutin often will be used with drug interaction	No
Mechanism of action – kills mycobacteria replicating in macrophages; exact mechanism is not known								
Pyrazinamide (PZA)	Tebrazid	• Tab: 15–30 mg/kg/day • Max: 2 g/day	• Acute gout • Severe hepatic damage	• Malaise • Anorexia • Hepatotoxicity	• LFTs • Uric acid levels • Sputum culture • Chest x-rays	Rifampin and pyrazinamide have been associated with hepatotoxicity	Typically used for the first 2 months of therapy	No
Mechanism of action – suppresses mycobacteria multiplication by interfering with RNA synthesis								
Ethambutol (EMB)	Myambutol	• Tab: 15–25 mg/kg/day • Max: 2.5 g/dose	Optic neuritis	• Myocarditis • Headache • Gout, abnormal LFTs	• Baseline and periodic (monthly) visual testing • Renal, hepatic, hematopoietic tests	• Decreased absorption with aluminum hydroxide. • Avoid antacids by 4 hours	Optic neuritis manifests as decreased red-green color perception, decreased visual field	No

Tuberculosis *(cont'd)*

Generic	Brand	Dose	Contra-indications	Primary Side Effects	Key Monitoring	Pertinent Drug Interactions	Med Pearl	Top 200
Mechanism of action – inhibits bacterial protein synthesis by binding directly to the 30S ribosomal subunit, causing faulty peptide sequence to form in the protein chain								
Streptomycin	Only available generically	• Inj: 15 mg/kg/day • Max: 1 g/day	Pregnancy	May cause neurotoxicity, nephrotoxicity	• Hearing (audiogram) • SCr and BUN • Serum concentration	Increased effect with depolarizing neuromuscular blockade agents	• Used as a substitute for ethambutol and for drug-resistant MTB • Does not penetrate the CNS and cannot be used for TB meningitis	No
Mechanism of action – inhibits bacterial RNA synthesis by binding to the beta subunit of DNA-dependent RNA polymerase, blocking RNA transcription								
Rifabutin	Mycobutin	• 300 mg/day	Hypersensitivity	Similar to rifampin	• Rash • Discoloration of urine • Neutropenia/leukopenia • Numbness • Flu-like symptoms • Platelets	Similar to rifampin	Used in place of rifampin for HIV patients	No

Storage and Administration Pearls

- Isoniazid: Tablets and oral solution must be protected from light

Patient Education Pearls

- A patient who is taking rifampin should report any tingling or numbness in the hands or feet.
- A patient who is taking streptomycin must maintain adequate hydration.

LEARNING POINTS

- Given an active case of TB, the clinician must ensure DOT to reduce bacterial resistance and exposure to other patients.
- Isoniazid is currently the drug of choice for a positive PPD and in combination-treatments for TB.

Medication Charts: Antibacterial Agents

Penicillins (β-Lactams)

Mechanism of action — inhibit bacterial cell wall synthesis; bactericidal

Generic	Brand	Dose/Dosage Forms	Spectrum of Activity	Contra-indications	Primary Side Effects	Pertinent Drug Interactions	Med Pearl	Top 200
Natural Penicillins								
Penicillin G	Pfizerpen	• 2–4 million units IV q4–6h • Injection	• *Strep. viridans* • *Strep. pyogenes* • *Strep. pneumoniae* (↑ resistance) • Mouth anaerobes	Allergy to penicillins, cephalosporins, or carbapenems	• Hypersensitivity reaction (rash, hives, dyspnea, throat swelling) • N/V/D • Interstitial nephritis • Hemolytic anemia (with prolonged administration)	• Probenecid may ↑ effects (may be used for this purpose) • May ↓ effects of oral contraceptives	• Adjust dose in renal dysfunction	No
Penicillin G benzathine	Bicillin LA	• 1.2–2.4 million units IM at specified intervals • Injection					• Penicillin G benzathine or procaine used for syphilis; benzathine a so used for Strep throat	No
Penicillin G procaine	Wycillin	• 1.2–4.8 million units IM/day at specified intervals • Injection						No
Penicillin VK	Veetids	• 250–500 mg PO q6h • Solution, tabs					• Take penicillin VK 1 hour before or 2 hours after meals	Yes
Penicillinase-Resistant Penicillins								
Dicloxacillin	Only available generically	• 125–500 mg PO q6h • Caps	• *Staph aureus* (methicillin-sensitive, MSSA) • *Streptococcus*	Same as natural penicillins	Same as natural penicillins	Same as natural penicillins	• No need to adjust dose in renal dysfunction (cleared by biliary excretion)	No
Nafcillin	Only available generically	• 500 mg–2 g IV q4–6h • Injection					• Take dicloxacillin 1 hour before or 2 hours after meals	No
Oxacillin	Only available generically	• 250 mg–2 g IV q4–6h • Injection					• Patients on nafcillin (IV) can be switched to dicloxacillin (PO)	No

Penicillins (β-Lactams) *(cont'd)*

Generic	Brand	Dose/Dosage Forms	Spectrum of Activity	Contra-indications	Primary Side Effects	Pertinent Drug Interactions	Med Pearl	Top 200
Aminopenicillins								
Amoxicillin	Moxatag	• Immediate-release (IR): 250–500 mg PO q8h or 500–875 mg PO q12h • Extended release (ER): 775 mg PO daily • Caps, suspension, chewable tabs, tabs (ER and IR)	• *Strep pneumoniae* • *H. influenzae* • *E. coli* • *Proteus mirabilis* • *Salmonella* • *Shigella*	Same as natural penicillins	Same as natural penicillins	Same as natural penicillins	• Amoxicillin can be used in three-drug regimen for *H. pylori* • Adjust dose in renal dysfunction • Take ampicillin 1 hour before or 2 hours after meals	Yes
Ampicillin	Principen	• 250–500 mg PO q6h • 250 mg–2 g IV q4–6h • Caps, injection, suspension						No
Aminopenicillins + β-Lactamase Inhibitors								
Amoxicillin-clavulanate	Augmentin	• IR: 250–500 mg PO q8h or 500–875 mg PO q12h • ER: 2,000 mg PO q12h • Chewable tabs, suspension, tabs (ER and IR)	• β lactamase-producing *Staph. aureus* (MSSA), *H. influenzae*, *M. catarrhalis*, *E. coli*, and *K. pneumoniae* • Anaerobes	Same as natural penicillins	Same as natural penicillins	Same as natural penicillins	• Adjust dose in renal dysfunction • Patients on ampicillin sulbactam (IV) can be switched to amoxicillin clavulanate (PO) • Good anaerobic coverage	Yes
Ampicillin-sulbactam	Unasyn	• 1.5–3 g IV q6h • Injection						No
Antipseudomonal Penicillins + β-Lactamase Inhibitors								
Piperacillin-tazobactam	Zosyn	• 3.375 IV q6h or 4.5 g IV q6–8h • Injection	• Same as amoxicillin-clavulanate and ampicillin-sulbactam • *Pseudomonas aeruginosa*	Same as natural penicillins	Same as natural penicillins	Same as natural penicillins	• Adjust dose in renal dysfunction • Primarily used for *Pseudomonas* infections • Good anaerobic coverage • Contain Na+ (use with caution in volume-overloaded patients)	No
Ticarcillin-clavulanic acid	Timentin	• 3.1 g IV q4–6h • Injection						No

Cephalosporins (β-Lactams)

Mechanism of action – inhibit bacterial cell wall synthesis; bactericidal

- As drugs move from 1st through 4th generation, ↑ activity against Gram (−) organisms and ↓ activity against Gram (+) organisms

Generic	Brand	Dose/Dosage Forms	Spectrum of Activity	Contraindications	Primary Side Effects	Pertinent Drug Interactions	Med Pearl	Top 200
First-Generation								
Cefadroxil	Duricef	• 500 mg–1 g PO q12h • Caps, suspension, tabs	• *Staph. aureus* • *Staph. epidermidis*	Allergy to penicillins, cephalosporins, or carbapenems (up to 10% risk of cross-sensitivity)	• Same as natural penicillins	• Same as natural penicillins	• Adjust dose in renal dysfunction • Patients on cefazolin (IV) can be switched to cephalexin (PO) • Cefazolin often used for surgical prophylaxis	No
Cefazolin	Ancef	• 250 mg–1 g IV q8h • Injection	• *Strep. pyogenes* • *Strep. pneumoniae* • *E. coli*					No
Cephalexin	Keflex	• 250–500 mg PO q6h • Caps, suspension, tabs	• *P. mirabilis* • *K. pneumoniae*					Yes
Second-Generation								
Cefaclor	Raniclor	• 250–500 mg PO q8h • Caps, chewable tabs, ER tabs, suspension	• Gram (+) activity similar to 1st-generation agents • Same Gram (−) activity as 1st-generation agents, but with added activity against *Acinetobacter, Citrobacter, Enterobacter, Neisseria, Serratia,* and *H. influenzae* • Anaerobic activity (cefotetan and cefoxitin only)	Same as 1st-generation agents	• Same as natural penicillins • Bleeding/bruising (with cefotetan and cefoxitin)	• Same as natural penicillins • Disulfiram-like reaction may occur if alcohol is used during treatment with cefotetan • Cefotetan and cefoxitin may ↑ effects of warfarin	• Adjust dose in renal dysfunction • Take cefaclor and cefuroxime suspension with food to ↑ absorption	No
Cefotetan	Cefotan	• 1–2 g IV q12h • Injection						No
Cefoxitin	Mefoxin	• 1–2 g IV q6–8h • Injection						No
Cefprozil	Cefzil	• 250–500 mg q12–24h • Suspension, tabs						Yes
Cefuroxime	Ceftin, Zinacef	• 250–500 mg PO q12h • 500 mg–1.5 g IV q8h • Injection, suspension, tabs						Yes

Cephalosporins (β-Lactams) *(cont'd)*

Generic	Brand	Dose/Dosage Forms	Spectrum of Activity	Contraindications	Primary Side Effects	Pertinent Drug Interactions	Med Pearl	Top 200
Third-Generation								
Cefdinir	Omnicef	• 300 mg PO q12h or 600 mg PO daily • Caps, suspension	• Limited Gram (+) activity • More extensive Gram (−) activity vs. 2nd-generation agents • *Pseudomonas aeruginosa* (ceftazidime only)	• Same as 1st-generation agents • Ceftriaxone should be avoided in neonates (↑ risk of hyperbilirubinemia, kernicterus)	• Same as natural penicillins • Bleeding/ bruising (with cefoperazone)	• Same as natural penicillins • Antacids and iron may ↓ absorption of cefdinir • Antacids and H₂ antagonists may ↓ absorption of cefpodoxime • Disulfiram-like reaction may occur if alcohol is used during treatment with cefoperazone • Cefoperazone may ↑ effects of warfarin • Ceftriaxone may cause precipitation if given with Ca²⁺-containing solutions	• Adjust dose for all, except cefoperazone and ceftriaxone, in renal dysfunction • Take cefpodoxime tabs with food to ↑ absorption • Take ceftibuten suspension 2 hours before or 1 hour after meals • Ceftriaxone often used for meningitis and STDs	Yes
Cefixime	Suprax	• 400 mg PO daily • Suspension, tabs						No
Cefoperazone	Cefobid	• 1–2 g IV q12h • Injection						No
Cefpodoxime	Vantin	• 100–400 mg PO q12h • Suspension, tabs						No
Cefotaxime	Claforan	• 1–2 g IV q8h • Injection						No
Ceftazidime	Fortaz, Tazicef	• 1–2 g IV q8–12h • Injection						No
Ceftibuten	Cedax	• 400 mg PO daily • Caps, suspension						No
Ceftriaxone	Rocephin	• 1–2 g IV daily • Injection						No
Fourth-Generation								
Cefepime	Maxipime	• 1–2 g IV q8–12h • Injection	• Gram (+) activity better than 3rd-generation agents • More extensive Gram (−) activity vs. 3rd-generation agents • *Pseudomonas aeruginosa*	Same as 1st-generation agents	Same as natural penicillins	Same as natural penicillins	Adjust dose in renal dysfunction	No

Cephalosporins (β-Lactams) *(cont'd)*

Generic	Brand	Dose/Dosage Forms	Spectrum of Activity	Contraindications	Primary Side Effects	Pertinent Drug Interactions	Med Pearl	Top 200
Fifth-Generation								
Ceftaroline	Teflaro	600 mg IV *q12h*, injection	*Staph. aureus* (MSSA and methicillin-resistant *Staph. aureus* [MRSA] [for skin infections only]), *Strep. pyogenes*, *Strep. pneumoniae*, *Klebsiella*, *E. coli*	Same as first-generation agents	Same as natural penicillins	Same as natural penicillins	Adjust dose in renal dysfunction	No

Carbapenems (β-Lactams)

Generic	Brand	Dose/Dosage Forms	Spectrum of Activity	Contraindications	Primary Side Effects	Pertinent Drug Interactions	Med Pearl	Top 200
Mechanism of action – inhibit bacterial cell wall synthesis; bactericidal								
Doripenem	Doribax	• 500 mg IV q8h • Injection	• Broad-spectrum (active against Gram (+), Gram (–), and anaerobic organisms) • All, except ertapenem, are active against *Pseudomonas aeruginosa*	Allergy to penicillins, cephalosporins, or carbapenems	• Same as natural penicillins • Seizures (esp. in patients with renal dysfunction or history of seizure disorder)	• Same as natural penicillins • May ↓ valproic acid levels	• Adjust dose in renal dysfunction • Risk of seizures is highest with imipenem/cilastatin	No
Ertapenem	Invanz	• 1 g IV daily • Injection						No
Imipenem-cilastatin	Primaxin	• 250 mg–1 g IV q6–12h • Injection						No
Meropenem	Merrem	• 500 mg–1 g IV q8h • Injection						No

Monobactam (β-Lactam)

Generic	Brand	Dose/Dosage Forms	Spectrum of Activity	Contra-indications	Primary Side Effects	Pertinent Drug Interactions	Med Pearl	Top 200
Mechanism of action – inhibit bacterial cell wall synthesis; bactericidal								
Aztreonam	Azactam, Cayston	• 500 mg–2 g IV q6–12h • Injection, nebulizer solution	Only effective against Gram (–) organisms, including *Pseudomonas aeruginosa*	None	Same as natural penicillins	None	• Can be used in patients allergic to penicillins, cephalosporins, or carbapenems • Adjust dose in renal dysfunction • Cayston used for cystic fibrosis patients (*Pseudomonas*)	No

Aminoglycosides

Generic	Brand	Dose/Dosage Forms	Spectrum of Activity	Contra-indications	Primary Side Effects	Pertinent Drug Interactions	Med Pearl	Top 200
Mechanism of action – inhibit bacterial protein synthesis by binding to the 30S subunit of the bacterial ribosome; bactericidal								
Amikacin	Amikin	• 15 mg/kg IV q24h or 5–7.5 mg/kg IV q8h • Injection	• Primarily used for Gram (–) organisms (*E. coli, Klebsiella, P. mirabilis, Enterobacter, Acinetobacter, Serratia, Pseudomonas aeruginosa*) • Provide synergistic activity against *Staph., Strep.,* or *Enterococcus* when used with penicillins or vancomycin • Streptomycin and amikacin active against *Mycobacteria* • Neomycin used as prep for bowel surgery or for hepatic encephalopathy	None	• Nephrotoxicity • Ototoxicity (both related to dose and duration of therapy; may be reversible)	• May ↑ effects of neuromuscular blocking agents • ↑ risk of nephrotoxicity when used with amphotericin B, loop diuretics, tacrolimus, cyclosporine, or cisplatin	• Bactericidal effect is concentration-dependent • Target serum concentrations (for traditional dosing): • Amikacin: Peak = 20–30 mcg/mL; Trough <6 mcg/mL • Gentamicin and tobramycin: Peak = 4–10 mcg/mL; Trough <1 mcg/mL • Target serum concentrations (for extended-interval dosing) (peaks not routinely monitored): • Amikacin: Trough <5 mcg/mL • Gentamicin and tobramycin: Trough <1 mcg/mL • TOBI used for cystic fibrosis patients (*Pseudomonas*)	No
Gentamicin	Gentak	• 5–7 mg/kg IV q24h or 1–2.5 mg/kg IV q8–12h • Injection, ophthalmic ointment/solution, topical cream/ointment						No
Kanamycin	Kantrex	• 5–7.5 mg/kg IV q8–12h • Injection						No
Neomycin	Neo-Fradin, Neo-Rx	• 500 mg–2 g PO q6–8h • Powder, tabs						No
Streptomycin	Only available generically	• 15 mg/kg/day IM • Injection						No
Tobramycin	AKTob, TOBI,	• 5–7 mg/kg IV q24h or 1–2.5 mg/kg IV q8–12h • Injection, nebulizer solution, ophthalmic ointment/solution						No

Macrolides and Ketolides

Mechanism of action – inhibit bacterial protein synthesis by binding to the 50S subunit of the bacterial ribosome; bacteriostatic

Macrolides

Generic	Brand	Dose/Dosage Forms	Spectrum of Activity	Contraindications	Primary Side Effects	Pertinent Drug Interactions	Med Pearl	Top 200
Azithromycin	Zithromax, Zmax	• 250–500 mg PO/IV q24h • Zmax: 2 g PO x 1 • Injection, ophthalmic solution, suspension (IR and ER), tabs	• Gram (+) organisms (esp. *Streptococcus*); azithromycin and clarithromycin have better activity against *Streptococcus* than erythromycin • Gram (–) organisms • Atypical organisms (e.g., *Chlamydia pneumoniae*, *Legionella*, *Mycoplasma pneumoniae*) • Azithromycin and clarithromycin active against *Mycobacteria*	QT interval prolongation or concurrent use with other drugs that prolong QT interval (clarithromycin and erythromycin)	• Prolonged QT interval (clarithromycin and erythromycin) • N/V/D • Phlebitis (erythromycin IV)	• Clarithromycin and erythromycin are major substrates and inhibitors of CYP3A4 (azithromycin least affected by CYP interactions) • CYP3A4 inhibitors may ↑ risk of side effects of clarithromycin and erythromycin	• Azithromycin ER suspension is not interchangeable with IR formulations • 400 mg erythromycin ethylsuccinate (EES) = 250 mg erythromycin base or stearate	Yes
Clarithromycin	Biaxin	• IR: 250–500 mg PO q12h • ER: 1,000 mg PO q24h • Suspension, tabs (IR and ER)				• CYP3A4 inducers may ↓ effects of clarithromycin and erythromycin • Clarithromycin and erythromycin may ↑ effect/toxicity of CYP3A4 substrates • ↑ risk of torsade de pointes (TdP) with other drugs that prolong QT interval (clarithromycin and erythromycin) • May ↑ effects of warfarin • May ↑ risk of digoxin toxicity	• Good alternative when patients allergic to penicillins • Take with food to ↓ gastrointestinal (GI) effects	Yes
Erythromycin	E.E.S., EryPed, Ery-Tab, Erythrocin, PCE	• 250–500 mg PO q6h • 500 mg–1 g IV q6h • Caps, injection, ophthalmic ointment, suspension, tabs, topical gel/ointment/solution					• Clarithromycin can be used in three-drug regimen for *H. pylori* • Erythromycin can be used for diabetic gastroparesis • Take ER azithromycin suspension 1 hour before or 2 hours after meals • Take ER clarithromycin tabs with food to ↑ absorption • Azithromycin or erythromycin preferred in pregnancy	No

Macrolides and Ketolides *(cont'd)*

Generic	Brand	Dose/Dosage Forms	Spectrum of Activity	Contraindications	Primary Side Effects	Pertinent Drug Interactions	Med Pearl	Top 200
Ketolide								
Telithromycin	Ketek	• 800 mg PO q24h • Tabs	• Greater activity (vs. macrolides) against resistant *Strep. pneumoniae* and *H. influenzae* • Atypical organisms	• History of hepatitis or jaundice with previous use of telithromycin or macrolides • Myasthenia gravis • QT interval prolongation • Concurrent use with other drugs that prolong QT interval	• N/V/D • ↑ LFTs/hepatitis • Visual disturbances (double vision, blurred vision, trouble focusing) • Loss of consciousness • Prolonged QT interval	• CYP3A4 inhibitors may ↑ risk of side effects • CYP3A4 inducers may ↓ effects • May ↑ effect/toxicity of CYP3A4 substrates • May ↑ effects of warfarin • May ↑ risk of digoxin toxicity • ↑ risk of TdP with other drugs that prolong QT interval	• Monitor LFTs and vision • Adjust dose in renal dysfunction	No

Tetracyclines

Mechanism of action – inhibit bacterial protein synthesis by binding to the 30S subunit of the bacterial ribosome; bacteriostatic

Generic	Brand	Dose/Dosage Forms	Spectrum of Activity	Contraindications	Primary Side Effects	Pertinent Drug Interactions	Med Pearl	Top 200
Demeclocycline	Declomycin	• 150 mg PO q6h or 300 mg PO q12h • Tabs	• Gram (+) organisms • Gram (–) organisms • Atypical organisms	Children ≤8 yr and pregnant or breast-feeding women (may cause permanent teeth discoloration and impaired teeth/bone growth)	• N/V/D • Photosensitivity • Phlebitis (IV) • Vertigo (minocycline)	• Absorption ↓ with antacids, dairy products, and products containing iron, magnesium, aluminum, calcium, or zinc (separate by 2 hr) • CYP3A4 inhibitors may ↑ risk of side effects • CYP3A4 inducers may ↓ effects • May ↑ effect/toxicity of CYP3A4 substrates • May ↑ effects of warfarin • May ↓ effects of oral contraceptives	• Good alternative for patients allergic to penicillin • Demeclocycline also used to treat syndrome of inappropriate antidiuretic hormone secretion (SIADH) • Tetracycline can be used in four-drug regimen for H. pylori • All except demeclocycline can be used for acne • Doxycycline is drug of choice for Lyme disease • Take demeclocycline and tetracycline 1 hour before or 2 hours after meals • Do not use after expiration date (can cause Fanconi syndrome) • Adjust dose for all, except doxycycline, in renal dysfunction	No
Doxycycline	Doryx, Vibramycin	• 100 mg IV/PO q12h • Caps, delayed-release caps/tabs, injection, suspension, syrup, tabs						Yes
Minocycline	Dynacin, Minocin	• 100 mg PO q12h • Injection, caps, tabs (IR and ER)						Yes
Tetracycline	Sumycin	• 250–500 mg PO q6–12h • Caps, suspension, tabs						No

Glycylcyclines

Mechanism of action – inhibits bacterial protein synthesis by binding to the 30S subunit of the bacterial ribosome (mechanism similar to tetracyclines); bacteriostatic

Generic	Brand	Dose/Dosage Forms	Spectrum of Activity	Contraindications	Primary Side Effects	Pertinent Drug Interactions	Med Pearl	Top 200
Tigecycline	Tygacil	• 100 mg IV x 1, then 50 mg IV q12h • Injection	Gram (+) organisms (MSSA, MRSA, vancomycin-sensitive Enterococcus faecalis)	Children ≤8 yr and pregnant/breast-feeding women (may cause permanent teeth discoloration and impaired teeth/bone growth)	• N/V/D • Infusion site reaction • Photosensitivity	May ↑ effects of warfarin	Structurally similar to tetracyclines	No

Oxazolidinones

Mechanism of action – inhibits bacterial protein synthesis by binding to bacterial 23S ribosomal RNA of the 50S subunit of the bacteria ribosome; bacteriostatic

Generic	Brand	Dose/Dosage Forms	Spectrum of Activity	Contra-indications	Primary Side Effects	Pertinent Drug Interactions	Med Pearl	Top 200
Linezolid	Zyvox	• 400–600 mg IV/PO q12h • Injection, suspension, tabs	Gram (+) organisms (vancomycin-resistant *Enterococcus faecium* [VRE], MRSA, resistant *Strep. pneumoniae*)	• Concurrent or recent (within 2 wk) use of MAO inhibitors (MAOI) • Patients with uncontrolled hypertension, pheochromocytoma, thyrotoxicosis, and/or taking sympathomimetic agents (e.g., pseudoephedrine), vasopressor agents (e.g., epinephrine), or dopaminergic agents (e.g., dopamine) • Concurrent use of selective serotonin reuptake inhibitors, tricyclic antidepressants, serotonin 5-HT1 receptor agonists (triptans), meperidine or buspirone	• N/V/D • Headache • Myelosuppression (more common if therapy >2 wk) • Peripheral/optic neuropathy (more common if therapy >4 wk) • Seizures	• Avoid taking with foods or beverages with high tyramine content (may ↑ risk of hypertensive crises) • Use with serotonergic agents may ↑ risk of serotonin syndrome; avoid concurrent use • Use with adrenergic agents (e.g., dopamine, epinephrine) may ↑ risk of hypertensive crises • Use with tramadol may ↑ risk of seizures	• Weak MAOI • Monitor CBC weekly if therapy >2 wk	No

Streptogramin

Mechanism of action – inhibits bacterial protein synthesis by binding to the 50S subunit of the bacterial ribosome; bactericidal

Generic	Brand	Dose/Dosage Forms	Spectrum of Activity	Contra-indications	Primary Side Effects	Pertinent Drug Interactions	Med Pearl	Top 200
Quinupristin-dalfopristin	Synercid	• 7.5 mg/kg IV q8–12h • Injection	Gram (+) organisms (MSSA and *Strep. pyogenes*)	None	• N/V/D • Infusion site reactions (pain, phlebitis) • Muscle/joint pain • ↑ bilirubin	May ↑ effect/toxicity of CYP3A4 substrates	• Flush line with D5W before and after infusion • If infusion reaction occurs, can ↑ volume of diluent or administer via central line	No

Fluoroquinolones

Generic	Brand	Dose/Dosage Forms	Spectrum of Activity	Contraindications	Primary Side Effects	Pertinent Drug Interactions	Med Pearl	Top 200
Mechanism of action – inhibit bacterial DNA topoisomerase and gyrase → inhibit bacterial DNA replication; bactericidal								
Ciprofloxacin	Cetraxal, Cipro, Cipro XR	• IR: 250–750 mg PO q12h • ER: 500 mg–1 g PO q24h • IV: 200–400 mg IV q8–12h • Injection, ophthalmic ointment/solution, suspension, tabs (ER and IR), otic solution	• Gram (+) organisms (levofloxacin, gemifloxacin, and moxifloxacin have greatest activity against *Streptococcus*) • Gram (−) organisms • Ciprofloxacin active against *Pseudomonas aeruginosa* • Atypical organisms	• Children <18 yr and pregnant/breast-feeding women (may cause impaired bone growth) • Concurrent use with other drugs that prolong QT interval	• Nausea/diarrhea • Photosensitivity • Tendinitis/tendon rupture • Hyper-/hypoglycemia • Peripheral neuropathy • Seizures • Prolonged QT interval	• Absorption ↓ with antacids, dairy products, and products containing iron, magnesium, aluminum, calcium, or zinc (separate by 2 hours) • Use with corticosteroids may ↑ risk of tendon rupture • Use with nonsteroidal anti-inflammatory drugs (NSAIDs) may ↑ risk of seizures • Ciprofloxacin and ofloxacin may ↑ effects of CYP1A2 substrates • Ciprofloxacin may ↓ phenytoin levels • May ↑ effects of warfarin • May ↑ effects of antidiabetic agents • ↑ risk of TdP with other drugs that prolong QT interval	• Ciprofloxacin ER and IR tabs are not interchangeable • Adjust dose for all, except moxifloxacin, in renal dysfunction • Take levofloxacin oral solution 1 hour before or 2 hours after meals • Patients with diabetes should monitor their blood glucose more frequently	Yes
Gemifloxacin	Factive	• 320 mg PO q24h • Tabs						No
Levofloxacin	Iquix, Levaquin, Quixin	• 250–750 mg IV/PO q24h • Injection, ophthalmic solution, solution, tabs						Yes
Moxifloxacin	Avelox, Moxeza, Vigamox	• 400 mg IV/PO q24h • Injection, ophthalmic solution, tabs						Yes
Ofloxacin	Floxin, Ocuflox	• 200–400 mg PO q12h • Ophthalmic solution, otic solution, tabs						No

Sulfonamides

Generic	Brand	Dose/Dosage Forms	Spectrum of Activity	Contraindications	Primary Side Effects	Pertinent Drug Interactions	Med Pearl	Top 200
Mechanism of action – inhibit incorporation of para-aminobenzoic acid (PABA) into DNA → inhibit folic acid production and bacterial growth; bacteriostatic								
Sulfadiazine	Only available generically	• 500 mg–1.5 g PO q6h • Tabs	• Gram (+) organisms (including MSSA, MRSA) • Gram (−) organisms • SMX/TMP is 1st-line drug to treat/prevent *Pneumocystis jiroveci* pneumonia (PJP) • Sulfadiazine used to treat toxoplasmosis	• Sulfa allergy • Porphyria • Megaloblastic anemia • Infants and pregnant/breast-feeding women (↑ risk of kernicterus) • G6PD deficiency	• N/V/D • Rash • Stevens-Johnson syndrome • Photosensitivity • Folate deficiency • Hypoglycemia (in patients with diabetes)	• May ↑ effects/toxicity of methotrexate • May ↑ effects of warfarin • May ↑ effects of antidiabetic agents	• Instruct patients to take with a full glass of water (to prevent crystalluria) • Adjust dose in renal dysfunction	No
SMX/TMP	Bactrim, Septra, Isulfatrim	• 1 double-strength tab PO q12h • 10–20 mg/kg/day of TMP IV in divided doses • Injection, suspension, tabs						Yes

Cyclic Lipopeptide

Generic	Brand	Dose/Dosage Forms	Spectrum of Activity	Contra-indications	Primary Side Effects	Pertinent Drug Interactions	Med Pearl	Top 200
Mechanism of action – bind to bacterial cell membranes and cause rapid depolarization → inhibit protein, DNA, and RNA synthesis; bactericidal								
Daptomycin	Cubicin	• 4–6 mg/kg IV q24h • Injection	Gram (+) organisms (MSSA, MRSA, vancomycin-sensitive *Enterococcus faecalis*, VRE)	None	• Nausea/diarrhea • Infusion site reactions • Muscle pain/weakness	Use with statins may ↑ risk of myopathy; consider discontinuing statin therapy throughout treatment	• Monitor creatine kinase levels weekly • Adjust dose in renal dysfunction	No

Miscellaneous Antibacterial Agents

Generic	Brand	Dose/Dosage Forms	Spectrum of Activity	Contra-indications	Primary Side Effects	Pertinent Drug Interactions	Med Pearl	Top 200
Mechanism of action – inhibits bacterial protein synthesis by binding to the 50S subunit of the bacterial ribosome; bacteriostatic								
Chloramphenicol	Only available generically	• 12.5–25 mg/kg IV q6h • Injection	• Gram (+) organisms (VRE) • Gram (–) organisms	Neonates (↑ risk of gray-baby syndrome)	• N/V/D • Myelosuppression (anemia, leukopenia, thrombocytopenia, aplastic anemia) • Gray-baby syndrome (vomiting, lethargy, respiratory depression, death) • Optic neuritis	• Phenobarbital and rifampin may ↓ effects • May ↑ effects of warfarin and phenytoin	• Only used for life–threatening infections • Monitor CBC frequently • Target serum concentrations: Peak = 15–25 mcg/mL; Trough = 5–10 mcg/ml	No
Mechanism of action – inhibits bacterial protein synthesis by binding to the 50S subunit of the bacterial ribosome; bacteriostatic								
Clindamycin	Cleocin, Clindesse, Evoclin	• 150–450 mg PO q6h • 300–900 mg IV q8h • Caps, injection, solution, topical foam/gel/lotion/pledgets/solution, vaginal cream/suppository	• Gram (+) organisms • Anaerobes	History of pseudo-membranous colitis or ulcerative colitis	• N/V/D • Pseudomembranous colitis (*Clostridium difficile*) (highest incidence)	None significant	• Also used for acne (topical) • Patients using intra-vaginally should avoid intercourse (↓ efficacy of condoms and diaphragms)	Yes
Mechanism of action – interferes with bacterial DNA synthesis; bactericidal								
Metronidazole	Flagyl, Metrogel, Noritate, Vandazole	• 250–500 mg PO q8–12h • 500 mg IV q8–12h • Caps, injection, tabs (ER and IR), topical cream/gel/lotion, vaginal gel	Anaerobes	Pregnancy (1st trimester)	• Nausea/diarrhea • Confusion • Dizziness • Peripheral neuropathy • Metallic taste	• Disulfiram-like reaction may occur if alcohol is used during treatment • May ↑ effects of warfarin and lithium • Phenobarbital and phenytoin may ↓ effects • Cimetidine may ↑ effects	• Can be used in four-drug regimen for *H. pylori* • Drug of choice for *Clostridium difficile* • Take ER tabs 1 hour before or 2 hours after meals	No

Miscellaneous Antibacterial Agents *(cont'd)*

Generic	Brand	Dose/Dosage Forms	Spectrum of Activity	Contra-indications	Primary Side Effects	Pertinent Drug Interactions	Med Pearl	Top 200
Mechanism of action – Inhibits bacterial cell wall synthesis; bactericidal								
Telavancin	Vibativ	• 10 mg/kg IV q24h • Injection	Gram (+) organisms (MSSA, MRSA, *Enterococcus faecalis*, *Streptococcus*)	Pregnancy	• Insomnia • Headache • Renal dysfunction • Red-man syndrome • Metallic taste • N/V/D • QT interval prolongation	↑ risk of nephro-toxicity when used with amphotericin B, loop diuretics, tacrolimus, cyclosporine, or cisplatin	• Adjust dose in renal dysfunction • Monitor renal function • If red-man syndrome occurs, ↓ infusion rate • May interfere with PT, INR, aPTT	No
Vancomycin	Vancocin	• 125–250 mg PO q6h • 500 mg–1 g q12h • Caps, injection	• Gram (+) organisms (MSSA, MRSA) • *Clostridium difficile*	None	• Red-man syndrome (flushing, hypotension, erythema, pruritus) • Nephrotoxicity • Ototoxicity	↑ risk of nephro-toxicity when used with amphotericin B, loop diuretics, tacrolimus, cyclosporine, or cisplatin	• Bactericidal effect is time-dependent • Adjust dose in renal dysfunction • Often used in patients with penicillin allergy • Use PO (NOT IV) to treat *Clostridium difficile* (PO not effective for any other type of infection) • If red-man syndrome occurs, ↓ infusion rate • Target serum concentrations (peaks not routinely monitored): Trough = 15–20 mcg/mL	No

Medication Charts: Antifungal Agents

Azole Antifungals

Generic	Brand	Dose/Dosage Forms	Spectrum of Activity	Contra-indications	Primary Side Effects	Pertinent Drug Interactions	Med Pearl	Top 200
Mechanism of action – inhibit synthesis of ergosterol (essential component of fungal cell membrane) • Imidazoles: butoconazole, clotrimazole, econazole, ketoconazole, miconazole, oxiconazole, sulconazole, tioconazole • Triazoles: fluconazole, itraconazole, terconazole, posaconazole, voriconazole								
Fluconazole	Diflucan	• 100–800 mg IV/PO q24h • Injection, tabs, suspension	• *Candida* spp. • *Coccidioides* spp. • *Histoplasma* spp. • *Cryptococcus* spp. • *Aspergillus* spp. (only itraconazole)	None	• Headache • N/V/D • Abdominal pain • Rash • ↑ LFTs • Prolonged QT interval	• May ↑ effect/toxicity of CYP2C9, CYP2C19, and CYP3A4 substrates • Rifampin may ↓ effects • ↑ risk of TdP with other drugs that prolong QT interval	• Adjust dose in patients with renal dysfunction • Conversion from IV to PO is 1:1 • Monitor LFTs	Yes
Itraconazole	Sporanox	• 100–400 mg/day PO • Caps, solution		• Concurrent use of dofetilide, ergot alkaloids, lovastatin, midazolam, pimozide, quinidine, simvastatin, or triazolam • HF	• Nausea • Abdominal pain • Rash • ↑ LFTs • Prolonged QT interval	• CYP3A4 inhibitors may ↑ risk of side effects • CYP3A4 inducers may ↓ effects • May ↑ effect/toxicity of CYP3A4 substrates • ↑ risk of digoxin toxicity • Absorption ↓ with antacids, H₂ antagonists, and proton pump inhibitors (acidic environment required for absorption) (separate by 2 hr) • ↑ risk of TdP with other drugs that prolong QT interval	• Caps and solution cannot be used interchangeably (bioavailability of solution > caps) • Potent negative inotrope • Monitor LFTs	No
Ketoconazole	Nizoral	• 200–400 mg PO q24h • Rx: Topical cream/ gel/shampoo/ aerosol, tabs • OTC: shampoo		Concurrent use of ergot alkaloids	• N/V • Gynecomastia • Sexual dysfunction • ↑ LFTs • Prolonged QT interval	Same as itraconazole	• May ↓ testosterone levels • Can also be used to treat prostate cancer • Monitor LFTs	Yes

Azole Antifungals *(cont'd)*

Generic	Brand	Dose/Dosage Forms	Spectrum of Activity	Contra-indications	Primary Side Effects	Pertinent Drug Interactions	Med Pearl	Top 200
Posaconazole	Noxafil	• 100–800 mg/day PO • Suspension	• *Candida* spp. • *Coccidioides* spp. • *Histoplasma* spp. • *Cryptococcus* spp. • *Aspergillus* spp.	Concurrent use of ergot alkaloids, quinidine, or pimozide	• Headache • N/V • Rash • Prolonged QT interval	• May ↑ effect/toxicity of CYP3A4 substrates • ↑ risk of TdP with other drugs that prolong QT interval	• Must be taken with full meal to ↑ absorption • Monitor LFTs	No
Voriconazole	Vfend	• *Loading dose:* 6 mg/kg IV q12h for 24 hr • *Maintenance dose:* 3–4 mg/kg IV q12h; 100–300 mg PO q12h • Injection, suspension, tabs		Concurrent use of pimozide, quinidine, long-acting barbiturates, carbamazepine, ergot alkaloids, rifampin, rifabutin, ritonavir (≥800 mg/day), St. John's wort, or sirolimus	• Visual disturbances (transient) (blurred vision, photophobia, altered perception of color) • Rash • Photosensitivity • ↑ LFTs • Hallucinations • N/V • Prolonged QT interval	• May ↑ effect/toxicity of CYP2C9, CYP2C19, and CYP3A4 substrates • CYP2C9 and CYP2C19 inducers may ↓ effects • May ↑ efavirenz levels • Efavirenz may ↓ effects • ↑ risk of TdP with other drugs that prolong QT interval	• ↓ dose of cyclosporine by 50% • When using with efavirenz, ↑ voriconazole dose and ↓ efavirenz dose • ↑ dose of voriconazole when using with phenytoin • Use PO when CrCl <50 mL/min (diluent in IV can accumulate) • Take PO 1 hour before or after meals • Monitor LFTs and vision	No

Echinocandins

Mechanism of action – inhibit synthesis of 1,3-β-d-glucan (essential component of fungal cell wall)

Generic	Brand	Dose/Dosage Forms	Spectrum of Activity	Contra-indications	Primary Side Effects	Pertinent Drug Interactions	Med Pearl	Top 200
Anidulafungin	Eraxis	• 100–200 mg IV on day 1, then 50–100 mg IV q24h • Injection	• *Candida* spp. • *Aspergillus* spp.	None	• N/V • Headache • Hypokalemia • Rash	None	• Monitor LFTs	No
Caspofungin	Cancidas	• 70 mg IV on day 1, then 50 mg IV q24h • Injection			• Fever • ↑ LFTs • Phlebitis	• Rifampin, carbamazepine, dexamethasone, efavirenz, nevirapine, and phenytoin may ↓ effects • May ↓ tacrolimus levels • Cyclosporine may ↑ risk of side effects	• ↑ dose of caspofungin to 70 mg/day when used with rifampin, carbamazepine, dexamethasone, efavirenz, nevirapine, or phenytoin • Adjust dose in moderate hepatic dysfunction • Monitor LFTs	No
Micafungin	Mycamine	• 50–150 mg IV q24h • Injection				None	Monitor LFTs	No

Amphotericin B

Mechanism of action — bind to ergosterol in cell membrane → produce a channel in cell membrane (↑ permeability) → allow K+ and Mg2+ to leak out of cell ("leaky membrane") → cell death

Generic	Brand	Dose/Dosage Forms	Spectrum of Activity	Contra-indications	Primary Side Effects	Pertinent Drug Interactions	Med Pearl	Top 200
Amphotericin B desoxycholate	Fungizone	• Test dose of 1 mg IV should be given over 20–30 min (monitor patient for 2–4 hr before starting infusion) • 0.5–1.5 mg/kg/day IV • Injection	• *Candida* spp. • *Coccidioides* spp. • *Blastomyces* spp. • *Histoplasma* spp. • *Cryptococcus* spp. • *Aspergillus* spp.	None	• Nephrotoxicity (less common with lipid-based formulations) • Infusion reactions (fever, chills, hypotension, nausea, tachypnea) • Phlebitis • Electrolyte disturbances (i.e., hypokalemia, hypomagnesemia)	↑ risk of nephrotoxicity when used with aminoglycosides, loop diuretics, tacrolimus, cyclosporine, or cisplatin	• May premedicate with acetaminophen, NSAIDs, diphenhydramine, and/or corticosteroid to prevent infusion reactions (give 30–60 min before infusion); meperidine may be used for rigors • Infusion reactions less common with lipid-based formulations (amphotericin B desoxycholate > ABCD > ABLC > L-Amb) • Infusion reactions ↓ after first few doses • Sodium loading (500 mL of 0.9% NaCl before and after infusion) may ↓ risk of nephrotoxicity with amphotericin B desoxycholate • Monitor blood urea nitrogen (BUN), serum creatinine (SCr), potassium, and magnesium	No
Amphotericin B lipid complex (ABLC)	Abelcet	• 5 mg/kg IV q24h • Injection						No
Liposomal amphotericin B (L-AmB)	AmBisome	• 3–6 mg/kg IV q24h • Injection						No
Amphotericin B colloidal dispersion (ABCD)	Amphotec	• 3–4 mg/kg IV q24h • Injection						No

Other Antifungals

Generic	Brand	Dose/Dosage Forms	Spectrum of Activity	Contra-indications	Primary Side Effects	Pertinent Drug Interactions	Med Pearl	Top 200
Mechanism of action – similar to amphotericin B								
Nystatin	Mycostatin	• Suspension: 400,000–600,000 units 4 times/day • Topical: Apply 2–3 times daily • Topical cream/ointment/powder, suspension, tabs, vaginal tabs	*Candida* spp.	None	• N/V/D • Abdominal pain	None	Suspension should be swished and swallowed	Yes
Mechanism of action – inhibits squalene epoxidase → inhibits synthesis of ergosterol								
Terbinafine	Lamisil	• PO: 250 mg q24h • Topical: Apply 1–2 times daily • Rx: Granules, tabs, topical solution • OTC: Topical/cream/gel/solution	*Trichophyton* spp.	• Liver disease • CrCl <50 mL/min	• Headache • N/V/D • ↑ LFTs	• May ↑ effect/toxicity of CYP2D6 substrates • May ↓ cyclosporine levels	• Oral used for onychomycosis or tinea capitis (scalp ringworm); topical used for tinea pedis (athlete's foot), tinea corporis (ringworm), or tinea cruris (jock itch) • Give for 6 wks for fingernail infection; 12 wk. for toenail infection • Monitor LFTs	Yes

Other Antifungals (cont'd)

Generic	Brand	Dose/Dosage Forms	Spectrum of Activity	Contra-indications	Primary Side Effects	Pertinent Drug Interactions	Med Pearl	Top 200
Mechanism of action – enters fungal cell wall → converted into 5-fluorouracil, which interferes with fungal RNA and protein synthesis								
Flucytosine	Ancobon	• 25–37.5 mg/kg PO q6h (administered with amphotericin B) • Caps	Candida spp. Cryptococcus spp.	None	• Confusion • Hallucinations • Ataxia • Headache • N/V/D • ↑ LFTs • Renal dysfunction • Bone marrow depression	None	• Should not be used as monotherapy • Adjust dose in patients with renal dysfunction • Monitor LFTs, BUN/SCr, and CBC • Flucytosine concentrations: Peak: 50–100 mcg/mL; Trough: 25–50 mcg/mL	No
Mechanism of action – inhibits fungal cell mitosis								
Griseofulvin	Grifulvin V, Gris-PEG, Fulvicin	• Microsize: 500–1,000 mg/day PO • Ultramicrosize: 375 mg/day PO • Microsize: Suspension, tabs • Ultramicrosize: Tabs	Trichophyton spp.	• Liver disease • Porphyria	• Rash/hives • N/V/D • Headache • Confusion • Photosensitivity	• Barbiturates may ↓ effects • May ↓ effects of cyclosporine and warfarin	• Monitor LFTs • Use with alcohol may cause disulfiram reaction • Administer with high-fat meal to ↑ absorption	No

KAPLAN MEDICAL

Medication Charts: Antiviral Agents

Drugs for Treatment of Herpes Simplex Virus and Varicella-Zoster Virus

Generic	Brand	Dose/Dosage Forms	Spectrum of Activity	Contra-indications	Primary Side Effects	Pertinent Drug Interactions	Med Pearl	Top 200
Mechanism of action – inhibit viral DNA polymerase → inhibit replication of viral DNA								
Acyclovir	Zovirax	• *Genital herpes (initial episode):* 200 mg PO 5 times/day x 7–10 days 5 mg/kg IV q8h x 5–7 days • *Herpes labialis (cold sores):* 400 mg PO 5 times/day x 5 days • *Varicella (chickenpox):* 800 mg PO q6h x 5 days 10 mg/kg IV q8h x 7 days • *Herpes zoster (shingles):* 800 mg PO 5 times/day x 7–10 days 10 mg/kg IV q8h x 7 days • Caps, injection, suspension, tabs, topical cream/ointment	• Herpes simplex virus (HSV)-1 (herpes labialis) and HSV-2 (genital herpes) • Varicella zoster virus (causes chickenpox and shingles)	None	• N/V/D • Headache • Phlebitis (IV acyclovir) • Renal dysfunction (IV acyclovir) • Seizures (esp. in patients with renal dysfunction)	None	• Adjust dose for all, except penciclovir, in renal dysfunction • To avoid renal damage with IV acyclovir (can crystallize), infuse slowly and keep patient hydrated	Yes
Famciclovir (prodrug of penciclovir)	Famvir	• *Genital herpes (initial episode):* 250 mg PO q8h x 7–10 days • *Cold sores:* 1,500 mg PO x 1 • *Herpes zoster:* 500 mg PO q8h x 7 days • Tabs						Yes
Penciclovir	Denavir	*Cold sores:* • Apply q2h while awake x 4 days • Topical cream						No
Valacyclovir (prodrug of acyclovir)	Valtrex	• *Genital herpes (initial episode):* 1 g PO q12h x 7–10 days • *Cold sores:* 2 g PO q12h x 1 day • *Herpes zoster:* 1 g PO q8h x 7 days • Caps						Yes

Drugs for Treatment of Cytomegalovirus

Generic	Brand	Dose/Dosage Forms	Spectrum of Activity	Contraindications	Primary Side Effects	Pertinent Drug Interactions	Med Pearl	Top 200
Mechanism of action — inhibit replication of viral DNA								
Cidofovir	Vistide	• 5 mg/kg IV once weekly x 2 wk, then q2 wk • Injection	• Cytomegalovirus • HSV (foscarnet) • Acute herpetic keratitis (ophthalmic gangiclovir)	• SCr >1.5 mg/dL, CrCl ≤55 mL/min, or proteinuria • Use of other nephrotoxic drugs within 7 days	• Nephrotoxicity • Neutropenia • Metabolic acidosis • ↓ intraocular pressure • Uveitis/iritis	Use of antiretroviral drugs may ↑ risk of side effects	• Monitor BUN/SCr • To minimize renal damage, administer 1 L of 0.9% NaCl before and after each infusion; also give 2 g of probenecid 3 hr before each infusion and then 1 g at 2 hr and 8 hr after each infusion • If SCr ↑ by 0.3–0.4 mg/dL above baseline, ↓ dose to 3 mg/kg; if SCr ↑ by ≥0.5 mg/dL, discontinue • Advise patients to use effective contraception	No
Foscarnet	Foscavir	• 60 mg/kg IV q8h or 90 mg/kg IV q12h x 14–21 days, then 90–120 mg/kg IV q24h • Injection		None	• Nephrotoxicity • N/V • Anemia • Electrolyte disturbances • Genital sores • Seizures	• ↑ risk of renal dysfunction when used with other nephrotoxic drugs • Zidovudine may ↑ risk of anemia	• Adjust dose in renal dysfunction • Monitor BUN/SCr • To minimize renal damage, administer 1 L of 0.9% NaCl with each infusion • Rapid infusion associated with seizures and arrhythmias	No
Ganciclovir	Cytovene, Vitrasert, Zirgan	• 1 g PO q8h • 5 mg/kg IV q12h x 14–21 days, then either 5 mg/kg/day IV 7 times/wk or 6 mg/kg/day IV 5 times/wk • 4.5 mg intraocularly q5–8 months • 1 drop 5 times/day until ulcer heals, then 1 drop 3 times/day/7 days • Caps, injection, intravitreal implant, ophthalmic gel		• Neutropenia • Thrombocytopenia • Anemia	• Myelosuppression • Fever • Rash • Phlebitis (IV) • ↑ LFTs • Nephrotoxicity • Seizures • N/V/D	• ↑ risk of myelosuppression when used with other immunosuppressive drugs • ↑ risk of renal dysfunction when used with other nephrotoxic drugs • May ↑ effects/toxicity of zidovudine	• For ganciclovir, IV route preferred (PO has poor bioavailability) • Adjust dose in renal dysfunction • Advise patients to use effective contraception during treatment and for at least 90 days after treatment • Take PO ganciclovir and valganciclovir with food	No
Valganciclovir (prodrug of ganciclovir)	Valcyte	• 900 mg PO q12h x 21 days, then 900 mg PO q24h • Tabs, solution						No

Drugs for Treatment of Influenza

Generic	Brand	Dose/Dosage Forms	Spectrum of Activity	Contra-indications	Primary Side Effects	Pertinent Drug Interactions	Med Pearl	Top 200
Mechanism of action – inhibit the enzyme (neuraminidase) responsible for releasing the newly formed mature virus from the host cell								
Oseltamivir	Tamiflu	*Prophylaxis:* 75 mg PO q24h x 10 days (6 wk for community outbreak) *Treatment:* 75 mg PO q12h x 5 days • Caps, suspension	• Influenza A and B • H1N1 influenza	None	• N/V/D • Headache • Neuropsychiatric events (e.g., confusion, delirium, hallucinations, self-injury)	None	• For prophylaxis, initiate therapy within 2 days of contact with infected person • For treatment, initiate therapy within 2 days of onset of symptoms • Adjust dose in renal dysfunction • ↓ flu severity and duration by ~ 1 day • Can be used in children ≥1 yr	Yes
Zanamivir	Relenza	*Prophylaxis:* 2 inhalations q24h x 10 days (28 days for community outbreak) *Treatment:* 2 inhalations q12h x 5 days • Powder for oral inhalation		Asthma/COPD	• Bronchospasm • Cough • Headache • Nausea/diarrhea • Neuropsychiatric events (e.g., confusion, delirium, hallucinations, self-injury)		• For prophylaxis, initiate therapy within 1.5 days (5 days in community setting) of contact with infected person • For treatment, initiate therapy within 2 days of onset of symptoms • ↓ flu severity and duration by ~ 1 day • Can be used in children ≥5yr (prophylaxis) or ≥7 yr (treatment)	No

LEARNING POINTS

- Compliance is a must with antiretroviral therapy. If a patient is going to stop the prescribed regimen, all the antiretrovirals must be stopped at the same time to prevent resistance.

- Patients receiving antibiotics should complete the entire course of therapy.

- Be aware of the patient's allergies when selecting antibiotic therapy (especially penicillin and sulfa allergies).

- Know agents to treat unique organisms:

  - MRSA: Vancomycin, linezolid, tigecycline, daptomycin, telavancin, ceftaroline

  - *Pseudomonas aeruginosa*: Piperacillin/tazobactam, ticarcillin/clavulanic acid, aztreonam, aminoglycosides, ciprofloxacin, ceftazidime, cefepime, carbapenems (except ertapenem)

  - Anaerobes: Metronidazole, clindamycin, piperacillin/tazobactam, ticarcillin/clavulanic acid, cefoxitin, cefotetan, carbapenems

- Know important/notable side effects and drug interactions of antibiotics:

  - Which ones cause nephrotoxicity?

  - Which ones are associated with QT interval prolongation?

  - Which ones cause myelosuppression?

  - Which ones are associated with a disulfiram reaction?

  - Which ones should be avoided with antacids or products containing di-/trivalent cations?

  - Which ones cause photosensitivity?

PRACTICE QUESTIONS

1. Which of the following medications should NOT be given to a 1-year-old child?

    (A) Amoxicillin
    (B) Cefuroxime
    (C) Clindamycin
    (D) Penicillin
    (E) Tetracycline

2. Which of the following medications would be appropriate for the treatment of *Pseudomonas aeruginosa*?

    (A) Ampicillin
    (B) Cefepime
    (C) Ceftriaxone
    (D) Erythromycin
    (E) Clindamycin

3. A patient admitted to the hospital is diagnosed with aspergillosis. Which of the following antimicrobial agents would be most appropriate to initiate in this patient?

    (A) Nystatin
    (B) Tigecycline
    (C) Chloramphenicol
    (D) Acyclovir
    (E) Caspofungin

4. Patients taking which of the following antimicrobial agents should be counseled to wear sunscreen because of the risk of photosensitivity?

    I. Cleocin
    II. Biaxin
    III. Factive

    (A) I only
    (B) III only
    (C) I and II only
    (D) II and III only
    (E) I, II, and III

5. Which of the following drugs used in the treatment of tuberculosis can cause orange-red discoloration of a patient's urine?

   (A) Isoniazid
   (B) Ethambutol
   (C) Rifampin
   (D) Pyrazinamide
   (E) Streptomycin

ANSWERS

1.   E

Tetracycline should not be given to children younger than 9 years of age, as it can cause enamel hypoplasia or permanent tooth discoloration, therefore choice (E) is correct. The other medications can be administered safely to children.

2.   B

Cefepime, a 4th-generation cephalosporin, is the only antibiotic listed that would treat an infection caused by *Pseudomonas aeruginosa*; therefore, choice (B) is correct.

3.   E

Aspergillosis is a serious fungal infection. Both caspofungin and nystatin (A) are considered antifungal agents; however, nystatin is used topically (as an oral suspension for thrush or as topical cream/ointment/powder) for local infections caused by *Candida* spp. Caspofungin is administered intravenously and can be used for the treatment of aspergillosis; thus, choice (E) is correct. Tigecycline (B) and chloramphenicol (C) are used for bacterial infections. Acyclovir (D) is an antiviral agent.

4.   B

Fluoroquinolones are associated with an increased risk of photosensitivity. Therefore, patients receiving Factive (gemifloxacin) should be counseled to wear sunscreen during the course of therapy. Neither Cleocin (clindamycin) nor Biaxin (clarithromycin) is associated with photosensitivity.

5.   C

Rifampin (C) can cause an orange-red discoloration of all bodily fluids (e.g., tears, saliva, urine). Rifabutin can also cause this discoloration of bodily fluids. Isoniazid (A), ethambutol (B), pyrazinamide (D), and streptomycin (E) do not cause discoloration of the urine.

Pulmonary Disorders

3

This chapter covers the following diseases:

- **Asthma**
- **Chronic obstructive pulmonary disease (COPD)**
- **Smoking Cessation**

 Suggested Study Time: **45 minutes**

ASTHMA

Definitions

Asthma is a disease of the airways characterized by airway inflammation and broncho-constriction of the smooth muscles. This hyperactivity is due to a wide variety of stimuli or triggers. The hallmark features of asthma include airflow obstruction that is reversible, bronchial hyperresponsiveness, and airway inflammation. The hyperactivity and inflammation lead to obstruction of the airways, cough, dyspnea, chest tightness, and wheezing. The inflammatory cell infiltration mainly consists of neutrophils (especially in sudden-onset, fatal asthma exacerbations, and in patients who smoke), eosinophils, lymphocytes, mast cell activation, and epithelial cell injury and is called remodeling.

Diagnosis

To diagnose asthma, a patient has to have episodes of airway obstruction or airway hyperresponsiveness and at least partially reversible airway obstruction, all alternative diagnoses excluded.

- Pulmonary function tests (PFTs) provide an objective means to diagnose asthma.

- PFTs are measured using spirometry and demonstrate an obstructive pattern of decreases in expiratory flow rates.

- Spirometry measures FVC and FEV1.
- FVC is the volume of air forcibly exhaled from the point of maximal inspiration; FEV1 is the volume of aired exhaled during the first second.
- The guidelines recommend that spirometry measurements of FEV1, FVC, and FEV1/FEV are used before and after the patient inhales a short-acting bronchodilator to assess bronchodilation. Improvements are defined as an increase of FEV1 by more than 12%, which is diagnostic of asthma.

Signs and Symptoms

- Shortness of breath and wheezing that lasts for hours
- May be completely symptom-free between attacks
- Triggered by acute exposure to irritants: pollen, dust, chemicals, changes in weather, perfumes, smoke, heartburn, mold
- Nasal polyps
- Excessive mucus and even mucus plugs

Guidelines

National Heart, Lung and Blood Institute, National Asthma Education and Prevention Program, Expert Panel Report 3: Guidelines for the Diagnosis and Management of Asthma—Full Report, 2007. http://nhlbi.nih.gov/guidelines/asthma/asthsumm.pdf.

Guidelines Summary

There are four components to asthma management:

- Measurement of assessment and monitoring
- Controlling environmental factors and comorbid conditions
- Education for asthma care
- Pharmacologic therapy

The goals of therapy are as follows:

- Patient education is a must.
- Daily usage of peak flow meter will provide an objective FEV1.
- Implementation of an action plan:
  - Green zone ("I feel good"), yellow zone ("I do not feel good"), red zone ("I feel awful")
  - Green zone = FEV1 >80% of personal best
  - Yellow zone = FEV1 >50–80% of personal best
  - Red zone = FEV1 <50% of personal best

- Attempt to identify triggers:
    - Consider subcutaneous allergen immunotherapy.
    - Management of gastrointestinal reflux disease (GERD) can greatly improve symptoms.
    - Avoid aspirin therapy due to prostaglandin inhibition; can cause bronchoconstriction.
    - Smoking cessation is recommended.
    - Consider clean home, dust, plastic case over mattress.
        - » Patient needs to be classified into mild, moderate, severe, or life threatening.
    - Identify frequency of symptoms and nighttime awakenings.
    - Identify use of short-acting beta-2 agonists and lung function.
        - » Ensure compliance with medications.
        - » Ensure proper inhaler technique.
        - » Use a stepwise approach to treatment.
        - » Long-term medications should include anti-inflammatory mechanism.

Asthma

Mechanism of action – glucocorticoid receptor agonist with an affinity for the receptor resulting in anti-inflammatory and immunosuppressive properties, and antiproliferative actions

Generic	Brand	Dose	Contra-indications	Primary Side Effects	Key Monitoring	Pertinent Drug Interactions	Med Pearl	Top 200
Fluticasone	• Flovent • Flovent HFA	44–440 mcg BID	Primary treatment for acute bronchospasm	• Throat irritation • Cough • Oral candidiasis • Lower respiratory tract infection	• FEV1 • Peak flow • Other PFTs • HPA axis suppression	None that are pertinent, due to topical administration at the lung tissue	• HFA formulation • Most potent corticosteroid	Yes
Budesonide	• Pulmicort • Respules	200–800 mcg BID					Respules are the only nebulized corticosteroid	Yes
Mometasone	Asmanex	220–440 mcg/day					True once daily	Yes
Beclomethasone	QVAR	40–320 mcg BID					HFA formulation	Yes
Flunisolide	AeroBid	500–2,000 mcg BID					AeroBid (M) has a mint flavor	No
Triamcinolone	Azmacort	150–400 mcg/day QID					• Built in spacer • Least potent corticosteroid	No
Ciclesonide	Alvesco	• 160 mcg/day • 80 mcg BID • *Max:* 320 mcg/day		• Bad taste • Throat hoarseness • Cough after inhalation			Drug is a solution aerosol so no shaking is required	No

Mechanism of action – long-acting beta-2 agonists

Generic	Brand	Dose	Contra-indications	Primary Side Effects	Key Monitoring	Pertinent Drug Interactions	Med Pearl	Top 200
Salmeterol	Serevent	• *Diskus:* 50 mcg/puff • *Max:* 2 puffs/day	• Use as an acute bronchodilator • Presence of tachyarrhythmias	• Headache • Hypertension • Dizziness • Chest pain	• FEV1 • Peak flow • Other pulmonary function tests	None	Long-acting beta-2 agonists may increase the risk of asthma-related deaths; should be used only in adjunct therapy with inhaled corticosteroids	No
Formoterol	Foradil	• *DPI:* 12 mcg/capsule • *Max:* 2 puffs/day				None		No

Asthma *(cont'd)*

Generic	Brand	Dose	Contra-indications	Primary Side Effects	Key Monitoring	Pertinent Drug Interactions	Med Pearl	Top 200
Mechanism of action – prevents the mass cells from releasing histamine and leukotrienes								
Cromolyn neb & inhaler	Intal	20–80 mg/day	Primary treatment for acute bronchospasms	• Cough and irritation • Unpleasant taste	Pulmonary function tests	None	• Safety is the primary advantage of this drug class • May take 4–6 weeks for full benefit • Approved to <2 yr of age	No
Nedocromil neb & inhaler	Tilade	1.75–14 mg/day		• Increase in sneezing				No
Mechanism of action – IgG monoclonal antibody which inhibits IgE receptor on mast cells and basophils.								
Omalizumab	XOLAIR	Subcutaneous 150–375 mg every 2–4 wk, based on weight and serum IgE	Acute bronchospasms	• Pain and bruising of injection sites • Anaphylaxis has been reported	Be prepared for anaphylaxis	None	Do not administer more than 150 mg per injection site	No
Mechanism of action – selective leukotriene-receptor antagonist of leukotrienes D4 and E4								
Montelukast	Singulair	4–10 mg/HS	Hypersensitivity	Rare Churg-Strauss syndrome		CYP450 inhibitor: 2C8 and 2C9	Approved as young as 1 year of age	Yes
Zafirlukast	Accolate	10–40 mg/day		Increase in LFTs	Must be taken on empty stomach	• CYP450 inhibitor: 1A2 • Warfarin		No
Mechanism of action – 5-lipoxygenase inhibitor limits neutrophil and monocyte aggregation								
Zileuton	Zyflo, Zyflo CR	600–2,400 mg/day	Acute liver disease	• Elevations in • LFTs	• LFT baseline every 2 months • Peak flow	CYP450 inhibitor: 1A2	QID dose is disadvantage	No
Mechanism of action – methylxanthine causes bronchodilation by increasing tissue concentrations of cyclic adenine monophosphate								
• Theophylline • Liquid, sustained-release tabs & caps	Theo-24, Uniphyl	10 mg/kg/day up to 800 mg/day	Allergy to corn-derived dextrose	• Tachycardia • N/V • CNS stimulation • Theophylline toxicity: persistent, repetitive vomiting	• Serum range: 5–15 mcg/mL • Serum levels <20 mcg/mL have few side effects	CYP450: inhibits 1A2, 3A4	Dosage adjustments should be in small increments (maximum 25%); elderly patients should be started on 25% reduction in the adult dose	No

Asthma *(cont'd)*

Generic	Brand	Dose	Contra-indications	Primary Side Effects	Key Monitoring	Pertinent Drug Interactions	Med Pearl	Top 200
Aminophylline	Only available generically	Diagnosis- and age-dependent	Hypersensitivity to theophylline and ethylendiamine		• Vital signs • In&Outs • Serum concentrations • CNS effects	CYP1F2, CYP3A4	IV only	No
Mechanism of action – relaxes bronchial smooth muscle by acting on beta-2 receptors								
Albuterol	Ventolin, Proventil	MDI: 90 mcg/puff Neb: 2.5 mg/mL	Patients with tachyarrhythmia risk	• Dose-dependent • Angina, atrial fibrillation, arrhythmias, chest discomfort, cough, tremor	• FEV1 • Peak flow • Blood pressure • Heart rate	Nonselective beta-adrenergic blockers decrease albuterol's effect	Excessive use can increase risk of death; nebulizer is compatible with budesonide, cromolyn, ipratropium	Yes
Levalbuterol	Xopenex, Xopenex HFA	MDI: 45 mcg/puff 200 puffs/canister Neb: 0.63/3 mL	Fewer cardiac side effects	Fewer cardiac side effects			Prime the inhaler by releasing 4 actuations prior to use	Yes
Pirbuterol	Maxair Autoinhaler	Autoinhaler: 200 mcg/puff NMI: 12 inhalations/day	Patients with tachyarrhythmia risk	• Dose-dependent • Angina, atrial fibrillation, arrhythmias, chest discomfort, cough, tremor			Autoinhaler is breath-actuated; child <4 years of age may not generate sufficient inspiratory flow	No
Combination		• See above for individual interactions • Synergistic effects are likely with combination products • Maximum dose of Advair is 1 puff BID; dosages: 100/50, 200/50, 500/50						
Fluticasone/salmeterol	Advair							Yes
Formoterol/budesonide	Symbicort							Yes
Mometasone/formoterol	Dulera							No
Ipratropium/albuterol	Combivent							Yes

Storage and Administration Pearls

- Metered-dose inhaler (MDI) requires hand coordination and proper technique.
- Dry powder inhaler (DPI) is breath-actuated and requires less coordination.
- Spacer with non–breath-actuated MDIs and mouth washing and spitting after inhalation decreases local side effects.
- Chlorofluorocarbons (CFCs) have been found to have an effect on the ozone layer in the earth's stratosphere.
- Hydrofluoroalkane (HFA) is an earth-friendly alternative to CFCs.
- Theophylline is incompatible with phenytoin.

Patient Education Pearls

- Patient should always use a spacer with inhaled corticosteroids for better deposition into the lungs and to prevent thrush.
- Patient should rinse and spit to avoid thrush from inhaled corticosteroids.
- Compliance is a must with all asthma medications.

CHRONIC OBSTRUCTIVE PULMONARY DISEASE (COPD)

Definitions

Chronic obstructive pulmonary disease (COPD) is characterized by persistent and largely irreversible airflow obstruction causing dyspnea, which does not fluctuate like asthma. Airflow obstruction is generally progressive and associated with abnormal inflammatory responses of lungs to noxious particles and gases. It is a disease entity with a spectrum of manifestation depending on the lung region affected. Chronic bronchitis affects the larger airways; emphysema affects the smaller airways, called alveolar sacs.

Diagnosis

If COPD is suspected, perform spirometry because diagnosis has to be confirmed with spirometry. FEV1 is the forced expiratory volume in 1 second. This percent is gathered from using spirometry and aids in determining the severity of COPD.

- History of cigarette smoking is a factor.
- α_1-antitrypsin deficiency in nonsmokers is a factor.
- Nocturnal symptoms are unusual.
- Chest x-ray often shows low and flattened diaphragms.
- FEV1 and all measurements of expiration airflow are reduced.
- FEV1 is the standard way to assess clinical course for response to therapy.
- FEV1/FVC <0.70 confirms diagnosis of airflow limitation that is not reversible.
- In smokers, the rate of decline in the FEV1 is approximately 60 mL/year.

Signs and Symptoms

- Tachypnea (rapid breathing)
- Pursed lips when breathing
- Cough and phlegm
- Chronic sputum production
- Wheeze and rhonchi
- Hyperinflation
- Use of accessory muscles to assist with respiration
- One or two acute exacerbations per year
- Blue bloater = chronic bronchitis
- Pink puffer = emphysema

Symptoms by Stage

- Stage I—Mild COPD: chronic cough and sputum production. These symptoms can be present for many years without airflow limitation. FEV1 ≥80% predicted.
- Stage II—Moderate COPD: dyspnea that interferes with daily activities. 80%<FEV1 <50% predicted.
- Stage III—Severe COPD: continued cough and sputum production, worsening dyspnea, respiratory failure, right heart failure, weight loss, and arterial hypoxemia may be seen in this stage. 30% ≤FEV1 <50% predicted.
- Stage IV—Very severe COPD: FEV1 <30% predicted or FEV1 <50% predicted plus chronic respiratory failure.

Guidelines

American College of Physicians 2008. www.acp.com.

Global Initiative for Chronic Obstructive Lung Disease. Global Strategy for the Diagnosis, Management, and Prevention of Chronic Obstructive Pulmonary Disease. 2010.

National Heart, Lung and Blood Institute, Expert Panel Report 3: Global Initiative for Chronic Obstructive Lung Disease (GOLD). www.goldcopd.org.

Guidelines Summary

- American College of Physicians – 2008
  - Spirometry should be used to diagnose airway obstruction only in symptomatic patients.
  - In patients with stable COPD, treatment should be reserved for those who are symptomatic with FEV1.

- Global Initiative for Chronic Obstructive Lung Disease (GOLD)
- Educate the patient in avoidance of risk factors (especially tobacco smoke) and start preventive efforts.
  - Smoking cessation for more than a year led to an improvement in lung function, with an FEV1 decline equal to that of nonsmokers (20–30 mL/year).
  - Consider flu and pneumonia vaccinations.
- Add a short-acting bronchodilator when needed.
- Add regular treatment with one or more long-acting bronchodilators and begin rehabilitation.
- Add inhaled glucocorticoids if the patient has repeated acute exacerbations.
- Start long-acting oxygen therapy if the patient is hypoxemic, and consider surgical treatments.

COPDs

Generic	Brand	Dose	Contra-indications	Primary Side Effects	Key Monitoring	Pertinent Drug Interactions	Med Pearl	Top 200
Mechanism of action – partial α4B2 nicotinic receptor agonist; prevents nicotine stimulation of mesolimbic dopamine system								
Varenicline	Chantix	0.5–2 mg/day	Hypersensitivity	• Insomnia • Headache • Abnormal dreams • Nausea		None	Start 1 week prior to target stop day with 0.5 mg/day	Yes
Mechanism of action – inhibits neuronal uptake of norepinephrine and dopamine								
Bupropion	Zyban	150–300 mg/day	• Seizure disorder • Anorexia/bulimia • Use of MAOI within 14 days	• Tachycardia • Headache • Insomnia	• Body weight • Mental status for depression • Suicidal ideation	• CYP450 inhibitor • 2D6 • MAOI	Can be co-administered with nicotine replacement patches	Yes
Mechanism of action – supplements nicotine which exhibits primary effects via autonomic ganglia stimulation								
Nicotine	Commit, NicoDerm, Nicorette	• Gum: max 24 pieces/day • Inhaler: max 16 cartridges/day • Patch: 1 patch per day • Lozenge: 2–4 mg; max 9/day • Spray: 80 sprays/day	• Smoking or chewing tobacco • Post-myocardial infarction • Life-threatening arrhythmias • Worsening angina	• Headache • Mouth or throat irritation • Dyspepsia • Cough	• Heart rate • Blood pressure • Nicotine toxicity (severe headache, dizziness, mental confusion)	CYP450 inhibits CYP2A4 and CYP2E1	Antidepressant medications may increase suicidal behavior in young adults	No
Mechanism of action – long-acting beta2-adrenergic agonist; relaxes bronchial smooth muscle								
Indacaterol	Arcapta	75 mcg/puff once daily	Patients with asthma without use of a long-term asthma control medication	• Cough • Oropharyngeal pain • Nasopharyngitis • Headache	• FEV1 • Peak flow • Other pulmonary function tests	• CYP450 3A4 • MAOIs • Beta blockers	• Not indicated as a treatment for asthma • Capsules should be only used with Neohaler device • Patients should be counseled on not swallowing the capsules	No

COPDs *(cont'd)*

Generic	Brand	Dose	Contra-indications	Primary Side Effects	Key Monitoring	Pertinent Drug Interactions	Med Pearl	Top 200
Mechanism of action – inhibits phosphodiesterase-4 leading to an accumulation of cyclic AMP								
Roflumilast	Daliresp	• 500 mcg/day	• Hepatic impairment (Child-Pugh class B or C)	• Diarrhea • Weight loss • Nausea	• Weight • Liver function parameters	• Cimetidine • CYP3A4 inducers • Ciprofloxacin • Rifampin	Not indicated for relieving acute bronchospasms or for use as monotherapy of COPD	No
Mechanism of action – blocks acetylcholine at the parasympathetic sites in bronchial smooth muscle, causing bronchodilation								
Ipratropium	• Atrovent • Atrovent HFA • Combivent (ipratropium & albuterol)	• MDI: 17 mcg/puff; max: 12 puffs/24 hours • Neb: 0.25 mg/mL	• Hypersensitivity • Peanuts allergy (due to soya lecithin) • Does not apply to Atrovent HFA	• Upper respiratory tract infection • Palpitation • Xerostomia • Pharyngeal irritation	• FEV1 • Peak flow • Other pulmonary function tests	CYP450 – substrate 2D6, 3A4	• Not recommended for initial treatment of acute episode of bronchospasm • Anticholinergic side effects are possible. Be careful in BPH, narrow-angle glaucoma, and myasthenia gravis	Yes
Tiotropium	Spiriva	DPI: 18 mcg/puff; max: 1 puff/day	Contains lactose					Yes
Mechanism of action – long-acting beta-2 agonists								
Formoterol	Perforomist	Neb: 20 mcg/2 mL	Same as above in asthma					No
Arformoterol	Brovana	15 mcg/2 mL					Black box warning—more asthma-related deaths than patients receiving salmeterol	No

STORAGE AND ADMINISTRATION PEARLS

- Nicotrol inhaler: Protect from light.
- Tiotropium: Do not store capsules in Handihaler device. Capsules should be used within 2 days of removal from blister pack.

Patient Education Pearls

- For improved outcomes, it is important to have consistent and regular interventions with the patient regarding smoking cessation education.
- When working with patient to stop smoking, it is recommended to use the 5 As: Ask, Advise, Assess, Assist, Arrange.

SMOKING CESSATION

Definitions

The dependence on tobacco is a chronic disease that often requires repeated intervention and multiple attempts to quit. Tobacco dependence is both physiological and psychological, so treatment interventions must be prepared to target both. Informing patients about the dangers of tobacco use is critical, as is educating patients about treatment options available.

Diagnosis

Patients are not always forthcoming about their use of tobacco, so it is important to assess patients' use status in every interaction possible.

Guidelines

Tobacco Use and Dependence Guideline Panel. Treating Tobacco Use and Dependence: 2008 Update. Rockville (MD): US Department of Health and Human Services; 2008 May.

Guidelines Summary

- The model for treatment and intervention of tobacco use and dependence is summarized by the "5 A's":
  - **ASK.** Identify and document tobacco use status for every patient and every visit.
  - **ADVISE.** Urge every tobacco user to quit in a strong and personalized manner.
  - **ASSESS.** Evaluate if your patient is willing to make a quit attempt.
  - **ASSIST.** For patients willing to make a quit attempt, offer treatment options and additional counseling; for those not willing, use motivational strategies to promote quitting.

- **ARRANGE.** Schedule follow-ups with those patients willing to make a quit attempt; for those not willing to make an attempt, address willingness to quit at the next visit.

■ Tobacco dependence is a chronic disease that often requires repeated intervention and multiple attempts to quit. Effective treatments exist, however, that can significantly increase rates of long-term abstinence.

■ It is essential that clinicians and health care delivery systems consistently identify and document tobacco use status and treat every tobacco user seen in a health care setting.

■ Tobacco dependence treatments are effective across a broad range of populations. Clinicians should encourage every patient willing to make a quit attempt to use the counseling treatments and medications recommended.

■ Brief tobacco dependence treatment is effective. Clinicians should offer every patient who uses tobacco at least the brief treatments shown to be effective.

LEARNING POINTS

■ Inhaled corticosteroids are the drug of choice when treating asthma. They prevent remodeling, improve symptoms, and prevent exacerbations as compared to the other medications.

■ Although peak flow meters are rarely dispensed in pharmacy, they are crucial to the maintenance of asthma. Peak flow meters should be used to determine a patient's personal best and used every morning to identify an early exacerbation.

■ Smoking cessation will help slow the progression of COPD and is the most important intervention when dealing with patients who have COPD.

PRACTICE QUESTIONS

1. What is Zyflo's mechanism of action?

   (A) Selective leukotriene-receptor antagonist of leukotrienes D4 and E4
   (B) 5-lipoxygenase inhibitor limits neutrophil and monocyte aggregation
   (C) Methylxanthine causes bronchodilation by increasing tissue concentrations of cyclic adenine monophosphate
   (D) Relaxes bronchial smooth muscle by acting on beta-2 receptors

2. The device used to measure forced vital capacity is called a

   (A) tonometer.
   (B) optomyometer.
   (C) sphygmomanometer.
   (D) spirometer.
   (E) gonioscope.

3. QVAR is indicated for which of the following scenarios?

   I. Asthma
   II. COPD
   III. Smoking cessation

   (A) I only
   (B) III only
   (C) I and II only
   (D) II and III only
   (E) I, II, and III

4. Which of the following have the same active ingredient?

   I. Flonase
   II. Flovent
   III. Veramyst

   (A) I only
   (B) III only
   (C) I and II only
   (D) II and III only
   (E) I, II, and III

ANSWERS

1. **B**

The challenging aspect of this question is that Zyflo is classified as a leukotriene modifier (A), like Accolate or Singular, but the two have different mechanisms of action. Zyflo's mechanism is an inhibitor of 5-lipoxygenase versus an antagonist at the receptor. Choice (C) is the mechanism of theophylline and choice (D) is the mechanism of albuterol.

2. **D**

A spirometer is a gasometer used for measuring respiratory gases, so (D) is correct. A tonometer (A) determines pressure or tension within the eye. An optomyometer (B) is an instrument for determining the relative power of the extrinsic muscles of the eye. A sphygmomanometer (C) measures arterial blood pressure. A gonioscope (E) measures the lens angle in relationship to the eye.

3. **A**

QVAR is an inhaled corticosteroid that is indicated only for the maintenance and pro-phylactic treatment of asthma, so (A) is the only correct answer.

4. **E**

Flonase, Flovent, and Veramyst all have the same active ingredient—fluticasone—so (E) is correct.

Endocrine Disorders

4

This chapter covers the following diseases:

- **Diabetes mellitus (DM) Type 1**
- **Diabetes mellitus (DM) Type 2**
- **Hypothyroidism**
- **Hyperthyroidism**
- **Polycystic ovarian syndrome (PCOS)**

 Suggested Study Time: **40 minutes**

DIABETES MELLITUS (DM) TYPE 1

Definitions

Diabetes mellitus type 1 accounts for fewer than 10% of all cases of diabetes, occurs in younger persons, and is caused by severe insulin deficiency that results from an immune-mediated destruction of the pancreatic-islet beta cells. Exogenous insulin is required to control blood glucose, prevent diabetic ketoacidosis (DKA), and preserve life. A transient period of insulin independence ("honeymoon phase") or reduced insulin requirement may occur early in the course of type 1 DM. When studying for the NAPLEX, be sure to recognize that DKA typically occurs in type 1 diabetes patients.

Diagnosis

- Impaired fasting glucose (IFG) is defined by a fasting plasma glucose between 100 and 125 mg/dL and is indicative of prediabetes.
- Impaired glucose tolerance (IGT) is defined by a 2-hour oral glucose tolerance test plasma glucose between 140 and 200 mg/dL and is indicative of prediabetes.

- An A1c ≥ 6.5% can also be used for diagnosis
- A plasma glucose of 126 mg/dL or greater after an overnight fast (and/or)
- Symptoms of diabetes and a random plasma glucose greater than 200 mg/dL (and/or)
- Oral glucose tolerance test indicating a plasma glucose of 200 mg/dL that is greater 2 hours after a 75-g glucose load.

Signs and Symptoms

- Polyuria is a sign, which is characterized by excessive excretion of urine
- Polyphagia is a sign, which is characterized by excessive eating
- Polydipsia is a sign, which is characterized by excessive thirst that is relatively prolonged
- Weight loss is due to excretion of glucose in the urine when blood sugars exceed 180 mg/dL. The excretion of glucose results in loss of calorie retention. In addition, the excessive polyuria leads to polyphagia and polydipsia.

Diabetes Complications

- Retinopathy
- Neuropathy
- Nephropathy
- Atherosclerosis

Guidelines

American Diabetes Association. *Diabetes Care*, no. 31 (Suppl 1) (2008): S4. www.diabetes.org

American Association of Clinical Endocrinologists. *Endocrine Practice*, no. 13 (Suppl 1) (May/June 2007). http://aace.com/pub/guidelines.

Guidelines Summary

- American Diabetes Association (ADA)
  - Goal blood glucose values between 80–120 mg/dL
  - A1c (average blood sugar for 3 months)
    - » Less than 7% (average blood sugar of 150 mg/dL)
      - 6% = 120 mg/dL; 7% = 150 mg/dL; 8% = 180 mg/dL
    - » A1c as close to 6% as possible without side effects of hypoglycemia
    - » LDL-C ≤100 mg/dL; TG ≤200 mg/dL

- American Association of Clinical Endocrinologists (AACE)
  - A1c (test that measures how much glucose has been sticking during the past 3–4 months to hemoglobin)
    - » Less than 6.5% (average blood sugar of 135 mg/dL)
  - Guidelines are more strict than ADA in glucose goals and triglycerides; goals: ≤150 mg/dL; LDL-C ≤100 mg/dL

Patient education is integral to successful management of diabetes. Diabetes education should be conducted through an interdisciplinary approach involving a provider, pharmacist, dietician, and nurse.

Dietary modifications should include education and instruction on carbohydrate counting. Men and women should limit carbohydrate intake between 45–60 g of carbohydrates per meal; 15 g of carbohydrates = 1 choice.

Exercise improves insulin sensitivity; reduces fasting and postprandial blood glucose; and offers numerous metabolic, cardiovascular, and psychological benefits. Exercise should consist of moderately intense cardio 30 min/day, 5 days a week; or vigorously intense cardio 20 min/day, 3 days a week, along with 8–10 strength-training exercise with 8–10 repetitions each, 2 day/week. These recommendations come from the American College of Sports Medicine.

DIABETES MELLITUS TYPE 2

Definitions

Diabetes mellitus type 2 accounts for more than 90% of all cases of DM. Usually a disease of adults, type 2 DM is increasingly being diagnosed in younger age groups. Obesity, insulin resistance, and relative insulin deficiency are characteristic findings. Insulin secretion may be sufficient to prevent ketosis under basal conditions, but DKA can develop during severe stress. When studying for the NAPLEX, be sure to understand the mechanism of actions of the medications. This will help with identifying duplications of drug therapy.

Diagnosis

- A1c ≥ 6.5%
- A1c 5.7%–6.4% has been renamed from prediabetes to categories of increased risk for diabetes.
- IFG is defined by a fasting plasma glucose between 100 and 125 mg/dL and is indicative of prediabetes.

- IGT is defined by a 2-hour oral glucose tolerance test plasma glucose between 140 and 200 mg/dL and is indicative of prediabetes.
- Plasma glucose of 126 mg/dL or greater after an overnight fast (and/or)
- Symptoms of diabetes and a random plasma glucose greater than 200 mg/dL (and/or)
- Oral glucose tolerance test indicating a plasma glucose of 200 mg/dL greater 2 hours after a 75-g glucose load.

Signs and Symptoms

- Polyuria is a sign, which is characterized by excessive excretion of urine
- Polyphagia is a sign, which is characterized by excessive eating
- Polydipsia is a sign, which is characterized by excessive thirst that is relatively prolonged
- Weight loss is due to excretion of glucose in the urine with blood sugars exceeding 180 mg/dL. The excretion of glucose results in loss of calorie retention. In addition, the excessive polyuria leads to polyphagia and polydipsia.

Guidelines

See Guidelines for DM type 1.

Guidelines Summary

See Guidelines Summary for DM type 1.

Drugs for Diabetes (Insulin)

Generic	Brand	Onset	Peak	Duration	Comments	Top 200
Rapid acting					• Hypoglycemia is the most common side effect. It is defined as blood sugar <70 mg/dL and must be treated as soon as recognized. • Insulin dosage is individually based due to sensitivity 0.51.0 units/kg/day for the average non-obese patient. • Duration of action is prolonged in renal failure.	
Aspart	NovoLog	5–15 min	30–90 min	<5 hrs		Yes
Lispro	Humalog	5–15 min	30–90 min	<5 hrs		Yes
Glulisine	Apidra	5–15 min	30–90 min	<5 hrs		No
Short-acting						
Regular	Humulin R (OTC)	30–60 min	2–3 hrs	5–8 hrs		No
Intermediate, Basal						
NPH (Neutral Protamine Hagedorn)	Humulin N (OTC)	2–4 hrs	4–10 hrs	10–16 hrs		Yes
Long-acting, basal						
Glargine	Lantus	2–4 hrs	No peak	20–24 hrs		Yes
Detemir	Levemir	3–8 hrs	No peak	6–24 hrs		Yes
Premixed						
75% Lispro protamine / 25% lispro	Humalog Mix 75/25	5–15 min	Dual	10–16 hrs		Yes
50% Lispro protamine / 50% lispro	Humalog Mix 50/50	5–15 min	Dual	10–16 hrs		No
50% Aspart protamine / 50% aspart	NovoLog Mix 50/50	5–15 min	Dual	10–16 hrs		No
70% Insulin aspart protamine / 30% aspart	NovoLog Mix 70/30	5–15 min	Dual	10–16 hrs		Yes
70% NPH / 30% regular	70/30 (OTC)	30–60 min	Dual	10–16 hrs		No

• OTC insulin is available without a prescription.
• Rapid-acting insulin should be given at time of meal ingestion, no more than 15 minutes from eating.
• Regular insulin should be given 30 minutes prior to meal due to delayed onset of action.

Drugs for Diabetes (Oral)

Generic	Brand	Dose & Max	Contra-indications	Primary Side Effects	Key Monitoring	Pertinent Drug Interactions	Med Pearl	Top 200
Sulfonylureas, first generation – stimulate insulin release from the pancreatic beta cells								
Tolbutamide	• Apo-tolbutamide • Orinase	0.5–2 g	• Type 1 DM • Sulfa allergy	• Hypoglycemia • Weight gain	Fasting plasma glucose and A1c at 3 months	• Cimetidine may increase hypoglycemia effects (CYP450) • Chronic ethanol ingestion may decrease hypoglycemic effect	Response plateaus after half maximum dose	No
Acetohexamide	Dymelor	0.25 mg–1.5 g						No
Tolazamide	Tolinase	0.1–1 g						No
Chlorpropamide	Diabinese	0.1–0.5 g						No
Sulfonylureas, second generation – stimulate insulin release from the pancreatic beta cells								
Glyburide	• Micronase • DiaBeta	1.25–20 mg	• Type 1 DM • Sulfa allergy	• Hypoglycemia • Weight gain	Fasting plasma glucose and A1c at 3 months	• Cimetidine may increase hypoglycemia effects (CYP450) • Chronic ethanol ingestion may decrease hypoglycemic effect	Response plateaus after half maximum dose	Yes
Glipizide	• Glucotrol • Glucotrol XL	2.5–40 mg						Yes
Glimepiride	Amaryl	1–8 mg						Yes
Meglitinides – stimulates insulin release from the pancreatic beta cells								
Repaglinide	Prandin	1–16 mg	Type 1 DM	• Hypoglycemia • Weight gain	Postprandial plasma glucose and A1c	• Decrease effect by CYP3A4, CYP2C8/9 inducers • Increase effect by CYP3A4 inhibitors	Faster acting and shorter duration than the traditional sulfonylureas, and recommended for postprandial blood sugars	Yes
Amino acid derivative – stimulates insulin release from the pancreatic beta cells								
Nateglinide	Starlix	180–360 mg	Type 1 DM	• Hypoglycemia • Weight gain	Postprandial plasma glucose and A1c	• Decrease effect by CYP3A4, CYP2C8/9 inducers • Increase effect by CYP3A4 inhibitors	Faster acting than the traditional sulfonylureas, and recommended for postprandial blood sugars	No

Drugs for Diabetes (Oral) *(cont'd)*

Generic	Brand	Dose & Max	Contra-indications	Primary Side Effects	Key Monitoring	Pertinent Drug Interactions	Med Pearl	Top 200
Biguanide – decreases hepatic glucose production, decreases intestinal absorption of glucose, improves insulin sensitivity								
Metformin	• Glucophage • Glucophage XR	500 mg–2.550 g	• SCr ≥1.5 male • SCr ≥1.4 female • Lactic acidosis • Contraindicated in severe heart failure, renal failure, radiographic dyes	GI intolerance (flatulence and diarrhea); lactic acidosis	• Serum creatinine • Fasting plasma glucose • A1c every 3 months	Cimetidine increases peak metformin plasma and whole blood concentration by 60%	Lactic acidosis black box warning.	Yes
Alpha-glucosidase inhibitors – inhibit pancreatic alpha-amylase and alpha-glucosidases, block carbohydrate hydrolysis to glucose								
Acarbose	Precose	75–300 mg	• Cirrhosis • Inflammatory bowel disease • Intestinal obstruction	• Abdominal pain and diarrhea • Flatulence	• LFTs q3 months x 1 year • Postprandial blood sugars and A1c	Hypoglycemia risk when given with sulfonylureas or insulin	Must treat hypoglycemia with simple carbo-hydrate such as glucose	No
Miglitol	Glyset	75–300 mg			• Postprandial blood sugars and A1c			No
Thiazolidinediones – PPAR-gamma activator, which improves insulin sensitivity								
Rosiglitazone	Avandia	2–8 mg	• History of liver disease • Unstable heart failure • Previous MI	Fluid retention and hepatotoxicity	Monitor LFTs, baseline and periodically	• Decrease effect by CYP3A4, CYP2C8 inducers • Decrease effect by CYP2C8 inhibitors	Rosi: potential link to an increase in cardiovascular events; however, very controversial	Yes
Pioglitazone	Actos	15–45 mg				• Decrease effect by CYP3A4, CYP2C8 inducers	Pio: thought to have a better lipid profile	Yes
Amylinomimetic – Amylin cosecreted with insulin reduces postprandial blood sugars, prolonging gastric emptying, reducing postprandial glucagon secretion, and caloric intake through centrally mediated appetite suppression								
Pramlintide	Symlin	15–120 mcg	• Gastroparesis • Hypoglycemia unawareness	• Nausea from delayed gastric emptying • Severe hypoglycemia	• Hypoglycemia • Blood sugars and A1c	• May delay absorption of other drugs due to increased gastric emptying time • Pramlintide: must reduce dose of insulin by 50% when starting	Administer medications 1 hour prior to the use of pramlintide and exenatide	No

Drugs for Diabetes (Oral) (cont'd)

GLP-1 inhibitors – glucagon-like peptide which increases insulin secretion, increases B-cell growth/replication, slows gastric emptying, decreases food intake

Generic	Brand	Dose & Max	Contra-indications	Primary Side Effects	Key Monitoring	Pertinent Drug Interactions	Med Pearl	Top 200
Exenatide	BYETTA	5–20 mcg	• Type 1 DM • Pancreatitis • DKA	• Nausea • Hypoglycemia • Decreased appetite	• Renal function • Blood sugars and A1c		Black box warning for acute pancreatitis	Yes
Liraglutide	Victoza	0.6–1.8 mg injection	• Family Hx of medullary thyroid carcinoma • Multiple endocrine neoplasia syndrome	• Headache • Nausea • Diarrhea • Antiliraglutide antibody formation	• Pancreatitis • Hypoglycemia • Thyroid tumors	Delays gastric emptying so it may impact absorption of concomitantly administered medications	It is a GLP-1 receptor agonist used to treat type 2 DM	No

Dipeptidyl-peptidase 4 inhibitors – prolong the active incretin levels of GLP and GIP

Generic	Brand	Dose & Max	Contra-indications	Primary Side Effects	Key Monitoring	Pertinent Drug Interactions	Med Pearl	Top 200
Sitagliptin	Januvia	25–100 mg	Type 1 DM	Headache	• Renal function • Blood sugars and A1c	May increase digoxin concentration	100 mg dose is preferred unless patient has renal impairment	Yes
Saxagliptin	Onglyza	5 mg/day	None	• URI • UTI • Headache • Peripheral edema • Hypoglycemia	A1C, absolute lymphocyte counts when clinically indicated	Coadministration with strong CYP3A4/5 inhibitors; these increase saxagliptins concentration and dose is decreased to 2.5 mg/day	Pregnancy category B	No

Drugs for Diabetes (Oral) *(cont'd)*

Generic	Brand	Dose & Max	Contra-indications	Primary Side Effects	Key Monitoring	Pertinent Drug Interactions	Med Pearl	Top 200
Combination								
Sitagliptin/ metformin	Janumet	• See above for individual interactions • Synergistic effects are likely with combination products • Maximum dose of metformin is 2,000 mg in combination products • Maximum dose for immediate release is 2,550 mg per day						Yes
Glyburide/ metformin	Glucovance							Yes
Rosiglitazone/ metformin	Avandamet							No
Rosiglitazone/ glimepiride	Avandaryl							No
Pioglitazone/ metformin	Actos Plus							No
Glipizide/ metformin	Metaglip							No

Storage and Administration Pearls

- Unopened containers of insulin should be stored in the refrigerator.
- If not refrigerated, use within 28 days and protect from heat and light.
- Do not freeze insulin.
- Once opened or in use, vials may be stored in refrigerator or at room temperature for up to 28 days.
- IV infusion: Must be kept stable for 24 hours at room temperature.
- Detemir's mechanism of action (MOA) is slightly different than the other insulin. It binds to albumin to extend its half-life.
- Detemir's storage life is 42 days outside of refrigerator.

Patient Education Pearls

- A patient who is on alpha-glycosidase inhibitors must use a simple sugar to treat hypoglycemia anytime.
- Rotate insulin injection sites.
- Mixing rule: "Clear, then cloudy" is the rule. It still applies to NPH (cloudy), regular (clear), fast-acting (clear).
- The exceptions: Never mix Detemir or glargine (clear) with anything.

HYPOTHYROIDISM

Definitions

Primary hypothyroidism accounts for more than 90% of cases. It is due to actual disease of the thyroid itself and not from a feedback or hypothalamus issue. Hashimoto's disease is the most common cause and may be associated with Addison's disease (chronic adrenocortical insufficiency) and other endocrine deficits.

Diagnosis

Plasma thyroid-stimulating hormone (TSH) is the best initial diagnostic test. A TSH that is markedly elevated (>20 mcgU/mL) confirms the diagnosis.

Signs and Symptoms

- Most symptoms are nonspecific and develop gradually.
- Typical symptoms are cold intolerance, fatigue, somnolence, poor memory, and depression.

- Atypical symptoms are constipation, menorrhagia, myalgias, and hoarseness.
- Physical exam will often show slow tendon reflexes, bradycardia, and facial and peri-orbital edema.

Guidelines

American Association of Clinical Endocrinologists. *Arch Intern Med*, no. 160 (2000): 1573–5. http://aace.com/pub/guidelines.

Guidelines Summary

The treatment and management of chronic thyroiditis and clinical hypothyroidism must be tailored to the individual patient. Many clinical endocrinologists treat the goiter of chronic thyroiditis with levothyroxine, even in patients with normal levels of TSH, and all physicians will treat clinical hypothyroidism with levothyroxine replacement therapy.

Drugs for Hypothyroidism

Generic	Brand	Dose	Contra-indications	Primary Side Effects	Key Monitoring	Pertinent Drug Interactions	Med Pearl	Top 200
Mechanism of action — T4 is converted to T3 and exerts many metabolic effects through control of DNA transcription and protein synthesis								
Levothyroxine (T4)	• Synthroid • Levoxyl • Levothroid • Unithroid	• Inj. powder: 0.2 and 0.5 mg • Tab: 25–300 mcg	• Recent myocardial infarction or thyrotoxicosis • Uncorrected adrenal insufficiency	• Angina • Anxiety • Alopecia • LFTs increased • Tachycardia	• TSH • T3 • T4 • Free T4 • Heart rate • Blood pressure • Weight	• Some drugs will decrease absorption: cholestyramine, aluminum-containing, sucralfate, Kayexalate, phenytoin, carbamazepine, rifampin may decrease levothyroxine levels	• T4: not the active compound; must be converted to T3 to become active • Thyroid treatment: used to augment depression treatment • Narrow therapeutic index drug • Often involved in drug errors	Yes
Liothyronine (T3)	Cytomel	• Inj. powder: 10 mcg/mL • Tab: 5–100 mcg	• Recent myocardial infarction or thyrotoxicosis • Uncorrected adrenal insufficiency					No
Desiccated thyroid T4 (80%) T3 (20%)	• Armour • Thyroid	Tab: 15–120 mg per day	• Hypersensitivity to beef or pork • Recent myocardial infarction or thyrotoxicosis • Uncorrected adrenal insufficiency				• Same as above • Origin: hog, cow, sheep • 80% T4 and 20% T3 is to mimic natural physiologic production	Yes
Liotrix	Thyrolar	5–50 mcg	• Uncorrected adrenal cortical insufficiency • Untreated thyrotoxicosis				Liotrix is LT4/LT3 which is T4:T3 ratio; this ratio is 4:1	No

Storage and Administration Pearls

- Levothyroxine: Administered on an empty stomach
- Levothyroxine tabs: Protect from light and moisture
- Levothyroxine injection at room temperature (59–86°F)
- IV solution not mixed with other IV infusion solutions
- Dilute vial with 5 mL of normal saline and inject immediately

Patient Education Pearls

- Thyroid supplementation is ineffective and potentially toxic for weight reduction.

HYPERTHYROIDISM

Definitions

Hyperthyroidism includes Graves' disease, which causes most cases of hyperthyroidism, especially in young patients. This autoimmune disorder may cause exophthalmos (protrusion of the eyes) and pretibial myxedema (nodules and plaques on skin). Toxic multinodular goiter is a common cause. Other causes can be drug-induced by amiodarone or radiographic contrast media and thyroid adenomas.

Diagnosis

- Plasma TSH is the best initial diagnostic test. The TSH will be markedly suppressed (<0.1 mcg/mL).

Signs and Symptoms

- Typical symptoms: Heat intolerance, insomnia, weight loss, weakness, palpitations, oligomenorrhea, and anxiety
- Sinus tachycardia, atrial fibrillation, and exacerbation of coronary artery disease
- Brisk tendon reflexes, fine tremor, proximal weakness, stare, and eyelid lag
- Thyroid storm: Presents as an acute life-threatening exaggeration of usual hyperthyroid symptoms

Guidelines

American Association of Clinical Endocrinologists. *Arch Intern Med*, no. 160 (2000): 1573–5. http://aace.com/pub/guidelines.

Guidelines Summary

Three types of therapy are available for Graves' disease: (*1*) Surgical intervention, (*2*) antithyroid drugs, and (*3*) radioactive iodine.

- In the United States, radioactive iodine is currently the treatment of choice for Graves' disease. Many clinical endocrinologists prefer an ablative dose of radioactive iodine, but some prefer use of a smaller dose in an attempt to render the patient euthyroid. Ablative therapy with radioactive iodine yields quicker resolution of the hyperthyroidism than does small-dose therapy, and thereby minimizes potential hyperthyroid-related morbidity.

- Although thyroidectomy for Graves' disease was frequently used in the past, it is now uncommonly performed in the United States unless coexistent thyroid cancer is suspected.

- Antithyroid medications methimazole and propylthiouracil have been used since the 1940s and are prescribed in an attempt to achieve a remission. The remission rates are variable, and relapses are frequent. Patients in whom remission is most likely to be achieved are those with mild hyperthyroidism and small goiters. Antithyroid drug treatment is not without the risk of adverse reactions, including minor rashes, and, in rare instances, agranulocytosis and hepatitis.

Drugs for Hyperthyroidism

Generic	Brand	Dose	Contra-indications	Primary Side Effects	Key Monitoring	Pertinent Drug Interactions	Med Pearl	Top 200
Mechanism of action – inhibits synthesis of thyroid hormones by blocking the oxidation of iodine in the thyroid gland								
Propylthiouracil	(PTU)	• Initial: 300–600 mg daily divided by TID or QID • Maintenance: 50–300 mg daily • Maximum: 1,200 mg daily	Breastfeeding	• Minor: therapy may still continue • Benign transient leukopenia (WBC <4,000/mm³, most common) • Pruritic maculopapular rashes, arthralgias, fevers	• WBC with differential • Granulocyte <250/mm³ (most severe) • LFT • TSH	Increase activity of anticoagulants	• Clinical improvement approx. 4–3 weeks • PTU is an error-prone abbreviation • Tapering doses may start once clinical improvement seen	No
Methimazole (MMI)	Tapazole	• Initial: 30–60 mg TID • Maintenance: 5–30 mg daily • Maximum: 120 mg daily	• Breastfeeding • Category D	• Greater frequency in higher doses and in children • Rashes may be treated with antihistamines • Severe side effect require discontinuation • Fever, malaise, gingivitis, sore throat, oropharyngeal infections • Aplastic anemia, lupus-like syndrome, polymyositis (rhabdomyolysis), GI intolerance, hepatotoxicity, hepatitis, hypoprothrombinemia, death	• T3 • T4	• CYP450 inhibitor • Moderate: CPY2D6 • Weak: CPY3A4, CPY1A2	• Alternate thiamide may be used, but cross-sensitivity is 50% • Correction of hyperthyroidism may alter disposition of beta-blockers, digoxin, and theophylline • PTU preferred in pregnancy	No

Storage and Administration Pearls

- Methimazole: Protect from light.
- On the NAPLEX and in the work force, PTU is an error-prone abbreviation and is not recommended for use on prescription pads, verbally, or within your computer system.

Patient Education Pearls

- If the patient is pregnant or is thinking about getting pregnant, it is recommended that she avoid taking propylthiouracil and methimazole; they cross the placenta and are found in breast milk. PTU is preferred over methimazole in pregnancy.

POLYCYSTIC OVARIAN SYNDROME (PCOS)

Definitions

Polycystic ovarian syndrome (PCOS) is a metabolic disorder involving infertility, hirsutism, obesity, and amenorrhea. The fundamental defect of PCOS is unknown but is thought to be from adrenal androgen excess of obesity, which results in enhanced extraglandular formation of estrogen. The dysfunctional uterine bleeding is usually due to estrogen excess.

Diagnosis

- History and physical examination, including the onset and duration of various signs of androgen excess; menstrual history; family history of diabetes and cardiovascular disease; lifestyle factors; evaluation of blood pressure, body mass index, and waist-hip ratio; and presence of acne, hirsutism, androgenic alopecia, and acanthosis nigricans
- Laboratory tests, including documentation of biochemical hyperandrogenemia (total testosterone and/or bioavailable or free testosterone); exclusion of other causes of hyperandrogenism, such as thyroid dysfunction, hyperprolactinemia, nonclassical congenital adrenal hyperplasia, and Cushing's syndrome; evaluation for metabolic abnormalities; and fasting lipid and lipoprotein level
- Optional tests to consider:
  - Ultrasound evaluation of ovaries
  - Gonadotropin determinations
  - Fasting insulin levels
  - 24-hour urine test

Signs and Symptoms

- Infertility: Inability to become pregnant
- Hirsutism: Caused by excess androgen levels
- Obesity: BMI > 29 kg/m^2
- Anovulation: Lack of ovulation; however, the woman may experience withdrawal bleeding after progestogen administration

Guidelines

American College of Obstetricians and Gynecologists, Medical Specialty Society. (December 2002). http://www.acog.org.

Guidelines Summary

Treatment is based on a symptoms approach for anovulation, amenorrhea, ovulation induction, and hirsutism.

Anovulation and Amenorrhea

- Combination oral contraceptives are often used to regulate or restore irregular or absent menses.
- Weight-reduction programs are important, and they affect and improve insulin resistance.
- Progestin, including medroxyprogesterone acetate, is often used to induce menses.
- Insulin-sensitizing agents, including metformin, pioglitazone, and rosiglitazone, are used to reduce insulin resistance.

Ovulation Induction

- Lifestyle modifications, especially weight loss, will assist with ovulation induction.
- Clomiphene citrate is used to induce ovulation for up to 6 months.
- Ovarian drilling with laser or diathermy can be considered but is not recommended.
- Insulin-sensitizing agents, such as metformin and thiazolidinediones, can induce ovulation.

Hirsutism

- Oral contraceptives can reduce hair growth.
- Antiandrogens, including spironolactone, flutamide, and insulin-sensitizing agents, and eflornithine can be used to reduce hair growth.
- Mechanical hair removal, such as shaving, plucking, waxing, depilatory creams, electrolysis, and laser vaporization, can also be used.

Drugs for Polycystic Ovarian Syndrome

Generic	Brand	Dose	Contraindications	Primary Side Effects	Key Monitoring	Pertinent Drug Interactions	Med Pearl	Top 200
Mechanism of action – inhibits secretion of pituitary gonadotropins, which prevents follicular maturation and ovulation; causes endometrial thinning								
Medroxyprogesterone	Provera	Amenorrhea: 5–10 mg x 10 days	• History of deep venous thrombosis, pulmonary embolism • Pregnancy	• Headaches • Weight changes • Edema • Menstrual irregularities	• Pregnancy should be ruled out • Symptoms of migraine	• CYP450 • Induces CYP3A4	Long-term use can lead to loss of bone mineral density	Yes
Mechanism of action – Enclomiphene is less potent in inducing ovulation; however, it is rapidly absorbed to be metabolized, allowing for the more potent zuclomiphene to act. Zuclomiphene – inhibits normal estrogen negative feedback, which results in release of luteinizing hormone (LH) and FSH; more potent than enclomiphene								
Clomiphene citrate* – zuclomiphene (38%) – enclomiphene (62%)	Clomid	50–100 mg	• Liver disease • Abnormal uterine bleeding • Ovarian cysts • Uncontrolled thyroid or adrenal dysfunction • Pregnancy category X	• Ovarian enlargement • Hot flashes • Breast discomfort • Nausea • Bloating	• Pregnancy test • Menstrual cycle		Dosages of 150 mg or greater do not improve symptoms for PCOS	No
Mechanism of action – competes with aldosterone receptor sites in the distal tubules								
Spironolactone	Aldactone	50–200 mg	• Acute renal failure • Hyperkalemia • Pregnancy category D	• Gynecomastia (men) • Hyperkalemia • Nausea, cramping	• Blood pressure • Renal function • Potassium	May reduce the inotropic (contraction) effect of digoxin and mitotane.	Needs to be renally adjusted	Yes
Mechanism of action – nonsteroidal antiandrogen that inhibits androgen uptake or inhibits binding to androgen in target tissue								
Flutamide	Eulexin	125–250 mg	• Severe hepatic impairment • Pregnancy category D	• Gynecomastia • Hot flashes • Breast tenderness • Galactorrhea • Libido decreased	LFTs monthly for 4 months, then periodically	• CYP450 • Inhibits CYP1A2	Black box warning for liver failure within 3 months of taking flutamide	No

Drugs for Polycystic Ovarian Syndrome *(cont'd)*

Generic	Brand	Dose	Contraindications	Primary Side Effects	Key Monitoring	Pertinent Drug Interactions	Med Pearl	Top 200
Mechanism of action – inhibitor of 5-alpha reductase which results in the inhibition of the conversion of testosterone to dihydrotestosterone								
Finasteride	• Proscar • Propecia	1–5 mg/day	Pregnancy category X Hirsutism	• Impotence • Ejaculation disturbances • Testicular pain	Absolute need for dual forms of birth control	• CYP450 • Substrate CYP3A4	• Category X in pregnancy (abnormalities of external male genitalia were reported in animal studies) • High-alert medication	Yes
Mechanism of action – inhibits ornithine decarboxylase (ODC), the rate-limiting enzyme in biosynthesis of putrescine, spermin, and spermidine (rapic dividing cell most susceptible)								
Eflornithine	VANIQA	Cream (facial hair)	Hypersensitivity	• Acne • Pruritus • Alopecia	CBC and platelets (systemic only)	Cream could interact with other creams		No

Storage and Administration Pearls

- Finasteride needs to be protected from light.
- Spironolactone needs to be protected from light.

Patient Education Pearls

- Prolonged use of medroxyprogesterone contraception injection may result in a loss of bone mineral density (BMD).

LEARNING POINTS

- The basic diagnoses for type 1 and type 2 DM are identical. However, patients with type 2 will go undiagnosed for as long as 10 years, whereas type 1 is usually diagnosed within 6 months. As a result, it is important to consider and assess risk factors for type 2 DM.
- For the NAPLEX, it is important that you understand the different mechanisms of action of the diabetes medications to ensure you can catch duplication of actions within the patient's drug profile.
- Hypothyroidism and hyperthyroidism have opposite side effects (i.e., somnolence with hypothyroid; insomnia with hyperthyroidism).
- PCOS has become more common as obesity rates have risen and as more women want to become pregnant.
- Remember, many women with diabetes may have PCOS and may be placed on an insulin sensitizer such as a glitazone. As a result, it is important to counsel the patient on an increased risk for ovulation if her uterus is still intact.

PRACTICE QUESTIONS

1. All of the following are used to treat conditions of hyperthyroidism EXCEPT

   (A) Propylthiouracil (PTU).
   (B) Methimazole (MMI).
   (C) Propranolol.
   (D) Lugol's solution.
   (E) Cytomel.

2. Patients with overactive thyroid may present with which of the following symptoms?

   (A) Weight loss
   (B) Heat intolerance
   (C) Heart palpitations
   (D) Goiter
   (E) All of the above

3. Which of the following statements is/are TRUE?

   I. T3 = Triiodothyronine = active form
   II. T4 = Thyroxine = converted to T3
   III. Thyroid peridoxase, tyrosine, and iodine all play a role in the thyroid hormone system.

   (A) I only
   (B) III only
   (C) I and II
   (D) II and III
   (E) I, II, and III

4. Which of the following conditions is/are associated with elevated thyroid hormone levels?

   I. Thyrotoxicosis
   II. Graves' disease
   III. Hashimoto's disease

   (A) I only
   (B) III only
   (C) I and II
   (D) II and III
   (E) I, II, and III

5. A patient comes to the pharmacy and tells you that her blood sugars were 126 and 127 mg/dL fasting on two occasions. She wants some advice because her doctor didn't have time to talk with her. What is the main point you will be addressing with this woman?

(A) This patient does not have diabetes because the doctor did the same test.
(B) This patient has diabetes but it's not bad and will not need medication.
(C) This patient has diabetes but does not need education; she should just watch what she eats and exercise more.
(D) This patient doesn't have diabetes but might develop it soon.
(E) This patient has diabetes, needs a formal diabetes education class, and is likely a candidate for a medication called metformin.

6. How many days can a Humalog stay out of the refrigerator and be considered safe to administer?

(A) 1 day
(B) 28 days
(C) 56 days
(D) 90 days
(E) 180 days

ANSWERS

1.   E

Cytomel, or T3, is the active form of thyroid hormone and should not be used if the patient has an overactive thyroid. It is used in hypothyroidism to stimulate thyroid hormone production. The other answer choices are all used in the treatment of hyperthyroidism.

2.   E

Weight loss, heat intolerance, heart palpitations, and goiter are all commonly seen symptoms with hyperthyroid disorders. Other common symptoms include nervousness, emotional lability, bowel frequency, irregular menses, and increased appetite.

3.   E

T3, or triiodothyronine, is the active form of thyroid hormone. T4, or thyroxine, is the bound form of thyroid hormone and must be converted into triiodothyronine to be active. Iodide + tyrosine + thyroid peroxidase is converted to iodotyrosine, which in turn forms triiodothyronine and thyroxine.

4.   C

Thyrotoxicosis, or hyperthyroidism, is caused by excessive levels of T3 or T4 or both. Graves' disease is an autoimmune disorder in which TSH is stimulated in the body. Hashimoto's disease (III), however, is the most common form of spontaneous hypothyroidism.

5.   E

This patient has diabetes and needs a formal diabetes education class. The newest guidelines suggest starting all eligible patients on metformin at the time of diagnosis. Choice (A) is not correct because this woman does have diabetes—her fasting blood sugar was verified and was ≥126 mg/dL. Although the doctor caught the disease early, the patient still needs to seek formal education as this will lead to the best management.

6.   B

Most unopened insulin preparations are stable at normal temperatures for 28 days. They should not be used if frozen or exposed to temperature greater than 98.6°F. Once opened (in use), vials may be stored in the refrigerator or for up to 28 days at room temperature.

Neurological Disorders

5

This chapter covers the following disease states:

- **Multiple sclerosis**
- **Epilepsy**
- **Parkinson's disease**
- **Migraine headache**

 Suggested Study Time: **45 minutes**

MULTIPLE SCLEROSIS

Definitions

Multiple sclerosis (MS) is a disease of the central nervous system (CNS) characterized by inflammation within the brain and spinal cord that results in areas of plaque formation and sclerosis and leads to neurological symptoms. The basic pathophysiological defect in MS is the demyelinization of the sheath surrounding the neurons in the CNS.

Diagnosis

The diagnosis of MS is primarily based on clinical presentation and requires two or more episodes of neurologic symptoms that: (*1*) cannot be attributed to another cause, (*2*) represent distinct areas of CNS involvement, and (*3*) occur at least 3 months apart. The McDonald criteria are often used to diagnose MS. These criteria do require two lesions separated by 3 months but allow for the use of magnetic resonance imaging (MRI) and cerebrospinal fluid analysis to be used as identification of a second attack. MRI is a useful tool for confirming diagnosis of MS because it is highly selective for MS lesions.

Signs and Symptoms

- The most common symptoms of early MS include weakness/numbness of limbs and visual disturbances. The clinical presentation of MS varies among patients and is classified as relapsing-remitting, primary progressive, or secondary progressive.

- Relapsing-remitting MS is most common (85%) and is characterized by frequent symptomatic episodes of ≥24 hours' duration followed by periods of remission of at least 30 days. During remission, residual symptoms and increasing clinical deficit are common.

- Primary progressive MS occurs in ~10% of patients and consists of persistently progressive disease from the time of disease onset that does not include remissions or relapses. This classification is associated with a poor prognosis.

- Secondary progressive MS occurs in about 5% of patients and consists of few exacerbations, no permanent disability, and gradual worsening of neurological symptoms. Many patients originally classified as relapsing-remitting may be reclassified as secondary progressive during the course of illness.

Guidelines

Medical Advisory Board of the National Multiple Sclerosis Society (2005). Disease Management Consensus Statement Expert Opinion Paper. http://www. nationalmssociety.org.

Guidelines Summary

The clinical management of MS should include consideration of treatment for acute exacerbations, retarding disease process, and alleviating ongoing symptoms related to the disease.

Disease-modifying drugs (DMDs) are used to alter the disease process and should be initiated as soon as possible after diagnosis. Therapies should be continued indefinitely except in the case of intolerable side effects, clear lack of benefit, or new therapy considerations.

Acute exacerbations — The cornerstone of therapy for acute exacerbations is intravenous (IV) corticosteroids. Methylprednisolone is most commonly used at 50–100 mg/day for 3 to 10 days. Oral prednisone may also be considered, but there is not strong evidence for this route. Although corticosteroids have been shown to be very effective in the treatment of acute exacerbations, they do not alter the disease process.

Altering disease process — DMDs are the therapy of choice in altering the MS disease process. There are currently six approved DMDs: interferon-β1a (Avonex and Rebif), interferon-β1b (Betaseron and Extavia), glatiramer acetate (Copaxone), natalizumab (Tysabri), mitoxantrone (Novantrone), and dalfampridine (Ampyra).

- The interferon agents and glatiramer acetate are considered first-line DMDs, whereas natalizumab is reserved for patients who do not respond to those therapies.
- Mitoxantrone is the only available agent that is approved to treat worsening relapsing-remitting MS and progressive MS.
- Patients are generally treated with one DMD at a time, but worsening disease can be treated with combination DMD + mitoxantrone pulse therapy.

Disease-Modifying Drugs

Generic	Brand	Dose & Max	Contra-indications	Primary Side Effects	Key Monitoring Parameters	Pertinent Drug Interactions	Med Pearls	Top 200
Disease-Modifying Drugs								
Mechanism of action — interferon β: anti-inflammatory and immunomodulatory effects are exerted through binding of interferon to human cell-surface receptors and subsequent decreased T-cell production of pro-inflammatory cytokines, decreased production of pro-inflammatory lymphocytes, and increased production of anti-inflammatory lymphocytes.								
Interferon-β1a	• Avonex intramuscular (IM) injection • Rebif subcutaneous (SC) injection	30 mcg IM 1 x week 8.8 mcg SC TIW–44 mcg SC TIW	• Hypersensitivity • Severe depression	Flu-like symptoms (fever, chills, fatigue, muscle aches); injection site reactions; mild anemia; thrombocytopenia; liver damage; depression	Liver transaminases periodically; response to therapy; presence of adverse effects; periodic complete blood count (CBC)	May decrease efficacy of vaccinations	• Acetaminophen or NSAIDs can decrease flu-like symptoms • Neutralizing antibodies may develop, rendering the drug less efficacious	No
Interferon-β1b	• Betaseron SC injection • Extavia SC injection	0.25 mg SC QOD	• Hypersensitivity • Severe depression	Flu-like symptoms (fever, chills, fatigue, muscle aches); injection site reactions; mild anemia; thrombocytopenia; liver damage; depression	Liver transaminases periodically; response to therapy; presence of adverse effects; periodic complete blood count (CBC)	May decrease efficacy of vaccinations	• Acetaminophen or NSAIDs can decrease flu-like symptoms • Neutralizing antibodies may develop, rendering the drug less efficacious • Extavia available in auto-injector	No
Mechanism of action — glatiramer acetate: influences immature CD4 cells to become less inflammatory, thereby suppressing demyelination and preventing nerve fiber damage								
Glatiramer acetate	Copaxone SC injection	20 mg SC daily	Hypersensitivity to the drug or to mannitol	Injection site reactions; postinjection reaction (chest pain, palpitations)	Response to therapy	None known	Does not produce neutralizing antibodies	No
Mechanism of action — fingolimod, decreases central inflammation by binding to sphingosine 1-phosphate receptors.								
Fingolimod	Gilenya	0.5 mg PO once daily	• Hypersensitivity • Resting heart rate <55 bpm	Bradycardia, hypertension, immunosuppression, macular edema, dyspnea, elevated liver enzymes, diarrhea, headache	Heart rate, blood pressure, CBC, ECG, ophthalmologic exam, decrease in relapse rate	Class IA and class III antiarrhythmics (may result in bradyarrhythmias, live vaccines, ketoconazole	Zoster vaccination prior to administration	No

Disease-Modifying Drugs *(cont'd)*

Generic	Brand	Dose & Max	Contra-indications	Primary Side Effects	Key Monitoring Parameters	Pertinent Drug Interactions	Med Pearls	Top 200
Mechanism of action – natalizumab: monoclonal antibody inhibits pro-inflammatory interactions within vascular endothelial cells and parenchyma brain cells.								
Natalizumab	Tysabri IV infusion	300 mg IV infusion every 4 wks	Hypersensitivity	• Infusion reactions are common (rash, drowsiness, fever, chills, hypotension, nausea, shortness of breath); headache, fatigue, urinary tract infection, joint pain, abdominal discomfort • Rare, potentially fatal ADE – progressive multifocal leukoencephalopathy (PML)	MRI at baseline, 3 mos, 6 mos; liver enzymes periodically	Interferon β products decrease natalizumab clearance; other DMDs increase risk of PML	• Reserved for patients who have not responded to other DMDs; should be used as monotherapy only; combining with other DMDs increases risk of PML • Available only through a restrictive prescribing program – TOUCH	No
Mechanism of action – Mitoxantrone decreases migration of T cells into the CNS by arresting the cell cycle and interfering with DNA repair and RNA synthesis								
Mitoxantrone	Novantrone IV infusion	12 mg/m² IV infusion every 3 mos; max cumulative dose of 140 mg/m²	LVEF <50%; hypersensitivity	Cardiac toxicity (heart failure, decreased LVEF); nausea; leukopenia; alopecia; menstrual irregularities; urinary and respiratory infections	• LVEF at baseline and prior to each IV infusion • Periodic CBC	Natalizumab (combination increases risk of PML)	Black box warning on cardiac risks and need for frequent LVEF monitoring	No
Mechanism of action – broad spectrum potassium channel blocker; increases action potential in demyelinated axons.								
Dalfampridine	Ampyra	10 mg PO BID	• History of seizures • Moderate-severe renal impairment (CrCl <50 mL/min)	Urinary tract infections, dizziness, insomnia, headache, back pain, nausea, constipation, balance disturbance, MS relapse, paresthesia	• Renal function periodically • Response to therapy	None known (limited data available)	• Indicated to improve walking (specifically speed) in patients with MS • Risk of seizure in patients with poor renal function	No

Storage and Administration Pearls

- Interferon β1a, interferon β1b, glatiramer acetate, natalizumab, and mitoxantrone should be refrigerated to 2–8°C (36–46°F). These products should not be frozen and should be protected from light.
- Interferon β1 products and glatiramer acetate are available in prefilled syringes.
- Interferon β1 products and glatiramer acetate can be self-administered. Natalizumab and mitoxantrone are administered via IV infusion by qualified healthcare professionals.

Patient Education Pearls

- For self-injectable therapies:
  - Use the auto-injector supplied by the manufacturer (when available).
  - Apply ice to the injection site prior to injection.
  - Allow the medication to reach room temperature prior to injection.
  - Rotate injection sites.
- For those newly initiated on therapy, a Natalizumab medication guide should be provided. Both patient and provider must be enrolled in TOUCH prescribing program.

EPILEPSY

Definitions

Epilepsy is a symptom of disturbed electrical activity within the brain. Epilepsy is a general term that encompasses a wide variety of symptomatic presentations that include periodic and recurrent seizures with or without convulsions. Seizures are classified as partial, generalized, or status epilepticus.

Partial seizures begin in one hemisphere of the brain and result in symptoms that are asymmetrical. Partial seizures can be classified as simple (no impairment of consciousness), complex (with impaired consciousness), or secondarily generalized (partial onset which becomes generalized).

Generalized seizures are bilateral/symmetrical in symptoms and can be classified as absence, myoclonic, clonic, tonic, tonic-clonic, atonic, or infantile spasms. The most common types are absence and tonic-clonic.

Diagnosis

The diagnosis of epilepsy is based on comprehensive history and physical, electroencephalography (EEG), and brain imaging by computed tomography (CT) scan or MRI. Differential diagnosis is important with exclusion of potential underlying causes of seizure including metabolic abnormalities (ruled out with evaluation of routine laboratory chemistries), traumatic head injury (determined by history), and presence of underlying structural abnormalities such as tumor (ruled out through brain imaging studies).

Signs and Symptoms

The clinical presentation of epilepsy is dependent on the classification of seizure type.

- Partial seizures result in asymmetrical alterations in motor function and in sensory or somatosensory symptoms, and may or may not involve a loss of consciousness. Nervous ticks, aberrations of normal behavior, and memory loss are also possible.
- Generalized seizures have symptoms that indicate involvement of both hemispheres of the brain. Motor symptoms are bilateral and there may be a loss of consciousness.
  - Absence seizures manifest as sudden interruption of ongoing activities, a blank stare, or an upward rotation of the eyes.
  - Tonic-clonic seizures consist of sharp tonic muscle contractions, rigidity, and clonic movement that are accompanied by a loss of consciousness and may be preceded by an aura.

Guidelines

Efficacy and tolerability of the new antiepileptic drugs I: treatment of new onset epilepsy: report of the Therapeutics and Technology Assessment Subcommittee and Quality Standards Subcommittee of the American Academy of Neurology and the American Epilepsy Society. *Neurology*, no. 62 (8) (2004): 1252–60. http://www.guideline.gov/summary/summary.aspx?ss=15&doc_id=5183&nbr=3565.

Guidelines Summary

- Goals of treatment include a lack of seizure activity, minimal medication side effects of treatment, and improved quality of life.
- Treatment with antiepileptic drugs (AEDs) is warranted for patients that experience multiple seizures or have significantly affected quality of life. AED choice is based on the specific seizure type, the patient's age, comorbidities, ability to adhere to the regimen, and insurance coverage.
- AED monotherapy is preferred, but some patients do require combination therapy.

- First-line AEDs for partial seizures include carbamazepine, phenytoin, lamotrigine, valproic acid, and oxcarbazepine.

- First-line AEDs for generalized absence seizures include valproic acid and ethosuximide.

- First-line AEDs for tonic-clonic seizures include phenytoin, carbamazepine, and valproic acid.

- Alternative AEDs include gabapentin, topiramate, levetiracetam, zonisamide, tiagabine, primidone, felbamate, lamotrigine, phenobarbital, lacosamide, and vigabatrin.

- In 2008, the FDA issued an alert regarding the relationship between the use of antiepileptic agents and suicidality (including suicidal behavior or ideation). Pooled analyses completed by the FDA indicated a significant increase of suicidality for patients treated with antiepileptic agents when compared to those given placebo. All antiepileptic agents appear to increase the risk similarly. Manufacturers of these agents are now required to include a boxed warning in their prescribing information and to include a medication guide for patients in their product labeling.

Anti-Epileptic Drugs

Generic	Brand	Dose & Max mg (frequency)	Contra-indications	Primary Side Effects	Key Monitoring Parameters	Med Pearls	Top 200
Mechanism of action – Carbamazepine inhibits voltage-gated sodium channels, thereby depressing electrical transmission in the nucleus ventralis anterior of the thalamus							
Carbamazepine	Tegretol	200–1,200 mg daily (BID)	Bone marrow suppression, porphyria, hypersensitivity	• Dizziness, drowsiness, unsteadiness, nausea, vomiting • Rare: aplastic anemia, agranulocytosis	CBC periodically; suicidality	First line for partial seizures and generalized tonic-clonic seizures	No
Mechanism of action – valproic acid: not fully understood, thought to increase gamma amino butyric acid (GABA) concentrations in the brain							
Valproic acid (divalproex sodium)	• Depakote • Depakote ER • Depakene • Depacon	10–60 mg/kg/day	• Hepatic dysfunction • Hypersensitivity • Urea cycle disorders	• Hepatic impairment • Thrombocytopenia • Hyperammonemia • Weight gain • Pancreatitis	• Serum drug concentrations (50–100 mcg/mL) • Liver function tests (LFTs), at baseline and periodically • Periodic CBC and serum ammonia levels • Suicidality	• First-line for partial, generalized, tonic-clonic, and absence seizures • Highly teratogenic • Available in oral capsules, tablets, extended-release tablets, sprinkle caps, oral syrup, and IV solution	Yes
Mechanism of action – Phenytoin: promotes neuronal sodium efflux, thereby stabilizing the threshold against hyperexcitability							
Phenytoin	Dilantin	300–600 mg daily (divided TID)	Hypersensitivity	• Nystagmus, ataxia, slurred speech, dizziness, insomnia, headache, tremor, gingival hyperplasia • Rare: Stevens-Johnson rash	• Serum drug concentrations (10–20 mcg/mL) corrected for serum albumin <4 g/dL • Suicidality	• First-line option for partial and generalized tonic-clonic seizures • Abrupt discontinuation should be avoided; this may precipitate status epilepticus • Takes 7–10 days to reach steady state	Yes
Mechanism of action – depresses motor cortex and elevates the threshold of the CNS to convulsive stimuli							
Ethosuximide	Zarontin	250–1,500 mg daily	Hypersensitivity	• Ataxia • Drowsiness • GI upset • Blood dyscrasias • Rash (Stevens-Johnson possible)	• Periodic CBC • Response to therapy • Presence of adverse effects • Suicidality	Available as capsules or syrup; used only for absence seizure	No

Anti-Epileptic Drugs (cont'd)

Generic	Brand	Dose & Max mg (frequency)	Contra-indications	Primary Side Effects	Key Monitoring Parameters	Med Pearls	Top 200
Mechanism of action – blocks voltage-sensitive sodium channels, resulting in stabilization of hyperexcitable neuronal membranes							
Oxcarbazepine	Trileptal tablets and oral suspension	600–2,400 mg daily (BID)	Hypersensitivity	Sedation, dizziness, ataxia, nausea, rash (Stevens-Johnson possible), hyponatremia	• Periodic Na, renal function; serum concentrations 12–30 mcg/mL • Suicidality	CrCl <30 mL/min requires half of initial dose	Yes
Felbamate	Felbatol	1,200–3,600 mg daily (TID–QID)	• Hypersensitivity • Blood dyscrasias • Liver dysfunction	• Aplastic anemia • Acute lever failure • Anorexia • Nausea, vomiting • Insomnia • Headache	• Frequent CBC • Frequent liver transaminases • Suicidality	• AST or ALT >2 x ULN requires discontinuation • Not a first-line agent; reserved for refractory cases	No
Lamotrigine	• Lamictal • Oral tablets, chewable tablets	25–700 mg daily (once to BID)	Hypersensitivity, history of Stevens-Johnson rash	Stevens-Johnson rash, other rash, diplopia, dizziness, headache	• Response to therapy, presence of side effects • Suicidality	• Risk of rash increased when combined with VPA • First-line option for partial seizures • Slow dose titration necessary	Yes
Lacosamide	Vimpat	• 50 mg PO BID; may be increased at weekly intervals by 100 mg/day • Maintenance dose: 200–400 mg/day • IV formulation available (equivalent dose)	None known	• Nausea/vomiting • Ataxia • Dizziness • Headache • Fatigue • Diplopia	• Patients with conduction problems or severe cardiac disease should have ECG tracing prior to start of therapy and when at steady-state • Suicidality	• Adjunctive therapy for partial-onset seizures • Only for adults (>17 year of age (yoa)) • Should not be abruptly discontinued	No
Mechanism of action – although structurally similar to GABA, pharmacological effects in epilepsy are not fully understood							
Gabapentin	• Neurontin • Tablets, capsules, oral solution	900–3,600 mg daily (TID)	Hypersensitivity	• Dizziness • Fatigue • Somnolence • Ataxia • Weight gain	• Response to therapy; presence of adverse effects • Suicidality	• No known drug interactions • Renal dose adjustment necessary when CrCl <60 mL/min	Yes

Anti-Epileptic Drugs *(cont'd)*

Generic	Brand	Dose & Max mg (frequency)	Contra-indications	Primary Side Effects	Key Monitoring Parameters	Med Pearls	Top 200
Mechanism of action – blocks voltage-dependent sodium channels, augments GABA activity, antagonizes glutamate receptors							
Topiramate	• Topamax • Tablets and sprinkle caps	25–400 mg daily (BID)	Hypersensitivity	Difficulty concentrating, psychomotor slowing, speech problems, somnolence, fatigue, dizziness, headache, weight loss, kidney stones	• Response to therapy, presence of side effects • Suicidality	• Adjunctive therapy in patients with partial seizures • Slow titration necessary to avoid adverse effects	Yes
Mechanism of action – not well understood							
Levetiracetam	• Keppra • Tablets, oral solution, parenteral solution	1,000–3,000 mg daily (BID)	Hypersensitivity	Dizziness, asthenia, behavioral disturbances (hostility, nervousness); somnolence, infection	Response to therapy, presence of side effects, renal function, suicidality	• No known drug interactions • Dose adjustment required in renal impairment (CrCl <80 mL/min) • Adjunctive therapy for partial seizures and for generalized tonic-clonic seizures	Yes
Mechanism of action – elevates seizure threshold by decreasing postsynaptic excitability through stimulation of postsynaptic GABA inhibitory responses							
Phenobarbital	• Solfoton • Tablets, capsules, elixir • Luminal IV injection	60–600 mg daily	Severe liver impairment, hypersensitivity, porphyria	Sedation, nystagmus, ataxia, hyperactivity, headache, nausea, blood dyscrasias (agranulocytosis, granulocytopenia), rash, behavior changes, intellectual blunting, mood change	Serum concentrations 10–40 mcg/mL, periodic CBC; periodic LFTs; suicidality	• Drug of choice for neonatal seizures; otherwise, adjunctive therapy for partial and generalized (other than absence) seizures • Frequency of side effects limits use • Titrate dose slowly to minimize adverse effects • Avoid abrupt discontinuation • Takes 3–4 wks to reach steady-state	No
Primidone	Mysoline	125–2,000 mg daily (TID–QID)			Serum concentrations, 5–10 mcg/mL; periodic CBC; periodic LFTs; suicidality	• Metabolized to phenobarbital • Avoid abrupt discontinuation	No

Anti-Epileptic Drugs *(cont'd)*

Generic	Brand	Dose & Max mg (frequency)	Contra-indications	Primary Side Effects	Key Monitoring Parameters	Med Pearls	Top 200
Mechanism of action – potent and specific inhibitor of GABA uptake into neuronal elements, thereby enhances GABA activity by decreasing its removal from the neuronal space							
Tiagabine	Gabitril	4–80 mg daily (BID–QID)	Hypersensitivity	Dizziness, fatigue, difficulty concentrating, nervousness, tremor, blurred vision, depression, weakness	Response to therapy, presence of adverse effects, suicidality	• Adjunctive therapy in partial seizures • Do not abruptly discontinue; taper dose	No
Mechanism of action – irreversible inhibition of gamma-aminobutyric acid transaminase (GABA-T), thereby increasing the levels of GABA within the brain.							
Vigabatrin	Sabril	• 500 mg twice daily initially, increase daily dose by 500 mg at weekly intervals • Recommended dose: 3 g/day	None	Permanent vision loss, fatigue, somnolence, tremor, nystagmus, blurred vision, memory impairment, weight gain, arthralgia, confusion, suicidality	Ophthalmologic exam, observe patient for excessive sedation, suicidality	• Used as adjunctive therapy for refractory complex-partial seizures • Should not be abruptly discontinued • Renal dose adjustment required • Boxed warning due to ocular effects • Available only through special, restricted distribution program (SHARE)	No
Mechanism of action – blocks voltage-dependent sodium and calcium channels, thereby reducing repetitive neuronal firing							
Zonisamide	Zonegran	100–600 mg daily	Hypersensitivity to zonisamide or sulfonamides	Sedation, dizziness, cognitive impairment, nausea, rash (Stevens-Johnson possible), oligohidrosis	Serum drug concentrations 10–40 mcg/mL (not routine)	• Adjunctive therapy in partial seizures • Takes up to 2 wks to achieve steady-state	No

AED Drug Interactions

AED	Interacting Medication	Effect
Carbamazepine	Felbamate	↓ Carbamazepine
	Phenobarbital	↓ Carbamazepine
	Phenytoin	↓ Carbamazepine
	Cimetidine	↑ Carbamazepine
	Erythromycin	↑ Carbamazepine
	Fluoxetine	↑ Carbamazepine
	Isoniazid	↑ Carbamazepine
	Propoxyphene	↑ Carbamazepine
	Oral contraceptives	↓ Contraceptives
	Doxycycline	↓ Doxycycline
	Theophylline	↓ Theophylline
	Warfarin	↓ Warfarin
VPA	Carbamazepine	↓ VPA
	Lamotrigine	↓ VPA
	Phenobarbital	↓ VPA
	Primidone	↓ VPA
	Phenytoin	↓ VPA
	Cimetidine	↑ VPA
	Salicylates	↑ VPA
	Oral contraceptives	↓ Contraceptives
Phenytoin	Carbamazepine	↓ Phenytoin
	Felbamate	↑ Phenytoin
	Phenobarbital	↑ or ↓ Phenytoin
	VPA	↓ Phenytoin
	Antacids	↓ Phenytoin
	Cimetidine	↑ Phenytoin
	Chloramphenicol	↑ Phenytoin
	Disulfiram	↑ Phenytoin
	Ethanol (acute)	↑ Phenytoin
	Ethanol (chronic)	↑ Phenytoin
	Warfarin	↑ Phenytoin
	Propoxyphene	↑ Phenytoin
	Fluconazole	↑ Phenytoin
	Isoniazid	↑ Phenytoin
	Oral contraceptives	↓ Contraceptives
	Folic acid	↓ Folic acid
	Quinidine	↓ Quinidine
Oxcarbazepine	Carbamazepine	↓ Oxcarbazepine
	Phenytoin	↓ Oxcarbazepine
	Phenobarbital	↓ Oxcarbazepine
	Oral contraceptives	↓ Contraceptives
Felbamate	Carbamazepine	↓ Felbamate
	Phenytoin	↓ Felbamate
	VPA	↑ Felbamate

AED Drug Interactions *(cont'd)*

AED	Interacting Medication	Effect
Lacosamide	Carbamazepine	↓ Lacosamide
	Phenobarbital	↓ Lacosamide
	Phenytoin	↓ Lacosamide
Lamotrigine	Carbamazepine	↓ Lamotrigine
	Phenobarbital	↓ Lamotrigine
	Phenytoin	↓ Lamotrigine
	Primidone	↓ Lamotrigine
	VPA	↑ Lamotrigine
Topiramate	Carbamazepine	↓ Topiramate
	Phenytoin	↓ Topiramate
	VPA	↓ Topiramate
	Oral contraceptives	↓ Contraceptives
Phenobarbital	Felbamate	↑ Phenobarbital
	Phenytoin	↑ Phenobarbital
	VPA	↑ Phenobarbital
	Acetazolamide	↑ Phenobarbital
	Oral contraceptives	↓ Contraceptives
Primidone	Carbamazepine	↓ Primidone, ↑ Phenobarbital
	Phenytoin	↓ Primidone, ↑ Phenobarbital
	VPA	↑ Primidone, ↓ Phenobarbital
	Isoniazid	↑ Primidone, ↓ Phenobarbital
	Nicotinamide	↑ Primidone, ↓ Phenobarbital
	Chlorpromazine	↓ Chlorpromazine
	Corticosteroids	↓ Corticosteroids
	Quinidine	↓ Quinidine
	Tricyclics	↓ Tricyclics
Tiagabine	Carbamazepine	↓ Tiagabine
	Phenytoin	↓ Tiagabine
Vigabatrin	CNS depressants	↑ CNS depressant effect
	Methotrimeprazine	↑ Methotrimeprazine, ↑ vigabatrin
	Phenytoin	↓ Phenytoin
	Ketorolac	↓ Vigabatrin
	Mefloquine	↓ Vigabatrin
Zonisamide	Carbamazepine	↓ Zonisamide
	Phenytoin	↓ Zonisamide
	Phenobarbital	↓ Zonisamide

Storage and Administration Pearls

- Valproic acid: Extended-release divalproex sodium should be swallowed whole and should not be chewed, crushed, or split. Divalproex sodium sprinkle caps may be swallowed whole or may be opened and sprinkled on a small amount (~ teaspoon) of soft food, such as pudding or applesauce.
- Phenytoin: Available in chewable tablets, capsules, extended-release capsules, oral suspension and parenteral solution (IM or IV).
- Oxcarbazepine oral suspension should be shaken well before administration and should be used within 7 weeks of opening the bottle.

Patient Education Pearls

- Antiepileptic medication should not be abruptly discontinued, as this may result in increased and emergent seizure activity.
- Any skin rash that develops should be reported to a healthcare provider immediately.
- When taking any new medications, patients should consult with their pharmacist, as multiple drug interactions are possible.
- Antiepileptic medications have been associated with an increased risk of suicidal thoughts and behaviors. Please discuss this with your healthcare provider and report any of these symptoms immediately.

PARKINSON'S DISEASE

Definitions

Parkinson's disease (PD) is a syndrome characterized by tremor, rigidity, bradykinesia, and/or postural instability caused by a progressive depletion of dopamine neurons in the substantia nigra of the basal ganglia. Symptoms are a result of the dopamine deficiency and subsequent relative acetylcholine excess.

Diagnosis

Diagnosis of PD is based on careful clinical history and physical exam. There are no agreed-upon objective or definitive lab or imaging criteria for diagnosis.

Signs and Symptoms

PD has an insidious onset and begins with nonspecific symptoms such as malaise and fatigue. Tremor is generally the first of the cardinal signs and is generally unilateral and occurring at rest rather than upon intention. Rigidity of the limbs manifests as resistance to passive movement of the joints, and bradykinesia as slow movements or difficulty moving. Symptoms generally begin unilaterally and progress asymmetrically.

Summary of Treatment Recommendations

▪ Initial therapy generally consists of either a dopamine agonist or carbidopa/levodopa.

- Patients ≥65 years of age or those with significant disability due to their PD should receive carbidopa/levodopa as initial therapy.

- Patients <65 years of age should receive a dopamine agonist as initial therapy.

- Inadequate response to maximum tolerable doses of initial therapy with a dopamine agonist or levodopa should result in the addition of the alternate medication.

- Subsequently, COMT inhibitors may be added to ongoing levodopa therapy, and adjunctive therapies such as amantadine or anticholinergics may be utilized.

- Anticholinergic agents are primarily useful for the treatment of tremor-predominant PD but should be used with caution in elderly patients and avoided in patients with pre-existing cognitive impairment.

- Because dopamine agonists and levodopa therapies are aimed at increasing the available dopamine in the CNS, side effects such as hallucinations and delusions are possible. Psychiatric side effects which occur at the lowest effective doses of these drugs may be treated with antipsychotic medications such as clozapine or quetiapine.

Drugs for Parkinson's Disease

Generic	Brand	Dose & Max	Contra-indications	Primary Side Effects	Key Monitoring Parameters	Pertinent Drug Interactions	Med Pearls	Top 200
Mechanism of action – antiviral that blocks the uncoating of influenza A virus, preventing penetration of virus into host								
Amantadine	Symmetrel	200–300 mg daily	Hypersensitivity	Confusion, nightmares, hallucinations, insomnia, nervousness, irritability	Response to therapy, presence of adverse effects	Quinidine and triamterene increase plasma amantadine concentrations	Renal dose adjustment necessary for CrCl <50 mL/min	No
Mechanism of action – monoamine-oxidase (MAO) B inhibitors: inhibit the catabolism of dopamine by selectively inhibiting the monoamine oxidase B enzyme								
Selegiline	• Eldepryl: tablets • Emsam: transdermal patch • Zelapar: disintegrating tablets	5–10 mg daily (once to BID)	Hypersensitivity; use of meperidine or other opioids	• Nausea, hallucinations, insomnia, depression, orthostasis, arrhythmia • Rare: hypertensive crisis (if high-tyramine foods are ingested)	Response to therapy, presence of adverse effects	• Avoid use with meperidine, other opioid analgesics, or dextromethorphan; may result in fatal increased activity of analgesics • Co-administration with other serotonergic agents increases risk of serotonin syndrome	• Avoid tyramine-containing foods • Discontinue 14 days prior to surgery if possible; should not te taken with general anesthesia	No
Rasagiline	Azilect	0.5–1 mg daily	Hypersensitivity	Flu-like syndrome, arthralgia, depression, dyspepsia, hypertension	Response to therapy, presence of side effects	• Avoid use with meperidine, opioid analgesics, or dextromethorphan; may result in fatal reaction • Co-administration with other serotonergic agents increases risk of serotonin syndrome • Ciprofloxaxin (and other CYP1A2 inhibitors) increases rasagiline plasma levels	• Should not be abruptly d scontinued • Avoid tyramine-containing foods	No

Drugs for Parkinson's Disease (cont'd)

Generic	Brand	Dose & Max	Contra-indications	Primary Side Effects	Key Monitoring Parameters	Pertinent Drug Interactions	Med Pearls	Top 200
Mechanism of action – levodopa is a direct precursor to dopamine and is converted to dopamine once it crosses the blood-brain barrier; carbidopa is a dopa decarboxylase inhibitor, and it is necessary to combine this with levodopa in order to prevent the peripheral degradation of levodopa prior to entry into the blood-brain barrier.								
Carbidopa/ levodopa	• Sinemet • Sinemet CR • Parcopa: Orally disintegrating tablets	• Carbidopa 75–300 mg daily (75 mg required, side effects if >300 mg day) • Levodopa 100–2,000 mg daily (individualized)	Hypersensitivity, narrow-angle glaucoma	Nausea, vomiting, orthostasis, confusion, hallucinations, wearing-off fluctuations, dyskinesias	Response to therapy, presence of side effects	• Nonselective MAO inhibitors should be avoided; may cause hypertensive crisis • Pyridoxine (vitamin B6) decreases effectiveness of levodopa	Immediate-release (IR) and controlled-release (CR) tabs often used simultaneously; IR tabs can treat wearing-off symptoms of CR tabs; CR is less bioavailable (~30% less) than IR	Yes
L-Dopa	Larodopa	Individualized (not more than 8 g/day)	Hypersensitivity; narrow-angle glaucoma	Nausea, vomiting, orthostasis, confusion, hallucinations, wearing-off fluctuations, dyskinesias		• Nonselective MAO inhibitors should be avoided; may cause hypertensive crisis • Pyridoxine (vitamin B6) decreases effectiveness of levodopa	Only used to supplement carbidopa/ levodopa therapy in patients that need a larger dose of levodopa than can be achieved with combination tablets	No
Mechanism of action – dopamine agonists: direct stimulation of striatal dopamine receptors								
Bromocriptine (Ergot-derivative)	Parlodel	1.25–40 mg daily (divided TID)	Uncontrolled hypertension, sensitivity to ergot alkaloids	• Cardiac valve fibrosis • Nausea, hallucinations, dizziness, drowsiness	Response to therapy, presence of adverse effects	Decrease levodopa dose by 20–30% when initiating	Cardiac side effects decrease clinical use; nonergot derivatives used much more commonly	No
Pramipexole (Nonergot derivative)	Mirapex Mirapex ER	1.5–4.5 mg daily	Dementia; hypersensitivity	Nausea, vomiting, constipation, orthostasis, hypersexuality, hallucinations, syncope	Renal function periodically, response to therapy, presence of adverse effects	Decrease levodopa dose by 20–30% when initiating; metoclopramide and phenothiazines decrease efficacy	• Renal dose adjustment required when CrCl <60 mL/min (pramipexole only) • Titrate dose slowly and taper upon discontinuation	Yes

Drugs for Parkinson's Disease *(cont'd)*

Generic	Brand	Dose & Max	Contra-indications	Primary Side Effects	Key Monitoring Parameters	Pertinent Drug Interactions	Med Pearls	Top 200
Ropinirole (Nonergot derivative)	• Requip • Tablets • Extended-release tablets	0.75–12 mg daily (divided TID)						Yes
Rotigotine	Neupro transdermal delivery system	2–8 mg daily (apply one patch daily)	Dementia; hypersensitivity	Application site reactions, nausea, vomiting, somnolence, insomnia, hallucinations, abnormal dreams	Response to therapy, presence of adverse effects	Decrease levodopa dose by 20–30% when initiating; metoclopramide and phenothiazines decrease efficacy	• Transdermal patch • Taper dose upon discontinuation	No

Mechanism of action – COMT inhibitors: inhibit the degradation of dopamine through inhibition of the catechol-O-methyltransferase enzyme

Generic	Brand	Dose & Max	Contra-indications	Primary Side Effects	Key Monitoring Parameters	Pertinent Drug Interactions	Med Pearls	Top 200
Tolcapone	Tasmar	300–600 mg daily (divided TID)	AST or ALT >2 x ULN, known liver disease, history or nontraumatic rhabdomyolysis	Liver failure; dyskinesias, nausea, vomiting, hallucinations	Frequent LFT monitoring	Nonselective MAO inhibitors; increased activity of drugs known to be metabolized by COMT (dopamine, dobutamine, isoproterenol, methyldopa)	• Reserved for third-line therapy in patients that do not respond adequately to levodopa and dopamine agonists • Only used as adjunct therapy with levodopa	No
Entacapone	Comtan	200–1,600 mg daily (divided up to 8x daily; administered with carbidopa/levodopa tablets)	Hypersensitivity	Dyskinesias, nausea, vomiting, hallucinations, urine discoloration	Response to therapy, presence of adverse effects, periodic LFTs	Increased activity of drugs known to be metabolized by COMT (dopamine, dobutamine, isoproterenol, methyldopa)	• Reserved for third-line therapy in patients that do not respond adequately to levodopa and dopamine agonists • Preferred over tolcapone, as no fatal liver injury has been reported with this agent	No

Drugs for Parkinson's Disease *(cont'd)*

Mechanism of action – anticholinergics: through diminished activity of acetylcholine, help to decrease the relative increase in activity compared to dopamine, thereby decreasing tremor

Generic	Brand	Dose & Max	Contra-indications	Primary Side Effects	Key Monitoring Parameters	Pertinent Drug Interactions	Med Pearls	Top 200
Benztropine	Cogentin	0.5–6 mg daily (BID)	Avoid in patients with cognitive impairment and in elderly (>75 yoa)	Dry mouth, blurred vision, constipation, urinary retention, confusion, memory impairment, hallucinations	Response to therapy, presence of adverse effects	Additive anticholinergic side effects when co-administered with other anticholinergic medications	Caution use in elderly patients who are at risk for mental status changes with anticholinergic medications; primarily used for tremor and/or drooling	No
Trihexyphenidyl	Artane	1–15 mg daily (BID–TID)	Hypersensitivity	Dry mouth, blurred vision, constipation, urinary retention, confusion, memory impairment, hallucinations	Response to therapy, presence of adverse effects	Additive anticholinergic side effects when co-administered with other anticholinergic agents	Caution use in elderly patients; primarily used for tremor and drooling	No

Storage and Administration Pearls

- Selegiline is available as a tablet, capsule, transdermal patch, and oral disintegrating tablet. Oral disintegrating tablets should be taken in the morning before any food or water. Tablets dissolve on the tongue, and food/drink should be avoided for 5 minutes after dose.

- Carbidopa/levodopa extended-release tablets can be taken as whole tablets or half tablets but should not be chewed or crushed. Extended-release tablets are less bioavailable than immediate-release tablets and patients may require up to a 30% dose increase to attain similar efficacy.

- Rotigotine patch should be worn continuously for 24 hours. Heat may increase absorption.

Patient Education Pearls

- Avoid concomitant alcohol with any antiparkinsonian agent.

- Rotigotine patch should be worn continuously for 24 hours. Heat may increase absorption. Patients should not take a hot bath or sauna or apply a heated pad while wearing patch.

- Hallucinations, delusions, or strange dreams should be immediately reported to a physician.

MIGRAINE HEADACHE

Definitions

Migraine headaches are defined as recurring headaches of moderate to severe intensity and are associated with gastrointestinal, neurological, and autonomic symptoms. Migraine headaches may or may not be preceded by an aura.

Diagnosis

Diagnostic criteria are established by the International Headache Society (IHS) and consist of distinct criteria for migraine with aura and migraine without aura.

Migraine with aura

- At least two attacks
- Aura symptoms that do not last more than 60 minutes
- Organic disorder ruled out or headaches do not relate temporally to organic disorder

Migraine without aura

- At least five attacks
- Headache lasts 4–72 hours

- Unilateral, pulsating, moderate/severe intensity, or aggravated by physical activity
- Nausea/vomiting, photophobia, or phonophobia
- Organic disorder ruled out or headaches do not relate temporally to organic disorder

Signs and Symptoms

Pain is the primary symptom of migraine headache. The pain is generally gradual in onset, peaks in intensity over minutes to hours, and lasts 4–72 hours if untreated. Intensity is often described as moderate to severe and generally stated as a 5 or greater on a 0–10 pain scale. Most commonly, pain occurs in the frontotemporal region and is most often unilateral and pulsating. Other symptoms that may accompany the pain include gastrointestinal symptoms of nausea/vomiting and neurological symptoms of photo- or phonophobia.

Guidelines

Treatment of primary headache: acute migraine treatment. Standards of care for headache diagnosis and treatment. National Headache Foundation; Chicago, IL. (2004): 27–39. http://www.guideline.gov/summary/summary.aspx?ss=15&doc_id=6579&nbr=4139.

Guidelines Summary

- Migraine treatment is divided into abortive treatment, rescue treatment, and prophylactic treatment. The majority of patients will respond to abortive treatment and can be controlled without the addition of rescue or prophylactic therapy.

- Abortive treatment options include analgesics (over-the-counter and prescription), NSAIDs (detailed in bone and joint chapter), ergotamine and dihydroergotamine, serotonin agonists, and butorphanol. Over-the-counter analgesics, prescription non-opioid analgesics, and NSAIDs are reserved for patients with mild symptoms.

- The serotonin agonists are the mainstay of abortive therapy options for patients with moderate to severe symptoms. Various dosage forms are available and there is only slight variability between the efficacy and safety of available agents. Patients may respond to one agent in this class and not to another; therefore, trial and error is often the approach taken.

- For patients who have >2 headaches/week or >8 headaches/month, or who do not have an adequate response to abortive therapy, prophylactic therapy may be warranted.

- Available prophylactic agents include antihypertensive medications such as propranolol, atenolol, and metoprolol (detailed in cardiovascular chapter); antidepressant medications such as amitriptyline, paroxetine, fluoxetine, and sertraline (detailed in psychiatric disorders chapter); and anticonvulsant medications such valproic acid, gabapentin, tiagabine, and topiramate (detailed earlier in this chapter). In general, migraine prophylactic doses are low compared to normal doses of these medications.

Drugs for Migraine

Generic	Brand	Dose & Max	Contra-indications	Primary Side Effects	Key Monitoring Parameters	Pertinent Drug Interactions	Med Pearls	Top 200
Analgesics								
Acetaminophen 250 mg/aspirin 250 mg/caffeine 65 mg	Excedrin Migraine	2 tablets PO at onset, then q6 hrs PRN	Hypersensitivity to any component	Minimal	Response to therapy, presence of adverse effects	Other acetaminophen-containing meds	Available OTC	No
Aspirin or acetaminophen with butalbital and caffeine	• Fiorinal • Fioricet	1–2 tabs PO q4–6 hrs PRN	Hypersensitivity to any component	Tachycardia, dizziness, drowsiness or insomnia, orthostatic hypotension	Response to therapy, presence of adverse effects	• Alcohol • Additive CNS depression with butalbital	• Limit to 4 tablets/day and use max of 2 days/week • Dependence may develop with continued use	Yes
Isometheptene 65 mg/dichloral-phenazone 100 mg/APAP 325 mg	Midrin	2 caps PO at onset, 1 cap q hour PRN	Glaucoma, severe renal or heart disease, hypertension	Dizziness, skin rash	Response to therapy, presence of adverse effects	MAOIs: potential for hypertensive crisis	Max 6 caps/day; 20 caps/month	No
Mechanism of action — ergotamine tartrate: exerts serotonergic agonist activity, resulting in vasoconstriction								
Ergotamine tartrate	Ergomar sublingual tablet	• 1 tab at onset and 1 tab q30 min PRN • Not to exceed 3 tabs/day	Peripheral arterial disease, heart disease, hypertension, impaired hepatic or renal function, hypersensitivity	Chest pain, hypertension, tachycardia, nausea, edema	Response to therapy, presence of adverse effects	Other meds with potential to increase blood pressure	Potential for dependence with long-term use	No
Mechanism of action — dihydroergotamine: serotonin agonistic activity, results in cerebral vasoconstriction								
Dihydroergotamine	DHE 45 SC, IM, or IV injection 1 mg/mL	1 mg at onset, repeated at 1-hr intervals (max = 2 mg/day IV or 3 mg/day SC or IM)	• Ischemic heart disease • Uncontrolled hypertension • Peripheral arterial disease	Hypertension, vasospasm, myocardial infarction, tachycardia	Blood pressure, heart rate, response to therapy, presence of side effects	Potent inhibitors of CYP3A4, including protease inhibitors and macrolide antibiotics	Use significantly limited by adverse effects	No
	Migranal nasal spray	1 spray (0.5 mg) in each nostril followed by repeat spray in each nostril >15 minutes (max = 3 mg/day)						

Drugs for Migraine *(cont'd)*

Mechanism of action – serotonin agonists (triptans); serotonin 5HT receptor agonists, resulting in vasoconstriction in the cerebral vasculature

Generic	Brand	Dose & Max	Contra-indications	Primary Side Effects	Key Monitoring Parameters	Pertinent Drug Interactions	Med Pearls	Top 200
Sumatriptan	Imitrex oral tablets	25–100 mg PO at onset, then q2 hrs PRN up to 200 mg/day	Ischemic cardiac disease, peripheral vascular disease, cerebrovascular disease	Fatigue, dizziness, flushing, neck/throat pressure	Response to therapy, presence of side effects	MAO – A inhibitors – increased triptan levels can lead to serotonin syndrome and cardiac side effects; sibutramine and SSRI coadministration – increased risk of serotonin syndrome	• First approved serotonin agonist for migraine • Also available in combination with naproxen (Treximet)	Yes
	Imitrex SC injection	4–6 mg SC; may repeat in 1 hour Max: 2 doses /day						
	Imitrex nasal spray	10–20 mg spray intranasally at onset; may repeat after 2 hrs • Max: 40 mg/day						
	• Sumavel Dosepro • Needle-free, SC injection	6 mg SC; may repeat in 1 hour						
Zolmitriptan	• Zomig • Oral tabs; rapid disintegrating tabs; nasal spray	1–5 mg at onset, redose >2 hrs if needed (max 10 mg/day)					Rapidly disintegrating tablets offer faster-onset option	No
Naratriptan	Amerge oral tablets	1–2.5 mg at onset; may re-dose >4 hrs if needed (max 5 mg/day)						No

Drugs for Migraine (cont'd)

Generic	Brand	Dose & Max	Contra-indications	Primary Side Effects	Key Monitoring Parameters	Pertinent Drug Interactions	Med Pearls	Top 200
Rizatriptan	Maxalt oral tabs	5–10 mg PO at onset; redose >2 hrs (max 30 mg/day)	Ischemic cardiac disease, peripheral vascular disease, cerebrovascular disease	Fatigue, dizziness, flushing, neck/ throat pressure	Response to therapy, presence of side effects	MAO – A inhibitors – increased triptan levels can lead to serotonin syndrome and cardiac side effects; sibutramine and SSRI coadministration – increased risk of serotonin syndrome	Rapidly disintegrating tablets offer faster-onset option	No
	• Maxalt • MLT rapid disintegrating tablets	5–10 mg dissolved followed by redose after 2 hrs if needed (max 30 mg/day)						
Almotriptan	Axert oral tablets	6.25–12.5 mg PO at onset; redose >2 hrs if needed (max 25 mg/day)						No
Eletriptan	Relpax oral tablets	20–40 mg PO at onset; redose >2 hrs if needed (max 80 mg/day)					• Metabolized by CYP3A4 • Dosage form is hydrobromide salt 24.2 mg (= 20-mg base) and 48.5 mg (= 40-mg base)	No
Frovatriptan	Frova oral tablets	2.5 mg PO at onset; redose >2 hrs if needed (max 7.5 mg/day)						No

Mechanism of action – butorphanol: mixed opioid agonist/antagonist with opioid analgesic properties

Generic	Brand	Dose & Max	Contra-indications	Primary Side Effects	Key Monitoring Parameters	Pertinent Drug Interactions	Med Pearls	Top 200
Butorphanol	Stadol nasal spray	1 mg (one spray) intranasally at onset; may repeat after 1 hour and then q3–4 hrs PRN	• Hypersensitivity, CrCl <30 mL/min • Patients with a history of narcotic dependence	Somnolence, dizziness, nausea, nasal congestion, insomnia	Response to therapy, presence of adverse effects	Concurrent use of other CNS depressants will have additive adverse effects and should be avoided	• Pharmacist often assembles nasal spray prior to patient use • Not routinely used for migraine • High addiction potential; controlled substance	No

Storage and Administration Pearls

- Store all preparations between 2–30°C (36–86°F). Protect from light.
- Place rapid disintegrating tablets directly on tongue and allow them to dissolve.
- Sumatriptan and zolmitran nasal sprays are sprayed into one nostril only.
- Sumatriptan injection is self-administered subcutaneously using prefilled syringes and an autoinjector.

Patient Education Pearls

- Rapid disintegrating tablets should be placed directly on the tongue and allowed to dissolve.
- Follow dosing recommendations carefully to decrease risk of adverse effects or dependence.

LEARNING POINTS

- Disease-modifying drugs are the agents of choice in treating MS.
- First-line choice of antiepileptic drug is based on seizure classification. Options include carbamazepine, phenytoin, lamotrigine, valproic acid, and oxcarbazepine.
- Antiepileptic drugs have a significant number of drug-drug interactions due to their impact on and metabolism by the cytochrome P450 enzyme system.
- Carbidopa/levodopa is the mainstay of therapy for PD and is available in numerous dosage forms. Controlled-and immediate-release tablets are often prescribed simultaneously.
- Anticholinergic agents should be avoided in elderly patients.
- Agents affecting dopamine, including dopamine agonists and carbidopa/levodopa, may elicit psychiatric side effects.
- Serotonin agonists are the mainstay of treatment for migraine headache and are available in numerous dosage forms.

PRACTICE QUESTIONS

1. What is recommended first-line for newly diagnosed multiple sclerosis?

   (A) Oral prednisone 50 mg PO daily for 1 week, then slowly tapered over 1 month
   (B) Betaseron
   (C) Methylprednisolone 100–500 mg/day for 3–10 days
   (D) Natalizumab
   (E) Rebif + mitoxantrone

2. What patient counseling should be provided when dispensing an interferon injectable prescription for multiple sclerosis?

   (A) If the medication cannot be used within 1 month, freeze the syringe to allow beyond-date use.
   (B) Apply heat to the injection site before and after the injection.
   (C) Try to use the same injection site each time.
   (D) If the medication reaches room temperature, it is no longer usable and must be discarded.
   (E) NSAIDs may decrease the flu-like symptoms.

3. Which of the following is NOT a first-line agent for treatment of generalized tonic-clonic seizures?

   (A) Tegretol
   (B) Topiramate
   (C) Depakote
   (D) Dilantin
   (E) Carbamazepine

ANSWERS

1. B

Interferon agents (such as Betaseron, Avonex, and Rebif) and glatiramer acetate (Copaxone) are considered first-line disease-modifying drugs (DMDs) for the treatment of MS. Therefore, (B) is correct. Natalizumab (D) is reserved for patients who do not respond to traditional therapy. Treatment is usually initiated one agent at a time and, as the disease progresses, treatment with DMD + mitoxantrone pulse therapy (E) may be used. Corticosteroids (A and C) are the cornerstone of acute exacerbations but will play no role in treating the disease itself.

2. E

Acetaminophen or NSAIDs can reduce the flu-like symptoms associated with the interferon injections. The injectables for multiple sclerosis should never be frozen (A) and should always be protected from light. To ease the discomfort of the injections, ice—not heat (B)—can be applied to the injection site prior to the injection, and the injection site should be rotated each time (making choice C incorrect). It is perfectly fine and recommended to allow the injectable to reach room temperature prior to the injection (D), but it should otherwise be stored in the refrigerator.

3. B

First-line treatment for tonic-clonic seizures includes phenytoin (D), valproic acid (C), and carbamazepine (E). Tegretol (A) is the generic for carbamazepine so it is also correct. Topiramate (B) is considered an alternate antiepileptic agent; it can be used as adjunctive therapy in partial seizures.

Gastrointestinal Disorders

6

This chapter covers the following diseases:

- **Gastroesophageal reflux disease/peptic ulcer disease**
- **Inflammatory bowel disease**

 Suggested Study Time: **45 minutes**

GASTROESOPHAGEAL REFLUX DISEASE/ PEPTIC ULCER DISEASE

Definitions

Gastroesophageal reflux disease (GERD) is a condition in which patients have symptoms or mucosal damage resulting from the abnormal reflux of stomach contents into the esophagus. If the esophagus is chronically exposed to these contents, inflammation of the esophagus can develop which is termed reflux esophagitis, and/or the esophageal mucosa can become ulcerated, leading to erosive esophagitis. Often, GERD results because of reduced lower esophageal sphincter (LES) pressures; however, this condition may also arise because of a delay in gastric emptying, use of certain medications or foods, or a hiatal hernia. Various medications may precipitate GERD symptoms either by decreasing LES pressure (e.g., anticholinergics, benzodiazepines, β-agonists, calcium channel blockers, dopamine agonists, estrogen, opioid narcotics, nicotine, nitrates, progesterone, theophylline) or by irritating the esophageal mucosa (e.g., nonsteroidal anti-inflammatory drugs [NSAIDs], bisphosphonates, salicylates, iron, potassium chloride).

Peptic ulcer disease (PUD) refers to the development of duodenal or gastric ulcers. The majority of PUD cases are caused by either *Helicobacter pylori* (*H. pylori*) infection or the use of NSAIDs, but can also be induced by stress. A number of risk factors exist that may predispose patients to NSAID-induced ulcers, including a prior gastrointestinal (GI) ulcer or hemorrhage; age >65 years; concurrent use of corticosteroids, antiplatelets, or anticoagulants; and chronic debilitating disorders, especially cardiovascular (CV) disease.

Patients taking NSAIDs can be categorized as being at high risk, moderate risk, or low risk for GI injury:

- High risk
  - History of previously complicated ulcer (especially recent)
  - Multiple (>2 risk factors) (see above)
- Moderate risk (1–2 risk factors)
  - Age >65 years
  - High-dose NSAID therapy
  - Previous history of uncomplicated ulcer
  - Concurrent use of aspirin (including low dose), corticosteroids, or anticoagulants
- Low risk
  - No risk factors

Diagnosis

Gastroesophageal Reflux Disease

- Diagnosis for uncomplicated cases is based primarily on description of symptoms and potential risk factors. Response to treatment can also be used as a diagnostic strategy.
- Endoscopy is recommended for the following patients:
  - Age >45 years
  - Presenting with atypical or alarm symptoms (see below)
  - Refractory to initial treatment
- Ambulatory pH testing can also be used if patients continue to have symptoms despite either normal endoscopic findings or appropriate therapy.

Peptic Ulcer Disease

- Clinical history (including symptoms and history of medication use) can be helpful in arriving at a preliminary diagnosis (not important to differentiate between duodenal and gastric ulcers).
- All patients with a suspected diagnosis of PUD should be tested for *H. pylori*.
  - Invasive tests (endoscopy): rapid urease tests (80–95% sensitive, 95–100% specific; false negatives can occur if patients previously on proton pump inhibitor [PPIs], H_2 receptor antagonist, or bismuth therapy; patient needs to be off these drugs for at least 1 week before performing this test)

- Noninvasive tests:
  - » Serological: 85% sensitive, 79% specific; not influenced by prior acid-suppressive therapy; can be used to confirm diagnosis but will not be helpful in determining eradication of infection
  - » Urea breath test: 97% sensitive, 95% specific; influenced by prior acid-suppressive and antibiotic therapy (↑ risk of false negative); can be used to confirm diagnosis and eradication
  - » Stool antigen test: 88–92% sensitive, 87% specific; influenced by prior acid-suppressive therapy; can be used to confirm diagnosis and eradication

Signs and Symptoms

Gastroesophageal Reflux Disease

- Typical symptoms: Heartburn (pyrosis), regurgitation, belching, water brash (↑ salivation)
- Atypical symptoms: Noncardiac chest pain, hoarseness, nausea, asthma-like symptoms, chronic cough, sore throat, dental erosions
- Alarm symptoms (indicate need for immediate evaluation): Dysphagia (difficulty swallowing), odynophagia (painful swallowing), bleeding, weight loss
- Long-term complications: Esophageal strictures, Barrett's esophagus, esophageal cancer

Peptic Ulcer Disease

- Abdominal pain (usually epigastric): The most common symptom
  - Can be described as burning, discomfort, or fullness
  - Duodenal ulcer: Pain often occurs 1–3 hours after a meal and is relieved with food
  - Gastric ulcer: Pain brought on by food
- Other symptoms: Heartburn, belching, bloating, nausea, anorexia
- Long-term complications: Upper GI bleeding, perforation

Guidelines

Gastroesophageal Reflux Disease

American College of Gastroenterology. *Am J Gastroenterol*, no. 100 (2005): 190–200.

Peptic Ulcer Disease

Guidelines for the treatment of Helicobacter pylori infection (American College of Gastroenterology). *Am J Gastroenterol*, no. 93 (1998): 2330–8.

Guidelines for treatment and prevention of NSAID-induced ulcers (American College of Gastroenterology). *Am J Gastroenterol*, no. 93 (1998): 2037–46.

Guidelines for prevention of NSAID-related ulcers complications (American College of Gastroenterology). *Am J Gastroenterol*, no. 104 (2009): 728–38.

Guidelines Summary

Gastroesophageal Reflux Disease

The goals of therapy are to relieve symptoms, promote healing of esophageal mucosa, prevent recurrence, and prevent complications.

- **Lifestyle modifications**
  - Unlikely to control symptoms, when used alone, in most patients
  - Dietary changes: Avoid foods that can worsen symptoms (alcohol, caffeine, chocolate, citrus juices, peppermint/spearmint, coffee, spicy foods, tomatoes, high-fatty meals, garlic, onions); avoid eating before bedtime; remain upright after meals
  - Weight loss
  - Smoking cessation
  - Head elevated off the bed by 6–8 inches
  - No tight-fitting clothes
  - No medications that can worsen symptoms
- **Pharmacological therapy**
  - Step 1: Antacids and over-the-counter (OTC) acid suppressants (H_2 receptor antagonists, omeprazole) can be used initially on an as-needed basis for intermittent or mild symptoms. If symptoms persist after 2 weeks, proceed to Step 2.
  - Step 2: PPI or H_2 receptor antagonist (can be used at higher prescription doses).
    » PPIs are considered more effective than H_2 receptor antagonists.
  - A promotility agent (e.g., metoclopramide) can be used as adjunctive therapy, if needed.

Peptic Ulcer Disease

The goals of therapy are to relieve symptoms, promote healing of the ulcer, eradicate *H. pylori* (if present), prevent recurrence, and prevent complications.

- **Lifestyle modifications:** Reduce stress, smoking cessation, discontinue NSAID use, avoid foods that can worsen symptoms
- **Pharmacological therapy**
  - *H. pylori* associated ulcers: PPI + two antibiotics (usually clarithromycin and amoxicillin); duration = 10–14 days. If this therapy fails, four-drug therapy should be used (PPI + bismuth + metronidazole + tetracycline); duration = 14 days.
  - NSAID-induced ulcers
    - » Treatment:
      - First-line therapy: PPI (duration of therapy = 6–8 weeks; may be longer if recurrent symptoms, heavy smoker, or continued NSAID use)
      - Second-line therapies: Misoprostol or H_2 receptor antagonist
    - » Primary prevention:
      - Recommendations based on whether patient is at low, moderate, or high risk for NSAID GI toxicity (see Definitions) and the patient's risk for CV disease; high CV risk is defined by the patient's need for low-dose aspirin to prevent future CV events

	Low GI Risk	Moderate GI Risk	High GI Risk
Low CV Risk	NSAID alone	NSAID + PPI/misoprostol	Alternative therapy, if possible; or, cyclooxygenase-2 inhibitor + PPI/misoprostol
High CV Risk	Naproxen + PPI/misoprostol	Naproxen + PPI/misoprostol	Avoid NSAIDS or cyclooxygenase-2 inhibitors; use alternative therapy

Antacids

Generic	Brand	Dose	Contra-indications	Primary Side Effects	Key Monitoring	Pertinent Drug Interactions	Med Pearl	Top 200
Mechanism of action – neutralize stomach acid and ↑ gastric pH								
Magnesium hydroxide/ aluminum hydroxide	Maalox, Mylanta	15 mL with meals and at bedtime	None	• Diarrhea (from magnesium [Mg^{2+}]) • Constipation (from aluminum [Al^{3+}] or calcium [Ca^{2+}])	S/S GERD	• May bind to numerous drugs (separate from other drugs by at least 2 hrs) • May ↓ absorption of drug whose absorption is pH-dependent (e.g., itraconazole, ketoconazole, iron, atazanavir)	Use Mg^{2+}- and Al^{3+}-containing products with caution in patients with renal dysfunction	No
Calcium carbonate	Tums, Rolaids, Maalox Chewables	1–2 tabs q2h as needed						No

H₂ Receptor Antagonists

Generic	Brand	Dose	Dosage Forms	Primary Side Effects	Key Monitoring	Pertinent Drug Interactions	Med Pearl	Top 200
Mechanism of action – reversibly inhibit histamine (H_2) receptors in the gastric parietal cells, which inhibits secretion of gastric acid								
Cimetidine	Tagamet	200–1,600 mg/day	• Rx: Tabs, solution • OTC: Tabs	• Headache • Fatigue • Dizziness • Confusion • Gynecomastia (cimetidine)	S/S GERD/PUD	• Cimetidine inhibits CYP enzymes to greater extent than the other drugs (inhibits CYP1A2, CYP2C19, CYP2D6, and CYP3A4) • May ↓ absorption of drugs whose absorption is pH-dependent (e.g., itraconazole, ketoconazole, iron, atazanavir)	• Adjust dose of all drugs in renal dysfunction • Pepcid Complete also contains calcium carbonate + magnesium hydroxide	No
Famotidine	Pepcid	20–80 mg/day	• Rx: Tabs, suspension, injection • OTC: Tabs, gelcaps					Yes
Nizatidine	Axid	150–300 mg/day	• Rx: Caps, solution • OTC: Tabs					No
Ranitidine	Zantac	75–300 mg/day	• Rx: Tabs, effervescent tabs, syrup, injection • OTC: Tabs					Yes

Proton Pump Inhibitors

Generic	Brand	Dose	Dosage Forms	Primary Side Effects	Key Monitoring	Pertinent Drug Interactions	Med Pearl	Top 200
Mechanism of action — irreversibly inhibit H$^+$/K$^+$-ATPase in gastric parietal cells, which inhibits secretion of gastric acid								
Dexlansoprazole	Dexilant	30–60 mg/day	Caps	• Diarrhea • Headache	S/S GERD/PUD	• May ↓ absorption of drugs whose absorption is pH-dependent (e.g., itraconazole, ketoconazole, iron, atazanavir) • May ↓ antiplatelet effects of clopidogrel	• Zegerid = omeprazole + sodium bicarbonate (available as caps or suspension) • Vimovo = omeprazole + naproxen • May be associated with: • Osteoporosis-related fractures • ↓ Mg^{2+} • ↑ risk of *Clostridium difficile*	No
Esomeprazole	Nexium	20–40 mg/day	Caps, granules for suspension, injection					Yes
Lansoprazole	Prevacid	15–30 mg/day	Caps, orally disintegrating tabs OTC: Caps					Yes
Omeprazole	Prilosec	20 mg/day	Rx: Caps, granules for subpension OTC: Tabs					Yes
Pantoprazole	Protonix	20–40 mg/day	Tabs, granules for suspension, injection					Yes
Rabeprazole	Aciphex	20 mg/day	Tabs					Yes

Promotility Drug

Generic	Brand	Dose	Contra-indications	Primary Side Effects	Key Monitoring	Pertinent Drug Interactions	Med Pearl	Top 200
Mechanism of action — dopamine antagonist; ↑ LES pressure and accelerates gastric emptying								
Metoclopramide	Reglan, Metozolv ODT	40–60 mg/day	Seizures	• Dizziness • Sedation • Diarrhea • Extrapyramidal symptoms (EPS)	• S/S GERD • EPS	Use with antipsychotic agents may ↑ risk of EPS	• Can also be used for diabetic gastroparesis; erythromycin is an alternative • ↓ dose in renal dysfunction	No

Mucosal Protectant Drug

Mechanism of action – nonabsorbable aluminum salt that forms bonds with damaged and normal GI tissue; complex forms protective cover over ulcerated area

Generic	Brand	Dose	Contra-indications	Primary Side Effects	Key Monitoring	Pertinent Drug Interactions	Med Pearl	Top 200
Sucralfate	Carafate	4 g/day	None	Constipation	S/S PUD	May bind to numerous drugs (separate from other drugs by at least 2 hrs)	• Use cautiously in patients with chronic kidney disease (↑ risk of Al^{3+} toxicity) • Limited value in treatment of GERD; more useful in treatment of PUD	Yes

Prostaglandin Analog

Mechanism of action – prostaglandin E1 analog; replaces protective prostaglandins inhibited by NSAID therapy

Generic	Brand	Dose	Contraindications	Primary Side Effects	Key Monitoring	Pertinent Drug Interactions	Med Pearl	Top 200
Misoprostol	Cytotec	400–800 mcg/day	Pregnancy (abortifacient) (Pregnancy Category X)	Diarrhea	S/S PUD	None	• Women of childbearing age should have pregnancy test before initiating therapy; educate regarding appropriate use of contraception • Can also be used for medical termination of pregnancy	No

Helicobacter pylori Treatment Regimens (for PUD)

Proton Pump Inhibitor	Drug #2	Drug #3	Drug #4	Comments
Three-Drug Regimen (PPI + two antibiotics; duration of therapy = 10–14 days; 14 days preferred)				
Esomeprazole 40 mg daily OR lansoprazole 30 mg 2x daily OR omeprazole 20 mg 2x daily OR pantoprazole 40 mg 2x daily OR rabeprazole 20 mg 2x daily	Amoxicillin 1,000 mg 2x daily	Clarithromycin 500 mg 2x daily		• Metronidazole (500 mg 2x daily) can be used instead of amoxicillin or clarithromycin in patients with penicillin or macrolide allergy, respectively • Rabeprazole regimen should be given for 7 days • Prevpac is a compliance package that contains individual units of lansoprazole, amoxicillin, and clarithromycin
Four-Drug Regimen (PPI + bismuth subsalicylate + metronidazole + tetracycline; duration of therapy = 14 days)				
Esomeprazole 40 mg daily OR lansoprazole 30 mg 2x daily OR omeprazole 20 mg 2x daily OR pantoprazole 40 mg 2x daily OR rabeprazole 20 mg daily	Bismuth subsalicylate 525 mg 4x daily	Metronidazole 500 mg 3x daily	Tetracycline 500 mg 4x daily	• Pylera contains bismuth, metronidazole, and tetracycline in each capsule • Helidac is a compliance package that contains individual units of bismuth, metronidazole, and tetracycline • Can alternatively use H₂ antagonist instead of PPI (4-drug regimen given for 2 weeks and then H₂ antagonist alone continued for additional 2 weeks)

Storage and Administration Pearls

- Esomeprazole
  - May be administered via nasogastric (NG) or orogastric (OG) tube
    » Capsules: Open the capsule and mix with water
    » Granules for oral suspension: Dilute granules in water
  - Capsules can be opened and mixed with applesauce (eat immediately)
- Lansoprazole
  - May be administered via NG or OG tube
    » Capsules: Open the capsule and mix with apple juice
    » Orally disintegrating tablets: Dilute tablet in water
  - Capsules can be opened and mixed with applesauce, Ensure, pudding, cottage cheese, or yogurt (eat immediately); can also mix in orange, apple, or tomato juice
- Dexlansoprazole
  - Capsules can be opened and mixed with applesauce (eat immediately)
- Omeprazole
  - May be administered via NG or OG tube
    » Capsules: Open the capsule and mix with sodium bicarbonate
    » Granules for oral suspension: Dilute granules in water
  - Capsules can be opened and mixed with applesauce (eat immediately)
- Pantoprazole
  - May be administered via NG or OG tube
    » Granules for oral suspension: Dilute in apple juice
  - Tablets: Should **not** be crushed; **cannot** be given via NG or OG tube
  - Granules for oral suspension can be mixed in apple juice or sprinkled on applesauce
- Rabeprazole
  - Tablets should **not** be crushed; **cannot** be given via NG or OG tube
- Misoprostol should be administered with meals.
- Sucralfate should be administered 1 hour before meals.

Patient Education Pearls

- Lifestyle changes should be continued throughout the course of therapy.
- Patient should separate the administration of antacids from other medications by at least 2 hours.

- PPIs should be taken 15–30 minutes before breakfast; if patient is taking two daily doses, final dose should be taken before dinner (not at bedtime).

- A patient who is being treated for *H. pylori* should complete the entire course of therapy to facilitate eradication of the infection.

INFLAMMATORY BOWEL DISEASE

Definitions

Inflammatory bowel disease (IBD) is a broad-based term used to describe two conditions: ulcerative colitis (UC) and Crohn's disease (CD). UC is a chronic inflammatory disease that consists of superficial mucosal lesions localized to the colon and rectum. CD is also a chronic inflammatory disease, but is characterized by transmural lesions that can occur anywhere along the GI tract. The etiology of both of these disorders is thought to be due to immunologic or infectious causes; however, environmental, psychological, or genetic factors may also contribute to the development of these diseases.

Diagnosis

Diagnosis is suspected on the basis of clinical presentation, but is confirmed through various studies, including sigmoidoscopy, colonoscopy, barium enema, and stool examination. A biopsy of the lesions is usually performed during the sigmoidoscopy or colonoscopy.

Signs and Symptoms

The following symptoms can occur with both UC and CD: fever, diarrhea, weight loss, rectal bleeding, and abdominal pain.

Clinical Findings Associated with Ulcerative Colitis or Crohn's Disease

Clinical Finding	Ulcerative Colitis	Crohn's Disease
Abdominal mass	No	Yes
Fistulas/strictures	No	Yes
Bowel involvement	Rectum/colon	Can affect anywhere from mouth to anus (often affects ileum)
Systemic complications (i.e., extraintestinal involvement)	Yes	Yes
Toxic megacolon	Yes	No
At risk for colorectal cancer	Yes	Rare
Pattern of inflammation	Continuous	Segmented ("cobblestone" appearance)

Severity of Disease: Ulcerative Colitis

- Mild: >4 stools/day (with or without blood), no systemic signs of toxicity, and normal erythrocyte sedimentation rate (ESR)
- Moderate: >4 stools/day and minimal signs of toxicity
- Severe: >6 stools/day (with blood) and evidence of toxicity (e.g., fever, tachycardia, anemia, or elevated ESR)

Severity of Disease: Crohn's Disease

- Mild-moderate: Ambulatory and able to tolerate oral intake without evidence of dehydration, systemic toxicity, abdominal tenderness, painful mass, intestinal obstruction, or >10% weight loss
- Moderate-severe: Fail to respond to treatment for mild-moderate disease or have fever, significant weight loss (>10%), abdominal mass/tenderness, intermittent nausea/vomiting (without findings of obstruction), or significant anemia
- Severe/fulminant: Persistent symptoms despite the initiation of treatment with corticosteroids or biologic agents as outpatients or presenting with high fevers, persistent vomiting, evidence of intestinal obstruction, significant peritoneal signs (e.g., rebound tenderness, cachexia, or evidence of abscess)

Guidelines

Guidelines for the treatment of ulcerative colitis (American College of Gastroenterology). *Am J Gastroenterol*, no. 105 (2010): 501–23.

Guidelines for the treatment of Crohn's disease (American College of Gastroenterology). *Am J Gastroenterol*, no. 104 (2009): 465–83.

GUIDELINES SUMMARY

The goals of therapy are to induce and maintain remission, to prevent and resolve complications and systemic symptoms, and to maintain quality of life. There is no pharmacologic cure for these diseases; therefore, treatment focuses on management of symptoms.

- **Nonpharmacologic therapy**
  - Lifestyle changes/diet: Avoid foods that may worsen disease symptoms
  - Possible surgery when complications (e.g., fistulas, strictures, perforation) develop or to manage refractory disease

- **Pharmacologic therapy**
  - Adjunctive therapies: antidiarrheals (e.g., loperamide), antispasmodics (e.g., dicyclomine, propantheline, hyoscyamine)
  - Ulcerative colitis:
    » Treatment based upon whether inflammation is distal (below the splenic flexure; topical therapy appropriate) or extensive (proximal to the splenic flexure; requires systemic therapy)
    » Mild/moderate distal disease:
      - Active disease: Topical mesalamine (enema or suppository preferred), oral aminosalicylate, topical corticosteroid
      - Maintenance of remission: Topical mesalamine or oral aminosalicylate
    » Mild/moderate extensive disease:
      - Active disease: Oral aminosalicylate (first-line), oral corticosteroids, azathioprine, 6-mercaptopurine, infliximab
      - Maintenance of remission: Oral aminosalicylate (first-line), azathioprine, 6-mercaptopurine, infliximab
    » Severe disease:
      - Infliximab (if urgent hospitalization not needed), intravenous (IV) corticosteroids (if urgent hospitalization needed), IV cyclosporine
  - Crohn's disease:
    » Mild/moderate active disease:
      - First-line: Oral aminosalicylate, budesonide (disease localized to ileum and/or right colon)
      - Second-line: Metronidazole, ciprofloxacin
    » Moderate/severe disease:
      - First-line: Prednisone
      - Second-line: Infliximab, adalimumab, certolizumab pegol, natalizumab, methotrexate (intramuscularly [IM] or subcutaneously [SC])
    » Severe/fulminant disease:
      - First-line: IV corticosteroids
      - Second-line: IV cyclosporine or IV tacrolimus
    » Maintenance therapy:
      - First line: Azathioprine, 6-mercaptopurine, methotrexate, infliximab, adalimumab, certolizumab pegol, or natalizumab

Aminosalicylates

Mechanism of action – ↓ inflammation in GI tract by inhibiting prostaglandin synthesis and subsequent production of various immune mediators; sulfasalazine is cleaved in colon to mesalamine (responsible for therapeutic effect) + sulfapyridine (causes side effects); olsalazine and balsalazide also contain mesalamine

Generic	Brand	Dose	Dosage Forms	Contra-indications	Primary Side Effects	Key Monitoring	MedPearl	Top 200
Sulfasalazine	Azulfidine, Azulfidine EN	• Induction: 3–4 g/day • Maintenance: 2 g/day	Tabs, delayed-release (enteric-coated) tabs	• Aspirin allergy • Sulfa allergy • G6PD deficiency • Pregnancy (near term)	• Stevens-Johnson syndrome • Photosensitivity • Nausea/vomiting (N/V) • Headache • Folate deficiency • Hemolytic anemia • Agranulocytosis • Hepatitis	• S/S IBD • Liver function tests (LFTs) (with sulfasalazine) • Complete blood count (CBC) (with sulfasalazine)	• Mesalamine, olsalazine, and balsalazide are not sulfa derivatives; are poorly absorbed from GI tract (better tolerated than sulfasalazine) • Folic acid should be given to patients on sulfasalazine • Sulfasalazine may ↑ effects of warfarin and oral hypoglycemics • All may ↓ absorption of digoxin	No
Mesalamine	Apriso, Asacol, Canasa, Lialda, Pentasa, Rowasa	• Oral: *Induction* 2.4–4.8 g/day; *Maintenance,* 1.5–4 g/day • Rectal enema (Rowasa): 4 g at bedtime • Rectal suppository (Canasa): 1 g at bedtime	Controlled-release caps, delayed-release tabs, rectal enema, rectal suppository	• Aspirin allergy • G6PD deficiency	• Nausea • Diarrhea • Headache • Malaise			Yes
Olsalazine	Dipentum	1–3 g/day	Caps					No
Balsalazide	Colazal	1.5–6.75 g/day	Caps					No

Corticosteroids

Generic	Brand	Dose	Dosage Forms	Contra-indications	Primary Side Effects	Key Monitoring	Med Pearl	Top 200
Mechanism of action – quickly ↓ inflammation during acute exacerbations of IBD								
Budesonide	Entocort EC	• Initial: 9 mg 1x daily for up to 2 mo • Maintenance: 6 mg 1x daily for up to 3 mo	Enteric-coated caps	None	• Hyperglycemia • ↑ appetite • Insomnia • Hypertension • Edema • Adrenal suppression • Osteoporosis • Cataracts • Delayed wound healing	• S/S IBD • Blood glucose • Blood pressure (BP) • Electrolytes	• Should only be used to treat acute exacerbation (4–8 wks) and then tapered • IV therapy given for severe exacerbations for 7–10 days, then switched to oral therapy • Budesonide has localized effect; has minimal systemic side effects	Yes
Methylprednisolone	Solu-Medrol	10–100 mg/day	Injection, tabs					Yes
Prednisone	Sterapred	20–60 mg/day	Tabs					Yes

Immunosuppressants

Generic	Brand	Dose	Contra-indications	Primary Side Effects	Key Monitoring	Pertinent Drug Interactions	Med Pearl	Top 200
Mechanism of action – ↓ production of inflammatory mediators (e.g., interleukins) through various mechanisms								
Azathioprine	Imuran	75–150 mg/day	• Pregnancy • Bone marrow suppression • Liver dysfunction	• Pancreatitis • Arthralgias • Nausea • Diarrhea • Rash • Bone marrow suppression • Hepatotoxicity	• Amylase/lipase (if symptoms) • CBC with differential • LFTs	• Allopurinol and febuxostat may ↑ risk of side effects (↓ azathioprine dose by 75% when used with allopurinol; avoid concomitant use with febuxostat) • Aminosalicylates may ↑ risk of side effects • May ↓ effects of warfarin	• 6-mercaptopurine is active metabolite of azathioprine • Adjust dose in patients with renal dysfunction	No
6-Mercaptopurine	Purinethol	50–100 mg/day						No
Cyclosporine	Sandimmune	4–8 mg/kg/day IV	Renal failure	• Hypertension • Nephrotoxicity • Hypomagnesemia • Infection • Anaphylaxis	• BP • Blood urea nitrogen (BUN)/serum creatinine (SCr) • Electrolytes • S/S infection • Cyclosporine levels	• Cyclosporine is a CYP3A4 substrate and inhibitor • CYP3A4 inhibitors may ↑ levels/toxicity • CYP3A4 inducers may ↓ effects • May ↑ effects of other CYP3A4 substrates	• Used only for severe disease that has not responded to corticosteroids • Used only for 7–10 days	No
Methotrexate	Rheumatrex	15–25 mg/wk IM or SC	• Pregnancy • Bone marrow suppression • Severe renal or hepatic dysfunction	• Hepatotoxicity • Bone marrow suppression • Pneumonitis • Rash • N/V • Diarrhea	• LFTs • CBC with differential • Chest x-ray (if symptoms)	• NSAIDs and salicylates ↑ risk of toxicity • Penicillins, sulfonamides, and tetracyclines may ↑ risk of toxicity	• Only effective for CD (useful for steroid-dependent and steroid-refractory CD) • Adjust dose in patients with renal dysfunction	Yes

Biological Agents

Mechanism of action – inhibits tumor necrosis factor

Generic	Brand	Dose	Contra-indications	Primary Side Effects	Key Monitoring	Pertinent Drug Interactions	Med Pearl	Top 200
Adalimumab	Humira	160 mg SC on day 1 or over 2 days, then 80 mg 2 wk later (day 15), then 40 mg every other wk beginning day 29	None	• Headache • Rash • Injection site reactions • Hypertension • Infection (especially tuberculosis or fungal infections) • Lymphoma • Heart failure exacerbation • Bone marrow suppression • Lupus-like syndrome	• S/S infection • S/S heart failure • CBC with differential	Do not administer live vaccines	• PPD should be done before initiating treatment • Only approved for moderately to severely active CD in patients who have not responded despite adequate therapy with a corticosteroid or immunosuppressant	No
Certolizumab pegol	Cimzia	400 mg SC at 0, 2, and 4 wks; then 400 mg every 4 wks	None	• Headache • Nausea • Hypersensitivity reactions • Hypertension • Infection (especially tuberculosis or fungal infections) • Lymphoma • Heart failure exacerbation • Bone marrow suppression • Lupus-like syndrome				
Infliximab	Remicade	5 mg/kg IV at 0, 2, and 6 wks; then every 8 wks	• NYHA class III or IV heart failure (for doses >5 mg/kg) • Active infection	• Infusion reactions (hypotension, fever, chills, urticaria, pruritus) • Delayed hypersensitivity (fever, rash, myalgia, headache, sore throat) • Infection (especially tuberculosis or fungal infections) • Heart failure exacerbation • Bone marrow suppression • Lymphoma • Hepatitis	• BP • LFTs • S/S infection • S/S heart failure • CBC with differential	Do not administer live vaccines	• Delayed hypersensitivity reaction may occur 3–12 days after administration • PPD should be done before initiating treatment • Approved for moderately to severely active CD in patients who have not responded despite adequate therapy with a corticosteroid or immunosuppressant • Also indicated for patients with UC who are steroid refractory or steroid-dependent despite conventional therapy	No

Biological Agents *(cont'd)*

Mechanism of action — ↓ inflammation by binding to α4-subunit of integrins; for patients with moderate to severely active CD who are refractory to or unable to tolerate conventional therapies and anti-TNF monoclonal antibody therapy

Generic	Brand	Dose	Contra-indications	Primary Side Effects	Key Monitoring	Pertinent Drug Interactions	Med Pearl	Top 200
Natalizumab	Tysabri	300 mg IV every 4 wks; discontinue if no response by week 12	Progressive multifocal leukoencephalopathy (PML); concurrent use of tumor necrosis factor inhibitors	• Headache • Fatigue • Depression • Rash • Nausea • Arthralgia • Infusion reactions • PML (may be fatal) • Infection • Hepatotoxicity	• S/S PML • Brain MRI (at baseline) • S/S infection • LFTs	Do not administer live vaccines	• Patients need to be enrolled in TOUCH program • Must be administered as monotherapy • Only approved for CD	No

STORAGE AND ADMINISTRATION PEARLS

- Patients receiving infliximab should be pretreated with antihistamines (H_1 and H_2 blockers), acetaminophen, and/or corticosteroid to prevent infusion-related reaction.
- Infliximab should be administered as an IV infusion over 2 hours.
- Natalizumab should be administered as an IV infusion over 1 hour.
- If switching from prednisone to budesonide, prednisone should be tapered over a period of 2 weeks.

PATIENT EDUCATION PEARLS

- Adherence to medication is very important as disease exacerbations can have a significant impact on quality of life.
- Mesalamine enemas and suppositories should be administered at bedtime to allow for direct contact of the drug with the rectal mucosa for at least 8 hours.
- Live vaccines should not be administered if a patient is receiving biological agents.
- Patients receiving azathioprine, 6-mercaptopurine, methotrexate, infliximab, adalimumab, or certolizumab pegol are at increased risk for infection. They should wash their hands frequently and avoid crowds or other persons who are sick.
- Patients taking sulfasalazine should wear sunscreen and protective clothing. Sulfasalazine should be taken with meals to minimize GI effects. Patients taking sulfasalazine should take folic acid (1 mg/day) to prevent folate deficiency. Sulfasalazine may cause an orange discoloration of body fluids (urine, tears), which may stain clothing and contact lenses.
- Women receiving azathioprine, 6-mercaptopurine, or methotrexate should be counseled on using appropriate contraceptive methods.
- NSAIDs and high-dose salicylates (not the doses of aspirin used for prevention of CV diseases) may increase the risk of methotrexate toxicity and should be avoided if the patient is receiving this immunosuppressant.

LEARNING POINTS

- **GERD/PUD**
  - Antacids should be separated from other medications by at least 2 hours because of the risk for binding and ↓ the absorption of these drugs.
  - The majority of PUD cases are caused by either *H. pylori* infection or NSAIDs.
  - Three-drug regimen (PPI + two antibiotics [usually clarithromycin and amoxicillin]) is recommended for treatment of *H. pylori* infection.

- The dosage of all H_2 antagonists needs to be adjusted in patients with renal insufficiency.
- Of all the H_2 antagonists, cimetidine is the most likely to be involved with drug interactions involving the CYP450 system.
- Of all the PPIs, only esomeprazole and pantoprazole are available as IV injection; also be familiar with the various dosage forms of the PPIs.

- **IBD**
  - Sulfasalazine should not be used in patients with sulfa allergies. The other aminosalicylates—mesalamine, olsalazine, and balsalazide—can be used in these patients.
  - Folic acid should be administered to patients receiving sulfasalazine to prevent folate deficiency.
  - Know the various dosage forms of the aminosalicylates.
  - Be familiar with the side effects of systemic corticosteroids.
  - Methotrexate is only effective for CD.
  - PPD should be performed prior to starting adalimumab, certolizumab pegol, or infliximab.
  - Infliximab is associated with infusion reactions; patients need to be pretreated with antihistamine, acetaminophen, and/or corticosteroid.
  - Natalizumab is associated with PML.

PRACTICE QUESTIONS

1. Remicade is the brand name for which of the following drugs?

    (A) Azathioprine
    (B) Budesonide
    (C) Cyclosporine
    (D) Infliximab
    (E) Balsalazide

2. Which of the following is a contraindication for the use of metoclopramide?

    (A) Hyperkalemia
    (B) Myasthenia gravis
    (C) Porphyria
    (D) Seizure disorder
    (E) Sulfa allergy

ANSWERS

1. **D**

Remicade is the brand name for infliximab. Imuran is the brand name for azathioprine (A). Entocort EC is the brand name for oral budesonide (B). Sandimmune, Gengraf, and Neoral are brand names for cyclosporine (C). Colazal is the brand name for balsalazide (E).

2. **D**

Seizure disorder is a contraindication for the use of metoclopramide; therefore, choice (D) is correct.

Oncology

7

This chapter covers the following topics:

- **Hematologic malignancies (lymphoma and leukemia)**
- **Solid tumors (lung, colorectal, breast, prostate, and ovarian cancers)**
- **Supportive care**

 Suggested Study Time: **2 hours**

Since many of the drugs used in chemotherapy are indicated for multiple types of cancer, the background information for all of the hematologic malignancies and solid tumors will be discussed first, with the drug therapies described in a chart at the end of the section. Because cancer therapy is generally protocol-driven, your focus should be mostly on toxicities and on certain cases where a specific drug is indicated on the basis of cell-surface markers such as CD20 or HER-2 overexpression. Supportive care (pain management, antinauseant and antiemetic agents, and colony-stimulating factors) is covered at the end of this chapter.

LYMPHOMA

Definitions

Lymphomas are tumors of the lymphoid cells. Hodgkin's lymphoma (or Hodgkin's disease, HD) is less common than other types of lymphoma and is marked by the presence of Reed-Steinberg cells. HD may have a genetic component and, while HD is not contagious, certain infections (particularly Epstein-Barr and human immunodeficiency virus [HIV]) may increase the risk of acquiring the disease. HD is more common in young adults (15–35 years) and those over 55.

Non-Hodgkin's lymphomas (NHLs) are a group of related cancers including follicular, diffuse large B-cell, and Burkitt's lymphoma. NHL is the seventh leading cause of cancer in the United States, and the incidence increases with age (median age of diagnosis is 50 years). Immunodeficiency and infections are risk factors for NHL, as is prior chemotherapy. The various types of NHL are typified by proliferation of malignant B or T lymphocytes. The cancer may be classified as either aggressive (fast-growing) or indolent (slow-growing).

Diagnosis

HD

- Lymph node biopsy → Presence of Reed-Sternberg cells
- Computed tomography (CT) scan, magnetic resonance imaging (MRI), position emission tomography (PET) scan, or bone marrow biopsy to determine staging

NHL

- Lab values:
  - Elevated white blood cells (WBCs)
  - Lactate dehydrogenase levels may be high
- Lymph node or tissue biopsy
- Flow cytometry — cell surface marker analysis

Staging is the same for HD and NHL. Each stage is subdivided into A and B; B denotes the presence of systemic symptoms, specifically night sweats, weight loss, and fever:

- Stage 1: present in one lymph node or one part of tissue or organ
- Stage 2: present in ≥2 lymph nodes on the same side of the diaphragm
- Stage 3: present in lymph nodes above and below the diaphragm
- Stage 4: present in several parts of ≥1 tissues, or in an organ and distant lymph nodes
- Recurrent: disease returns after remission

Signs and Symptoms

HD

- Painless enlargement of lymph nodes, especially in the neck
- Fever, night sweats, and/or weight loss
- Malaise
- Possible bone pain

NHL

- Swollen lymph nodes on neck, underarms, and groin
- Fever, weight loss, and night sweats
- Fatigue
- Weakness

Guidelines

National Comprehensive Cancer Network, Clinical Practice Guidelines in Oncology, Version 1.2012: Hodgkin Lymphoma – Full Report, 2012. www.nccn.org/professionals/physician_gls/PDF/hodgkins.pdf.

National Comprehensive Cancer Network, Clinical Practice Guidelines in Oncology, Version 2.2012: Non-Hodgkin's Lymphoma – Full Report, 2012. www.nccn.org/professionals/physician_gls/PDF/nhl.pdf.

Guidelines Summary

HD

- Gold standard: ABVD (Adriamycin [doxorubicin], bleomycin, vinblastine, dacarbazine)
- Also used:
  - Stanford V (mechlorethamine, doxorubicin, etoposide, vincristine, vinblastine, bleomycin, prednisone)
    - » Dose-intense, but cumulative doses are lower
    - » Reduces risks of infertility, secondary neoplasms, cardiac and pulmonary toxicity

NHL

- Gold standard—combination chemotherapy:
  - CHOP (cyclophosphamide, doxorubicin [hydroxydaunorubicin], vincristine [Oncovin], prednisolone), or
  - CVP (no doxorubicin)
- Rituximab used if CD20 antigen is expressed (>90% of B-cell lymphomas)
  - Pretreat with diphenhydramine, steroids, H_2 antagonist
  - May be added to CHOP or CVP
  - Ibritumomab tiuxetan and tositumomab iodine 131 also target CD20
- Radiation therapy: Standard of care for early-stage follicular lymphoma, localized diffuse large B-cell lymphoma
- Relapsing cases: May require bone marrow transplantation

- Single-agent chemotherapy: May work for indolent cases (alkylating agents, purine nucleoside analogs).

Specific dosing depends on disease stage.

LEUKEMIA

Definitions

The leukemias are a group of blood malignancies characterized by unregulated growth of blood-forming cells in the bone marrow. These immature white cells crowd out normal cells in the bone marrow, leading to low red cell, white cell, and platelet counts. Four major types of leukemia exist: Acute lymphocytic (ALL), acute myeloid (AML), chronic lymphocytic (CLL), and chronic myeloid (CML) leukemias. Acute leukemias worsen rapidly; chronic leukemias worsen slowly. Exposure to radiation and chemicals (particularly benzene and formaldehyde) can increase leukemia risk.

Although the overall incidence of acute leukemias is low, they are the most common cancers in children, and ALL is the leading cause of cancer-related death in those under 35 years. AML occurs with increasing frequency in the elderly.

Diagnosis

- Bone marrow biopsy → Send for morphologic examination
- AML diagnosis requires 20% blasts

Signs and Symptoms

- Weight loss, fatigue, malaise
- Palpitations and dyspnea on exertion
- Fever and chills; night sweats
- Bruising
- Bone pain

Guidelines

National Comprehensive Cancer Network, Clinical Practice Guidelines in Oncology, Version 2.2011: Acute Myeloid Leukemia – Full Report, 2011. www.nccn.org/professionals/physician_gls/PDF/aml.pdf.

National Comprehensive Cancer Network, Clinical Practice Guidelines in Oncology, Version 2.2012: Chronic Myelogenous Leukemia – Full Report, 2012. www.nccn.org/professionals/physician_gls/PDF/cml.pdf.

Guidelines Summary

AML

- Anthracyclines (i.e., idarubicin, daunorubicin) and cytarabine are the most active agents.
- Duration of remission is generally short; postremission therapy to prevent or delay relapse includes:
  - High-dose cytarabine
  - Allogenic or autologous hematopoietic stem cell transplantation (HSCT, bone marrow transplant)

CML

- Philadelphia chromosome: abnormality characteristic of CML.
  - Results in *bcr-abl* fusion gene
  - Bone marrow makes tyrosine kinase enzyme; causes too many stem cells to form into WBCs
- Tyrosine kinase inhibitors (imatinib, nilotinib, or dasatinib):
  - Target *bcr-abl* fusion gene
  - First-line treatment
- Interferon and conventional chemotherapy no longer considered first-line
- Allogenic HSCT (alloHSCT): curative in many CML patients
  - Mortality is high
  - Busulfan and interferon-α increase post-transplant complications
  - Matched donor and younger age (<50 years) required
  - No longer considered first-line

The National Comprehensive Cancer Network does not give guidelines for lymphocytic leukemias. Although protocols vary, methotrexate and cytarabine are commonly used in ALL. CLL is not currently considered curable; however, due to its often indolent time course, patients may live for years after diagnosis. Several biologic therapies targeting antigens expressed on B lymphocytes may be useful in appropriate cases of lymphocytic leukemia.

- Rituximab: Targets CD20
- Alemtuzumab: Targets CD52

LUNG CANCER

Definitions

Lung cancer is the leading cause of cancer death in men and women. Most lung cancers are non-small cell (NSCLC); while this type of cancer is slow-growing, it does not respond well to chemotherapy and only about 14% of patients can be cured. Small-cell lung cancer (SCLC) is very aggressive and, though it is chemotherapy-sensitive, most patients die within 2 years of diagnosis. Smoking is the primary risk factor for lung cancer; over 80% of patients have a history of smoking. Occupational exposure to asbestos, radon, and other agents may also increase risk, as can certain genetic abnormalities and family history of the disease.

Diagnosis

- Chest x-ray, CT scans, and PET scan to detect lesions and determine extent of disease
- Pathological confirmation by sputum cytology or tumor biopsy

Signs and Symptoms

- Cough—most common
- Other lung-related symptoms (sputum production, dyspnea, wheezing); often misattributed to concomitant pulmonary conditions
- Weight loss, fever, bone pain
- Paraneoplastic syndromes:
  - Occur in 10% of cases; may be first sign or symptom
  - Inappropriate secretion of antidiuretic hormone (SIADH)
  - Hypercalcemia
  - Eaton-Lambert myasthenic syndrome: muscle weakness and autonomic dysfunction

Guidelines

National Comprehensive Cancer Network, Clinical Practice Guidelines in Oncology, Version 2.2012: Non-Small Cell Lung Cancer–Full Report, 2012. www.nccn.org/professionals/physician_gls/PDF/nscl.pdf.

National Comprehensive Cancer Network, Clinical Practice Guidelines in Oncology, Version 2.2010: Small Cell Lung Cancer–Full Report, 2010. www.nccn.org/professionals/physician_gls/PDF/sclc.pdf.

Guidelines Summary

- Early-stage NSCLC: Surgical resection is the treatment of choice
- Radiation and chemotherapy: May also be used, and preferred with SCLC
- Advanced disease:
  - Cisplatin-based combination therapy
  - Bevacizumab is used in cases with vascular endothelial growth factor (VEGF) overexpression
  - Erlotinib used if patients have epidermal growth factor receptor (EGFR) mutation
  - Crizotinib used if patients are anaplastic lymphoma kinase (ALK) positive
- Recurrent disease:
  - Docetaxel or pemetrexed
  - Erlotinib in cases with EGFR overexpression; works only in small subset of patients

COLORECTAL CANCER

Definitions

Colorectal cancer is the third leading cause of cancer death in the United States. Incidence is highest in industrialized countries and may be linked to a higher-fat, lower-fiber diet in such locations. Genetic predisposition also plays a role in 5–10% of cases. Primary prevention strategies involve dietary change (increase calcium, fiber, and antioxidants and decrease fat).

Diagnosis

- Fecal occult blood testing (FOBT) may decrease cancer mortality by one-third, but has a high false-negative rate as many early stage tumors do not bleed.
- FOBT plus immunochemical assays lead to improved specificity and sensitivity.
- Flexible sigmoidoscopy can detect lesions in distal and sigmoid colon; early detection and excision can decrease mortality by 60%.
- Colonoscopy is preferred screening method as it shows entire colon, but it requires more bowel preparation.
- Double-contrast barium enema plus flexible sigmoidoscopy may be used instead of colonoscopy.

Signs and Symptoms

- Change in bowel habits (diarrhea, constipation, stools narrower than usual)
- Rectal bleeding/blood in the stool
- Nausea, vomiting, and abdominal discomfort (gas pains or cramps, bloating)

- Fatigue (generally related to anemia)
- Weight loss
- Leg edema (result of lymph node involvement)
- Hepatomegaly and jaundice

Guidelines

National Comprehensive Cancer Network, Clinical Practice Guidelines in Oncology, Version 3.2012: Colon Cancer – Full Report, 2012. www.nccn.org/professionals/physician_gls/PDF/colon.pdf.

Guideline Summary

- Surgical resection is treatment of choice (Stages I–III)
  - Complete resection of tumor and adjacent sections of tumor-free bowel; regional lymphadenectomy
- Adjuvant radiation therapy and chemotherapy: may be indicated for Stage II; standard therapy for Stage III
- Most common: 5-fluorouracil (5-FU) with leucovorin to enhance cytotoxicity
  - Alternative therapies include oxaliplatin + leucovorin + 5-fluorouracil OR capecitabine
- Biologic therapies gaining popularity:
  - Bevacizumab: Targets VEGF
  - Cetuximab or panitumumab: Targets EGFR

BREAST CANCER

Definitions

Breast cancer is the most common cancer in women and is second only to lung cancer as a cause of cancer death in women. Family history plays a large role in the development of breast cancer, with mutations in the *BRCA1/BRCA2* tumor suppressor genes leading to high risk. Long-term progestin use and other endocrine factors (early menarche, late menopause, advanced age at first pregnancy) and lifestyle factors (high fat intake, alcohol consumption, obesity) also increase risk of developing breast cancer. Prognosis is poor in younger (<35 years) and premenopausal patients, African Americans, and those with *HER2/neu* overexpression.

Diagnosis

- Palpable mass on physical examination
- Breast imaging techniques: mammography and/or ultrasound
- Biopsy if mass or cluster of calcifications is detected

Signs and Symptoms

- May be asymptomatic
- Painless lump: Initial sign in 90% of patients
- Stabbing or aching pain is initial sign in remaining 10%
- Nipple discharge, retraction, dimpling
- Scaly, red, or swollen skin of breast or nipple
- Advanced disease: Bone pain, difficulty breathing, jaundice, abdominal enlargement, mental status changes

Guidelines

National Comprehensive Cancer Network, Clinical Practice Guidelines in Oncology, Version 1.2012: Breast Cancer – Full Report, 2012. www.nccn.org/professionals/physician _gls/PDF/breast.pdf.

Guideline Summary

- Early-stage treatment: Surgery and chemotherapy, with possible radiation therapy
- Adjuvant chemotherapy:
  - Anthracyclines: Most active against breast cancer
  - Taxanes
- Adjuvant endocrine therapy:
  - Antiestrogens: Tamoxifen gold standard in premenopausal women
  - Aromatase inhibitors: Anastrazole, letrozole, exemestane (more effective than tamoxifen in postmenopausal women)
- In metastatic cancer, endocrine therapy given first, then chemotherapy.
- Biologic therapy:
  - Trastuzumab: If tumor overexpresses *HER2/neu*; do not give with anthracyclines (additive cardiotoxicity)
  - Lapatinib: Targets *HER2/neu* and EGFR

PROSTATE CANCER

Definitions

Prostate cancer is the most common cancer in men, and the second most common cause of cancer death in men. One-third to one-half of men present with advanced disease, for which there is no cure. High-fat diet and hormonal factors are two of the primary risk factors; as prostate cancer is androgen-dependent, high levels of testosterone can fuel tumor growth. This may explain the increased incidence in African-American men, who generally have testosterone levels 15% higher than Caucasian men.

Diagnosis

- Transrectal ultrasound or cystoscopy
- Biopsy: Only sure method of diagnosis

Signs and Symptoms

- Elevated prostate-specific antigen (PSA)
- Nodule on digital rectal exam of the prostate
- Localized disease: Generally asymptomatic; symptoms of prostatic enlargement may indicate cancer, benign prostatic hyperplasia, or infection; further investigation warranted
  - Urinary difficulty
  - Difficulty in having an erection
  - Blood in the urine or semen
- Advanced disease:
  - Bone pain
  - Anemia and fatigue
  - Weight loss
  - Back pain
  - Edema of the legs

Guidelines

National Comprehensive Cancer Network, Clinical Practice Guidelines in Oncology, Version 1.2012: Prostate Cancer – Full Report, 2012. www.nccn.org/professionals/physician _gls/PDF/prostate.pdf.

Guideline Summary

- Radiation therapy
- Prostatectomy
- Bilateral orchiectomy (removal of testes): Reduces androgen levels but unacceptable to many patients
- Endocrine therapy: Used to reduce androgen levels
- Luteinizing hormone-releasing hormone (LH-RH) agonists
  - Monotherapy is effective
  - Lower side effect profile
- Antiandrogens
  - Monotherapy is less effective than LH-RH agonists
  - No sexual dysfunction; more accepted by younger patients
- Combined hormonal blockade; small survival advantage, but large financial cost and additional toxicities

OVARIAN CANCER

Definitions

Ovarian cancer typically occurs postmenopause. Risk factors include family history of ovarian or breast cancer, personal history of other types of cancer, nulliparity, and long-term estrogen therapy (without progesterone). Genetics also play a role; breast cancer and ovarian cancer are linked to mutation in *BRCA1/BRCA2*, along with other genetic alterations.

Diagnosis

- Ovarian size/contour on pelvic exam
- Elevation of CA-125 (antigen common to most ovarian cancers)
- Pelvic ultrasound
- Biopsy

Signs and Symptoms

Symptoms may be vague and nonspecific, but may include:

- Fatigue
- Back pain
- Bloating, constipation, abdominal pain
- Palpable abdominal mass, abdominal distention
- Hepatic and renal function abnormalities

Guidelines

National Comprehensive Cancer Network, Clinical Practice Guidelines in Oncology, Version 2.2012: Ovarian Cancer – Full Report, 2012. www.nccn.org/professionals/physician _gls/PDF/ovarian.pdf.

Guideline Summary

- Surgery and chemotherapy are used; radiation therapy is not often included unless the cancer is confined to one or both ovaries.
- Drug treatment generally involves taxane (paclitaxel or docetaxel) and/or platinum therapy (carboplatin or cisplatin).

Oncology Drugs

Generic	Brand/Route of Administration	Contraindications	Primary Side Effects	Key Monitoring	Pertinent Drug Interactions	Med Pearl	Top 200
Mechanism of action – alkylating agents: alkylate DNA, making it more prone to breakage; most effective against rapidly dividing cells							
Cyclophosphamide	Cytoxan (IV and PO)	Hypersensitivity to any alkylating agent	• Alopecia • Hemorrhagic cystitis • Infertility • Nausea, vomiting (N/V), mucositis, stomatitis • Bone marrow suppression	• Complete blood count (CBC) with differential • Blood urea nitrogen (BUN)/serum creatinine (SCr) • Uric acid (UA)	CYP3A4 inducers may ↑ levels of active metabolite (acrolein)	• Maintain adequate hydration to avoid hemorrhagic cystitis; can also use mesna • Higher emetogenic potential • Tablets should be taken with food	No
Chlorambucil	Leukeran (PO)		• Bone marrow suppression • Infertility • Secondary leukemias • Seizures • Stevens-Johnson syndrome • Hepatotoxicity	• CBC with differential • LFTs	None	• Take on empty stomach • Avoid alcohol	No
Carmustine	• BiCNU (IV) • Gliadel (intracranial implant)		• Bone marrow suppression • Pulmonary fibrosis • Severe N/V • Hypotension (IV) • Secondary leukemias (with long-term use) • Reversible elevation of liver function tests (LFTs)	• CBC with differential • Pulmonary function tests • LFTs • Blood pressure (BP) (during IV administration)	IV solution contains ethanol; do not give aldehyde-dehydrogenase inhibitors	Very high emetogenic potential	No

Oncology Drugs *(cont'd)*

Mechanism of action – platinum-based agents: crosslink DNA, causing it to break

Generic	Brand/Route of Administration	Contraindications	Primary Side Effects	Key Monitoring	Pertinent Drug Interactions	Med Pearl	Top 200
Cisplatin	Platinol AQ (IV)	• Hypersensitivity to any platinum-containing compounds • Renal insufficiency • Pre-existing hearing impairment (cisplatin)	• Anaphylaxis • Dose-related myelosuppression • N/V • Ototoxicity (cisplatin) • Nephrotoxicity with cumulative doses (esp. cisplatin) • Peripheral neuropathy	• BUN/SCr • Electrolytes • Neurologic exam • CBC with differential • Urine output	• Administration with taxane derivatives may ↑ myelosuppression and ↓ efficacy of platinum agents • May ↓ digoxin levels (oxaliplatin)	• Do not administer doses exceeding 100 mg/m^2 every 3 wks • High emetogenic potential	No
Carboplatin	Paraplatin (IV)					Moderate emetogenic potential	No
Oxaliplatin	Eloxatin (IV)					• Moderate emetogenic potential • Warn patients to wear a scarf if being treated during cold weather to prevent laryngeal spasms	No

Mechanism of action – enzyme inhibitors: target enzymes responsible for DNA replication and repair

Generic	Brand/Route of Administration	Contraindications	Primary Side Effects	Key Monitoring	Pertinent Drug Interactions	Med Pearl	Top 200
Irinotecan	Camptosar (IV)	Concurrent therapy with ketoconazole or St. John's wort	• Bone marrow suppression • Severe, life-threatening diarrhea	• CBC with differential • Electrolytes (esp. if diarrhea)	• CYP3A4 substrate • CYP3A4 inhibitors may ↑ risk of toxicity • CYP3A4 inducers may ↓ effects	• Diarrhea may be early or late onset • High emetogenic potential	No
Etoposide	VePesid (IV and PO)	None	• Bone marrow suppression • Hepatotoxicity	• CBC with differential • LFTs	CYP3A4 substrate	• Do NOT give IV push (may cause hypotension) • Do NOT give IM (necrosis)	No

Oncology Drugs *(cont'd)*

Mechanism of action – antimitotics (spindle poisons): interfere with mitotic spindle; prevent chromosome segregation and lead to cell death

Generic	Brand/Route of Administration	Contraindications	Primary Side Effects	Key Monitoring	Pertinent Drug Interactions	Med Pearl	Top 200
Vincristine	Oncovin (IV)	None	• Peripheral neuropathy (dose-limiting) • Paralytic ileus (secondary to neurologic toxicity) • Hepatotoxicity	• Neurologic exam • LFTs • Change in frequency of bowel movements	None	• Do NOT give intrathecally (IT) (fatal) • All patients should be on a prophylactic bowel management regimen • Avoid extravasation (vesicant) • Should NOT exceed 2 mg/dose	No
Vinblastine	Velban (IV)	None	• Peripheral neuropathy • Bone marrow suppression (dose-limiting)	• CBC with differential • Neurologic exam	None	• Do not give intrathecally (fatal) • Avoid extravasation (vesicant)	No
Paclitaxel	Taxol (IV)	• Hypersensitivity to Cremophor • Absolute neutrophil count (ANC) <1,500/mm³ (ovarian, lung, or breast cancer) • ANC ≤1,000/mm³ (Kaposi's sarcoma)	• Bone marrow suppression (dose-limiting) • Peripheral neuropathy • Cardiac rhythm abnormalities • Hepatotoxicity • Mucositis, stomatitis (severe)	• CBC with differential • Electrocardiogram (ECG) • LFTs • Neurologic exam	• CYP2C8 and CYP3A4 substrate • Administer prior to platinum derivatives to limit myelosuppression and enhance efficacy	Pretreat with dexamethasone, diphenhydramine, and H₂-receptor antagonist	No
Paclitaxel protein-bound particles	Abraxane (IV)	Baseline neutrophils <1,500/mm³				No need for pretreatment	No
Docetaxel	Taxotere (IV)	• Hypersensitivity to polysorbate 80 • Baseline neutrophils <1,500/mm³ • Severe hepatic impairment	• Significant, dose-dependent fluid retention • Bone marrow suppression • Hypersensitivity reactions	• CBC with differential • LFTs • Weight, signs of edema	• CYP3A4 substrate • Administer prior to platinum derivatives to limit myelosuppression and enhance efficacy	• Avoid doses >100 mg/m² • Pretreat with corticosteroids for 1–5 days to prevent fluid retention and hypersensitivity reactions	No

Oncology Drugs *(cont'd)*

Generic	Brand/Route of Administration	Contraindications	Primary Side Effects	Key Monitoring	Pertinent Drug Interactions	Med Pearl	Top 200
Mechanism of action – antimetabolite nucleoside analogs							
Cytarabine	Cytosar-U (IV)	None	• Severe bone marrow suppression • Cytarabine syndrome: myalgia, bone pain, rash, conjunctivitis, and fever	CBC with differential	May ↓ levels of digoxin	• Pretreat with corticosteroid; may prevent cytarabine syndrome • May also be administered IM or subcutaneously (SC) • Moderate emetogenic potential	No
	DepoCyt (IT)	Active meningeal infection	• Chemical arachnoiditis (N/V, headache, and fever) • Neurotoxicity	Monitor closely for signs of immediate reactions and neurotoxicity	None reported; limited systemic exposure	• Co-administer dexamethasone to lessen chemical arachnoiditis • Moderate emetogenic potential	No
5-Fluorouracil	Adrucil (IV)	Dihydropyrimidine dehydrogenase (DPD) deficiency	• Hand-and-foot syndrome • N/V, diarrhea, mucositis, stomatitis • Bone marrow suppression	CBC with differential	May ↑ effects of warfarin	• Leucovorin ↑ effectiveness and toxicity; dose of fluorouracil may need to be ↓	No
Mechanism of action – antimetabolite folic acid antagonist							
Methotrexate	Trexall (PO) Generic (IV, IM, IT)	None	• Nephrotoxicity • Bone marrow suppression • Stevens-Johnson syndrome • Severe diarrhea and ulcerative stomatitis • Neurotoxicity • Hepatotoxicity	• CBC with differential • SCr • LFTs	NSAIDs may ↑ risk of toxicity	• Give leucovorin rescue 24 hrs after dosing to limit toxicity; do not administer concurrently • Can be given IT for leukemias • Also used SC as DMARD for rheumatoid arthritis	Yes

Oncology Drugs (cont'd)

Mechanism of action – anthracyclines: intercalate DNA and generate reactive oxygen species

Generic	Brand/Route of Administration	Contraindications	Primary Side Effects	Key Monitoring	Pertinent Drug Interactions	Med Pearl	Top 200
Daunorubicin	Cerubidine (IV)	Pre-existing severe myocardial insufficiency or arrhythmia	• Dose-related cardiotoxicity • Severe bone marrow suppression • Red coloration of body fluids	• CBC with differential • ECG • Left ventricular ejection fraction (LVEF)	↑ risk of cardiotoxicity with trastuzumab, cyclophosphamide, and taxane derivatives	• Greatest risk of irreversible myocardial damage at cumulative dose >550 mg/m² • Moderately emetogenic	No
Doxorubicin	Adriamycin (IV)		• Dose-related cardiotoxicity • Severe bone marrow suppression • Secondary leukemias • Red coloration of body fluids				

Oncology Drugs *(cont'd)*

Mechanism of action – hormonal agents: treat cancers in which growth is accelerated by hormones

Generic	Brand/Route of Administration	Contraindications	Primary Side Effects	Key Monitoring	Pertinent Drug Interactions	Med Pearl	Top 200
Leuprolide	Lupron (SC)	• Spinal cord compression • Undiagnosed abnormal vaginal bleeding	• Abnormal menses • Exacerbation of endometriosis	• Leutinizing hormone (LH) and follicle-stimulating hormone (FSH) levels • Serum testosterone (males), estradiol (females) • Bone mineral density	None	• Administered daily • Rotate injection sites	No
	Lupron depot (IM)		• Hot flashes/sweats • ↓ bone mineral density (if used >6 mo)			• Administered every 1–6 mo, depending on dosage • Rotate injection sites	No
	Eligard (SC depot formulation)		• Spinal cord compression and urinary tract obstruction in prostate cancer • Tumor flare • Depression, mood disturbaces				
Tamoxifen	Nolvadex (PO)	• Concurrent warfarin therapy • History of deep vein thrombosis (DVT) or pulmonary embolism	• Thromboembolic events • ↑ risk of endometrial cancer • Hot flashes • Altered menses • Mood disturbances, depression	Annual gynecologic exams	• CYP3A4 substrate • May ↑ effects of warfarin	• Bone pain may indicate a good therapeutic response; manage with mild analgesic • Used in premenopausal women with breast cancer • Should not exceed 5 years of therapy	No
Anastrozole	Arimidex (PO)	None	• ↓ bone mineral density • Hyperlipidemia • Mood disturbances	• Bone mineral density • Low-density lipoprotein (LDL) and total cholesterol	None	Used in postmenopausal women with breast cancer	Yes
Letrozole	Femara (PO)	None	• ↓ bone mineral density • Hyperlipidemia • Hot flashes	• Bone mineral density • LDL and total cholesterol	None	Used in postmenopausal women with breast cancer	No

Chemotherapy Agents: Common Adverse Effects

- Cardiotoxicity
  - Doxorubicin
  - Daunorubicin
  - Idarubicin
  - Mitoxantrone
  - Trastuzumab
- N/V
  - Cisplatin
  - Carboplatin
  - Cytarabine
  - Doxorubicin
  - Cyclophosphamide
- Mucositis
  - Cytarabine
  - Cyclophosphamide
  - 5-FU
  - Methotrexate
- Neuropathy
  - Vincristine
  - Vinblastine
  - Oxaliplatin
  - Paclitaxel
- Renal dysfunction
  - Cisplatin
  - Cyclophosphamide
  - Ifosfamide
- Pulmonary fibrosis
  - Bleomycin
  - Busulfan
- Infusion reactions
  - Monoclonal antibodies
  - Paclitaxel

Targeted and Biologic Agents

Monoclonal Antibodies

- Alemtuzumab (Campath) (IV)
  - Used for B-cell CLL (targeted against CD52 antigen)
  - Major toxicities: Infusion-related reactions, myelosuppression (prolonged)
  - Premedicate with diphenhydramine and acetaminophen
- Ibritumomab tiuxetan (Zevalin) (IV)
  - Used for CD20-positive, B-cell NHL (including rituximab-resistant)
  - Linked to a radioisotope that targets B cells, including malignant ones
  - Used in combination with rituximab as part of a two-step process using indium-111 (step 1) and yttrium-90 (step 2) ibritumomab tiuxetan
  - Major toxicities: Infusion-related reactions, myelosuppression (prolonged), secondary leukemia, myelodysplastic sydrome, Stevens-Johnson syndrome, toxic epidermal nectolysis, exfoliative dermatitis
  - Premedicate with diphenhydramine and acetaminophen
- Rituximab (Rituxan) (IV)
  - Used for CD20-positive, B-cell NHL
  - Also used for rheumatoid arthritis
  - Major toxicities: Infusion-related reactions, tumor lysis syndrome, Stevens-Johnson syndrome, toxic epidermal necrolysis, cardiotoxicity
  - Premedicate with diphenhydramine and acetaminophen
- Tositumumab (Bexxar) (IV)
  - Used for CD20-positive, follicular, NHL refractory to rituximab
  - Linked to a radioisotope (I-131) that targets B cells, including malignant ones
  - Adminstration involves two-step process
  - Major toxicities: Infusion-related reactions, myelosuppression (prolonged), secondary malignancy, hypothyroidism
  - Premedicate with diphenhydramine and acetaminophen

EGFR Inhibitors

- Cetuximab (Erbitux) (IV)
  - Used for squamous cell cancer of head and neck and colorectal cancer (EGFR positive)
  - Major toxicities: Infusion-related reactions, rash (can be severe)
  - Premedicate with diphenhydramine

- Erlotinib (Tarceva) (PO)
  - Used for locally advanced/metastatic NSCLC or locally advanced, surgically unresectable, or metastatic pancreatic cancer
  - Major toxicities: Rash (can be severe), diarrhea
  - CYP3A4 substrate
- Lapatinib (Tykerb) (PO)
  - Used for metastatic breast cancer with tumor overexpression of HER2
  - Major toxicities: Diarrhea, hepatotoxicity, rash (can be severe), QT interval prolongation
  - CYP3A4 substrate
- Trastuzumab (Herceptin) (IV)
  - Used for HER2-positive metastatic breast cancer
  - Major toxicities: Cardiotoxicity, infusion-related reactions (can be treated with diphenhydramine, acetaminophen, and meperidine), myelosuppression
  - Should not be used with anthracyclines (↑ risk for cardiotoxicity)

VEGF Inhibitors

- Bevacizumab (Avastin) (IV)
  - Used for metastatic colorectal cancer, locally advanced, recurrent or metastatic nonsquamous NSCLC, glioblastoma, and metastatic renal cell carcinoma
  - Major toxicities: Thromboembolic events, hypertension, bleeding
- Sunitinib (Sutent) (PO)
  - Used for gastrointestinal stromal tumor (GIST), renal cell carcinoma, and pancreatic neuroendocrine tumors
  - Major toxicities: Diarrhea, rash, hypertension, heart failure
  - CYP3A4 substrate
- Sorafenib (Nexavar) (PO)
  - Used for advanced renal cell carcinoma and unresectable hepatocellular carcinoma
  - Major toxicities: Diarrhea, rash, hypertension, hand-foot syndrome
  - CYP3A4 substrate

Tyrosine Kinase Inhibitors

- Dasatinib (Sprycel) (PO)
  - Used for CML and Philadelphia-positive (Ph+) ALL
  - Major toxicities: Myelosuppression, fluid retention
  - CYP3A4 substrate

- Imatinib (Gleevec) (PO)
  - Used for Ph+ CML, Kit (CD117)-positive GIST, Ph+ ALL, and a variety of other disorders
  - Major toxicities: Fluid retention, Stevens-Johnson syndrome
  - CYP3A4 substrate and inhibitor; CYP2D6 inhibitor

Storage and Administration Pearls

- Do not administer live vaccines during chemotherapy cycles.

Patient Education Pearls

- Patient should not breastfeed or attempt to become pregnant while taking chemotherapy.
- Because Bexxar and Zevalin contain radioactive isotopes, patients should be instructed on proper handwashing, special disposal of bodily waste, and other ways to limit exposure to family members postdischarge.

SUPPORTIVE CARE

Nausea and Vomiting

About 55% of cancer patients experience nausea and vomiting during the first week of chemotherapy. 5HT3 antagonists are useful in most cases, but should be used only for prevention of nausea and vomiting. Corticosteroids should be given unless contraindicated, as they are synergistic with the 5HT3 antagonists; other drug therapies depend on the type of nausea and vomiting experienced.

- Benzodiazepines: Treatment of choice for anticipatory nausea and vomiting (caused by the sights and smells of the chemotherapy environment)
- Aprepitant: Useful for delayed nausea and vomiting caused by drugs with high emetic potential (cisplatin, cyclophosphamide, doxorubicin)
- Prochlorperazine or metoclopramide: May be used in less severe cases

Pain Management

Pain is one of the most common symptoms associated with cancer and occurs in up to 75% of advanced cases, greatly affecting quality of life. Cancer pain frequently requires much higher analgesic doses than pain from other causes. As a result, cancer pain is often undertreated.

For uncontrolled pain, drug choice depends on prior opioid use and severity of pain. If opioids have not been used:

- Severe pain: Rapid titration with short-acting opioids
- Moderate pain: Slower titration with short-acting opioids
- Mild pain: NSAID, acetaminophen, or slow titration with short-acting opioids

Morphine, codeine, oxycodone, oxymorphone, hydromorphone, and fentanyl are the most commonly used opioids for cancer pain; all are short-acting agents unless given in a controlled-release dosage form. Controlled-release formulations are recommended only for non–opioid naïve patients, as they cannot be easily titrated. Methadone is occasionally used in cancer pain, and has a longer half-life and duration of action. Patients taking controlled-release formulations should also receive a prescription for a short-acting, fast-onset analgesic for breakthrough pain. Likewise, patient-controlled analgesia devices should have on-demand bolus doses available for acute pain, with a lockout setting to reduce the risk of overdose.

Management of Neutropenia and Anemia

Neutropenia and its major complication, neutropenic fever, are major concerns in many types of cancer. The nadir, or lowest, concentration of WBCs in the peripheral blood usually occurs 1–2 weeks following the administration of chemotherapy and is typically proportional to the dose. Subsequent chemotherapy is delayed until the ANC recovers, which explains the 3- to 4-week cycle length of most chemotherapy regimens. Classification of ANC is:

- Normal: 3,000–7,000 neutrophils/mm^3
- Mild neutropenia: 500–1,000/mm^3
- Moderate neutropenia: 100–500/mm^3
- Severe neutropenia: <100/mm^3

Colony-stimulating factors (CSF) such as filgrastim have been shown to shorten the duration of neutropenia, but they have little effect on mortality and are very expensive. CSFs do decrease hospitalizations, however, and clinical judgment should be used to determine which patients are most likely to benefit. Because infection leads to death in a large percentage of neutropenic patients (possibly up to 30%), anti-infective therapy is frequently needed. Broad-spectrum bactericidal antibiotics are generally used (third- and fourth-generation cephalosporins, carbapenems, or fluoroquinolones with or without aminoglycosides or β-lactams), with antipseudomonal activity being particularly important. If antifungal therapy is needed, amphotericin B is the drug of choice.

Anemia is also common in cancer patients. Treatment of anemia is currently the subject of much controversy; use of erythropoiesis-stimulating agents, including erythropoietin and darbepoetin, is no longer supported in myeloid malignancies (these agents have been associated with increase in mortality compared to patients not receiving erythropoietin). The hypothesis is that the drug may be stimulating cancer growth. These drugs should NOT be used in patients with myeloid malignancies who are receiving chemotherapy when the anticipated outcome is a cure. This finding may not apply to solid tumors; more information is needed.

Antiemetic Drugs

Generic	Brand	Dose	Contraindications	Primary Side Effects	Key Monitoring	Pertinent Drug Interactions	Med Pearl	Top 200
Mechanism of action – 5HT3 antagonists; prevent release of serotonin in GI mucosa								
Ondansetron	Zofran	16–24 mg PO or 8–12 mg IV	Current nausea and vomiting (useful only for prevention)	• Headache • Constipation or diarrhea	None	CYP3A4 substrate	• Single dose prior to chemotherapy; repeat doses do not ↑ effect • Palonosetron effective in preventing delayed N/V • Ondansetron also available as orally-disintegrating tabs (ODT) and oral films • Granisetron also available as transdermal patch (Sancuso)	Yes
Granisetron	Kytril	2 mg PO or 1 mg IV		• Fatigue • Dry mouth				No
Dolasetron	Anzemet	100 mg IV/PO		• Transient elevations in LFTs				No
Palonosetron	Aloxi	0.25 mg IV		• QT interval prolongation				No
Mechanism of action – neurokinin-1 (NK-1) antagonist; blocks substance P from NK-1 receptor								
Aprepitant	Emend	Day 1: 125 mg PO Days 2–3: 80 mg PO	None	• Asthenia • Fatigue • Diarrhea • Hiccups • Dizziness • Dehydration	Monitor levels of chemotherapy agents metabolized by CYP3A4	• Inhibits CYP3A4 • Induces CYP2C9	• Use in combination with 5HT3 antagonist and dexamethasone • Prevents delayed N/V	No
Mechanism of action – corticosteroids; potentiate antiemetic properties of 5HT3 antagonists								
Dexamethasone	Decadron	8–40 mg daily PO/IV	Systemic fungal infections	• Hyperglycemia • Immunosuppression • Adrenal suppression • Insomnia • Mood changes, anxiety • GI irritation • Weight gain	• Hemoglobin/hematocrit • Serum potassium • Glucose	CYP3A4 substrate	• Synergistic with 5HT3 antagonists • Can use as single agents for mild chemotherapy-induced N/V	No
Methylprednisolone	Solu-Medrol	40–125 mg daily PO/IV						Yes
Mechanism of action – dopamine-2 antagonists								
Metoclopramide	Reglan	10–20 mg PO/IV q2h PRN	Seizures	• Dizziness • Sedation • Diarrhea • Extrapyramidal symptoms (EPS)	EPS	Antipsychotic agents may ↑ risk of EPS	Should not drive or operate heavy machinery while taking this drug	No

Cancer Pain Drugs

Mechanism of action: narcotic opioid analgesics; stimulate the mu(μ) opioid receptor, inhibiting pain pathways

Generic	Brand	Dose	Contraindications	Primary Side Effects	Key Monitoring	Pertinent Drug Interactions	Med Pearl	Top 200
Codeine	Generic (tabs, injection)	15–60 mg q4–6h	• ↑ intracranial pressure • Severe respiratory depression • Severe or acute asthma • Paralytic ileus	• Drowsiness • Dizziness • Hypotension • N/V • Constipation • Xerostomia • Respiratory depression	• Pain relief • Respiratory status • Mental status • BP	• Central nervous system (CNS) depression with alcohol or sedative/hypnotics • Mixed agonist/antagonist analgesics (could precipitate withdrawal) • Cimetidine may ↑ effect • Use of monoamine oxidase inhibitors (MAOI) within 14 days may ↑ risk of severe reactions (↓ morphine dose by 25%)	• Often used in combination with aspirin, acetaminophen, or NSAIDs • Poor metabolizers of CYP2D6 cannot convert to morphine and receive no pain relief; start immediately on another drug	Yes (combination products)
Morphine	Roxanol (liquid)	2.5–5 mg IV/IM q3–4hr 0.8–10 mg/hr continous infusion					• Drug of choice for severe pain • Use IR products to titrate and to control breakthrough pain • Do not crush controlled-release (CR) products; Kadian and Avinza may be opened • Do not give Kadian through nasogastric (NG) tube	Yes
	Generic (injection immediate-release [IR] tabs, suppository) rectal	• 5–30 mg PO q4h • 10–20 mg rectally q4h						
	Extended release tabs/caps: • MS Contin • Avinza • Kadian • Oramorph	Varies widely in opioid-tolerant patients; no max dose in chronic pain						

Cancer Pain Drugs *(cont'd)*

Generic	Brand	Dose	Contraindications	Primary Side Effects	Key Monitoring	Pertinent Drug Interactions	Med Pearl	Top 200
Hydromorphone	Dilaudid (tabs, liquid, injection, suppository)	• 2.5–10 mg (PO) q3–6h • 1–2 mg SC or IM q4–6h	• ↑ intracranial pressure • Severe respiratory depression • Severe or acute asthma • Paralytic ileus	• Drowsiness • Dizziness • Hypotension • N/V • Constipation • Xerostomia • Respiratory depression	• Pain relief • Respiratory status • Mental status • BP	• CNS depression with alcohol or sedative/hypnotics • Mixed agonist antagonist analgesics (could precipitate withdrawal) • Cimetidine may ↑ effects • Use of MAOIs within 14 days may ↑ risk of severe reactions	• More potent than morphine • Short half-life; requires frequent dosing	Yes
Oxycodone	• Generic (1 R tabs/caps, liquid) • OxyContin (ER tabs) • Percocet (with acetaminophen)	• 10–30 mg q4h (IR) • 10 mg q12h (CR); titrate dosage upward as needed					Do not crush CR tabs	Yes
Fentanyl	Actiq, (transmucosal lozenge)	200 mcg per episode (limit to ≤4 units/day)					• Actiq, Fentora, Lazanda, Abstral, and Onsolis should be used for breakthrough pain only; they are not interchangeable • Duragesic should be used only for chronic pain in patients who are opioid-tolerant	No
	Fentora (buccal tab)	100–200 mcg per episode						
	Duragesic (transdermal)	25–100 mcg/hr						Yes
	Onsolis (buccal film)	200 mcg per episode						
	Lazanda (nasal spray)	100–200 mcg per episode						
	Abstral (sublingual tab)	100 mcg per episode						
Hydrocodone (available only in combination products)	With acetaminophen: • Vicodin • Lortab • Lorcet • Anexsia With ibuprofen: • Vicoprofen • Reprexain	• 1 tab (5–10 mg) q4–6h • Maximum of 5 tabs/24 hrs					Combination with other drugs (i.e. ibuprofen, acetaminophen) limit ability to titrate upward	Yes

Colony-Stimulating Factors

Generic	Brand	Dose	Contra-indications	Primary Side Effects	Key Monitoring	Pertinent Drug Interactions	Med Pearl	Top 200
Mechanism of action – stimulate production of WBCs								
Filgrastim	Neupogen	300–480 mcg SC daily	Hypersensitivity to *E. coli*	• Bone pain • Hypertension • Swelling • Redness • Hypersensitivity reactions • Can act as tumor growth factor	CBC with differential	Use lithium with caution, as it can potentiate neutrophil release	• Requires daily administration • Neutrophil-specific	No
PEG-Filgrastim	Neulasta	6 mg SC with each chemo-therapy cycle					• PEG unit increases half-life; can give 1x per chemotherapy cycle • Neutrophil-specific	No
Sargramostim	Leukine	250–500 mcg SC daily	• Hypersensitivity to yeast • Excessive leukemic myeloid blasts in bone marrow	• Fever, chills • Bone pain • Myalgia • Hypertension • Hypersensitivity reactions			• Requires daily administration • Stimulates formation of all WBCs except lymphocytes	No

Storage and Administration Pearls

- Dolasetron injection may be diluted in apple or apple-grape juice and taken orally; stable for 2 hours.
- Zofran ODT contains phenylalanine; sensitive patients may take IV solution orally.

Patient Education Pearls

- Kadian and Avinza may be opened and sprinkled on applesauce; do not chew, crush, or let dissolve or too much drug will be absorbed too quickly.
- Patient should take morphine with food if it causes stomach upset.
- Patient should not take echinacea if he/she is taking corticosteroids.

LEARNING POINTS

- Chemotherapy protocols vary tremendously; do NOT spend your time memorizing drugs of choice for the various cancers (pharmacists usually do not play a role in selecting drug therapies as treatment is usually protocol driven).
  - Focus more on the toxicity profile of the most commonly used drugs and less on dosing and specific drug combinations.
- Because of the increasing importance of pharmacogenomics, you should know which drugs target specific receptors (Trastuzumab, HER2 receptor; Cetuximab, EGFR; Rituximab, CD20 cell surface protein, etc.).
- Leucovorin is used as a rescue agent in patients receiving methotrexate but enhances the effect of 5-fluorouracil.
- To treat N/V, most patients should receive a corticosteroid, a 5HT3 antagonist, and possibly a benzodiazepine. For severe cases, aprepitant should be added.
- Short-acting opioids are the pain management drugs of choice for cancer pain. As severity increases, titration should be performed more quickly.

PRACTICE QUESTIONS

1. Effective antiandrogen therapy in prostate cancer consists of which of the following?

    I. An LH-RH agonist
    II. Bilateral orchiectomy
    III. Atestosterone antagonist

    (A) I only
    (B) III only
    (C) I and II only
    (D) II or III only
    (E) I, II, and III

2. Which of the following chemotherapeutic agents is associated with profound acute- and late-onset diarrhea?

    (A) Irinotecan
    (B) Doxorubicin
    (C) Daunorubicin
    (D) Trastuzumab
    (E) Methotrexate

3. The mechanism of action of Emend is

    (A) 5HT3 receptor antagonist.
    (B) neurokinin-1 receptor antagonist.
    (C) D2 receptor antagonist.
    (D) benzodiazepine receptor agonist.
    (E) histamine receptor antagonist.

ANSWERS

1. **C**

Either an LH-RH agonist (I) or a bilateral orchiectomy (II) is considered adequate anti-androgen therapy in prostate cancer. Therefore, (C) is correct. Testosterone antagonists (III) are not generally considered as solo agents and, in most studies, have been shown to provide limited (if any) survival benefit when added to LH-RH agonist therapy. The major use for testosterone blockers is to prevent adverse effects from the initial testosterone surge that accompanies the initiation of LH-RH agonist therapy.

2. **A**

Of the drugs listed, only irinotecan exhibits major GI adverse effects. The other drugs are more likely to lead to cardiomyopathy (trastuzumab, doxorubicin, and daunorubicin) or neuro-, nephro-, and hepatotoxicity (methotrexate).

3. **B**

Emend (aprepitant) is a highly selective emetogenic agent that works against the neurokinin-1 receptor. It has little to no affinity for the other receptor targets of chemotherapy-induced or postoperative nausea and vomiting.

Psychiatric Disorders

8

This chapter covers the following disease states:

- **Depression**
- **Anxiety**
- **Bipolar disorder**
- **Schizophrenia**
- **Alzheimer's disease**

 Suggested Study Time: **45 minutes**

DEPRESSION

Definition

Depression, or major depressive disorder, is a complex mood disorder that has many subtypes and is due to multiple etiologies. Depression can be classified as single-episode, recurrent, or chronic and as depression with or without psychotic features, with typical or atypical symptoms, etc.

Diagnosis

The diagnosis of depression is based on the *Diagnostic and Statistical Manual of Mental Disorders*, 4th Edition (DSM IV). Criteria for diagnosis are based primarily on symptoms. Five or more of the following symptoms must have been present during the same 2-week period and must represent a change from previous functioning; at least one of the symptoms is either (*1*) depressed mood or (*2*) loss of interest or pleasure.

- Depressed mood most of the day, nearly every day
- Markedly diminished interest or pleasure in all, or almost all, activities

- Significant weight loss when not dieting, or weight gain
- Insomnia or hypersomnia nearly every day
- Psychomotor agitation or retardation nearly every day
- Fatigue or loss of energy nearly every day
- Feelings of worthlessness or of excessive or inappropriate guilt
- Diminished ability to think or concentrate, or indecisiveness
- Recurrent thoughts of death (not just fear of dying), recurrent suicidal ideation without a specific plan, or a suicide attempt or a specific plan for committing suicide

Signs and Symptoms

Signs and symptoms are detailed in the diagnostic criteria.

GUIDELINES

American Psychiatric Association practice guideline for the treatment of patients with major depressive disorder. Third edition. www.psych.org/guidelines/mdd2010.

GUIDELINES SUMMARY

- The primary goal of therapy is remission of symptoms.
- There are various antidepressant medications available. Clinical evidence indicates that, in general, efficacy is similar between classes.
- Initial choice of pharmacotherapy agent is based on anticipated side effects, tolerability of these side effects for an individual patient, patient preference, quantity and quality of clinical evidence, and cost.
- First-line options for most patients include selective serotonin reuptake inhibitors (SSRIs), desipramine, nortriptyline, bupropion, and venlafaxine. Because of the potential for serious side effects and drug interactions, monoamine oxidase inhibitors (MAOIs) should be reserved for patients who do not respond to other therapies.
- An adequate therapy trial requires at least 6–8 weeks. Dose adjustments or treatment changes are made at 6- to 8-week intervals at the earliest.
- There is significant interpatient variability in response to antidepressants. Patients may respond to classes/agents that have been effective in the past or that have been effective for family members. Bupropion has a lower incidence of sexual side effects and may be preferred in patients presenting with this complaint related to therapy.
- In 2005, the FDA required that all product labeling for antidepressants include a boxed warning regarding the potential for increased risk of clinical worsening and suicidality in children, adolescents, and young adults taking these agents.

Antidepressants

Generic	Brand	Dose & Max mg (frequency)	Contra-indications	Primary Side Effects	Key Monitoring Parameters	Pertinent Drug Interactions	Med Pearls	Top 200
Mechanism of action – SSRIs: inhibit reuptake of serotonin, allowing more serotonin availability in synapses								
Citalopram	Celexa	10–60 mg daily	MAOI, pimozide, hypersensitivity	• Lightheadedness • Syncope • Sweating • Diarrhea • Nausea • Xerostomia • Confusion • Dizziness • Somnolence • Tremor • Hallucinations • Disorder of ejaculation • Impotence • Rhinitis • Fatigue	• Reduction or resolution of symptoms • Withdrawal symptoms from abrupt discontinuation • Abnormal bleeding • Worsening of depression, suicidality, or unusual behavior at initiation of therapy or when changing dose	• Other serotonergic medications, such as MAOI, SSRI, triptans, linezolid, St. John's wort, tramadol	Racemic mixture R and S isomer	Yes
Escitalopram	Lexapro	10–20 mg daily					Only contains the S isomer of citalopram	Yes
Fluoxetine	• Prozac • Prozac Wkly • Sarafem • Rapiflux	20–60 mg daily or 80 mg wkly				• Other serotonergic medications such as MAOI, SSRI, triptans, linezolid, St. John's wort, tramadol, phenytoin • Drugs metabolized by cytochrome P450	Allow 5 wks washout prior to MAOI due to long half-life	Yes
Fluvoxamine	Luvox	50–300 mg daily	MAOI, pimozide, thioridazine, alosetron, astemizole, terfenadine, tizanidine, hypersensitivity					No
Paroxetine	Paxil	20–60 mg daily	MAOI, pimozide, thioridazine, hypersensitivity			Other serotonergic medications such as MAOI, SSRI, triptans, linezolid, St. John's wort, tramadol		Yes
Sertraline	Zoloft	50–200 mg daily	MAOI, pimozide, disulfiram-like compounds (oral concentrate), linezolid, hypersensitivity				Oral concentrate contains alcohol	Yes
Mechanism of action – Selective serotonin reuptake inhibitor, partial 5HT1A receptor agonist								
Vilazodone	Viibryd	10–40 mg PO once daily	MAOI	• Diarrhea • Nausea • Xerostomia • Dizziness • Insomnia	• Reduction or resolution of symptoms • Worsening of depression/suicidality	• Other serotonergic medications such as MAOI, SSRI, triptans, linezolid, St. John's wort, tramadol • Warfarin, NSAIDs, antiplatelet agents—increased risk of bleeding	• Should be taken with food • Avoid abrupt discontinuation • Risk of bleeding is unique among antidepressants	No

Antidepressants *(cont'd)*

Mechanism of action – tricyclic antidepressants (TCAs): increased synaptic concentration of norepinephrine and serotonin

Generic	Brand	Dose & Max mg (frequency)	Contra-indications	Primary Side Effects	Key Monitoring Parameters	Pertinent Drug Interactions	Med Pearls	Top 200
Amitriptyline	• Elavil • Vanatrip	50–300 mg daily (q day–TID)	• MAOI • Post-myocardial infarction (MI) acute recovery • Hypersensitivity	• Anticholinergic symptoms • Weight gain • Bloating • Blurred vision • Xerostomia • Constipation • Asthenia • Dizziness • Somnolence • Headache • Fatigue	• Reduction or resolution of symptoms • Withdrawal symptoms from abrupt discontinuation • Worsening of depression, suicidality, or unusual behavior at initiation of therapy or when changing dose • Blood pressure (BP) • Electrocardiogram (ECG) in patients with cardiac disease or hyperthyroidism	Other serotonergic medications such as MAOI, SSRI, triptans, linezolid, St. John's wort, tramadol	• Dangerous in overdose situations • Avoid in patients with high suicidality • Avoid dispensing large quantities • Also used for sleep disorders	Yes
Amoxapine	Ascendin	50–600 mg daily (BID–TID)						No
Clomipramine	Anafranil	75–250 mg daily (divided TID)						No
Desipramine	Norpramin	100–300 mg daily (q day or divided doses)						No
Doxepin	• Sinequan • Prudoxin • Zonalon	25–300 mg daily (q day–TID)						No
Imipramine	Tofranil	100–300 mg daily (q day–divided)						No
Nortriptyline	• Pamelor • Aventyl	25 mg TID–QID; max: 150 mg daily						No
Protriptyline	Vivactil	15–60 mg daily (TID–QID)						No
Trimipramine	Surmontil	75–300 mg daily (q day–TID)						No

Antidepressants *(cont'd)*

Mechanism of action – selective serotonin and norepinephrine reuptake inhibitors (SSNRI): inhibit the reuptake of serotonin and norepinephrine to allow higher available synaptic concentrations

Generic	Brand	Dose & Max mg (frequency)	Contra-indications	Primary Side Effects	Key Monitoring Parameters	Pertinent Drug Interactions	Med Pearls	Top 200
Duloxetine	Cymbalta	30–120 mg daily (q day)	• MAOI • Hypersensitivity • Uncontrolled narrow-angle glaucoma	• Palpitations • Diaphoresis • Constipation • Decreased appetite • Diarrhea • Nausea • Xerostomia • Asthenia • Dizziness • Insomnia • Somnolence • Vertigo • Blurred vision • Polyuria • Reduced libido • Cough • Nasopharyngitis • Fatigue	• Reduction or resolution of symptoms • Withdrawal symptoms from abrupt discontinuation • Worsening of depression	Other serotonergic medications such as MAOI, SSRI, Triptans, Linezolid, St. John's wart, Tramadol;	Doses greater than 60 mg did not provide additional benefit in generalized anxiety disorder	Yes
Venlafaxine	• Effexor • Effexor XR	37.5–375 mg daily (q day–TID)	• MAOI • Hypersensitivity	• Hypertension • Sweating • Weight loss • Constipation • Loss of appetite • Nausea • Xerostomia • Insomnia or somnolence • Erectile dysfunction	• Reduction or resolution of symptoms • Withdrawal symptoms from abrupt discontinuation • Worsening of depression • BP			Yes

Antidepressants (cont'd)

Generic	Brand	Dose & Max mg (frequency)	Contra-indications	Primary Side Effects	Key Monitoring Parameters	Pertinent Drug Interactions	Med Pearls	Top 200
Nefazodone	Serzone	200–600 mg daily (BID)	• Previous nefazodone-induced hepatic damage • Hypersensitivity • Astemizole • Carbamazepine • Cisapride • Triazolam • Terfenadine • Pimozide	• Lightheadedness • Constipation • Indigestion • Nausea • Xerostomia • Asthenia • Confusion • Dizziness • Headache • Insomnia • Memory impairment • Somnolence	• Reduction or resolution of symptoms • Withdrawal symptoms from abrupt discontinuation • Worsening of depression			No
Desvenlafaxine	Pristiq	50–400 mg PO daily	• Hypersensitivity • MAOI therapy	• Orthostatic hypotension (elderly) • Nausea • Dizziness • Insomnia • Hyperhidrosis • Constipation • Somnolence • Decreased appetite • Anxiety • Male sexual dysfunction	• Renal function • Response to therapy • BP • Worsening of depressive symptoms • Suicidality	• MAOI serotonergic agents increase risk of serotonin syndrome • Increased risk of bleeding when used in combination with warfarin (NSAIDs, aspirin)	• Renal dose adjustment required • Should not be abruptly discontinued	Yes

Antidepressants *(cont'd)*

Mechanism of action – MAOIs: increase epinephrine, norepinephrine, dopamine, and serotonin

Generic	Brand	Dose & Max mg (frequency)	Contra-indications	Primary Side Effects	Key Monitoring Parameters	Pertinent Drug Interactions	Med Pearls	Top 200
Isocarboxazid	Marplan	20–60 mg daily (BID–QID)	• Cardiovascular disorder • Hypertension • Cerebrovascular disorder • Concurrent administration of interacting medications • General anesthesia • History of headache • Hypersensitivity • Pheochromocytoma • Severe renal function impairment	• Weight gain • Constipation • Xerostomia • Dizziness • Headache • Insomnia • Somnolence • Blurred vision • Anxiety • Mania	• Reduced depression and associated symptoms • BP • Liver function • Worsening of depression, suicidality, or unusual changes in behavior	• Other serotonergic medications such as SSRI, triptans, linezolid, St. John's wort, tramadol • Concurrent administration of antihistamine, sedative, or anesthetic substances • Bupropion • Buspirone • Narcotics • Barbiturates • Ethanol • Dextromethorphan • Excessive caffeine • Foods containing high concentrations of tyramine • Meperidine • SSRI • Sympathomimetic drugs • MAOI • Tricyclic antidepressants (TRAs) • Maprotiline • Carbamazepine • Cyclobenzaprine	Used very infrequently due to poor side effect profile and frequency of drug interactions	No
Phenelzine	Nardil	45–90 mg daily (TID–QID)	• Cardiovascular disorder • Hypertension • Cerebrovascular disorder • Concurrent administration of interacting medications • General anesthesia • History of headache • Hypersensitivity • Pheochromocytoma • Severe renal function impairment					No
Tranylcypromine	Parnate	30–60 mg daily (divided doses)						No

Antidepressants *(cont'd)*

Generic	Brand	Dose & Max mg (frequency)	Contra-indications	Primary Side Effects	Key Monitoring Parameters	Pertinent Drug Interactions	Med Pearls	Top 200
Selegiline	Emsam	6 mg daily transdermal patch (q day)	• Cardiovascular disorder • Hypertension • Cerebrovascular disorder • Concurrent administration of interacting medications • General anesthesia • History of headache • Hypersensitivity • Pheochromocytoma • Severe renal function impairment			• Other serotonergic medications such as SSRI, triptans, linezolid, St. John's wort, tramadol • Concurrent administration of antihistaminic, sedative, or anesthetic substances • Bupropion • Buspirone • Narcotics • Barbiturates • Ethanol • Dextromethorphan • Excessive caffeine • Foods containing high concentrations of tyramine • Meperidine • SSRI • Sympathomimetic drugs • MAOI • TCA • Maprotiline • Carbamazepine • Cyclobenzaprine	Used primarily for Parkinson's disease and less frequently for depression	No

Antidepressants *(cont'd)*

Generic	Brand	Dose & Max mg (frequency)	Contra-indications	Primary Side Effects	Key Monitoring Parameters	Pertinent Drug Interactions	Med Pearls	Top 200
Mechanism of action – SSNDRI: inhibits the reuptake of both serotonin and norepinephrine, increasing available concentrations in the synapse								
Bupropion	• Wellbutrin • Wellbutrin SR • Wellbutrin XL • Zyban	100–450 mg daily (q day–QID)	• MAOI • Bulimia or anorexia • Patients in withdrawal from alcohol • Seizure disorders	• Taste disturbance • Agitation • Increased seizure activity	• Reduction or resolution of symptoms • Withdrawal symptoms from abrupt discontinuation • Worsening of depression • Seizure activity	MAOI	• Also used for smoking cessation • Mostly dopamine reuptake activity	Yes
Mechanism of action – tetracyclic antidepressants: increase available synaptic concentrations of norepinephrine, serotonin, or both								
Maprotiline	Ludiomil	75–225 mg daily (BID–TID)	• MAOI • Hypersensitivity • Seizure disorder • Post-MI acute recovery period	• Hypotension • Tachyarrhythmia • Rash • Weight gain • Constipation • Nausea • Pancreatitis • Reduced salivation • Vomiting • Xerostomia	• Reduction or resolution of symptoms • Withdrawal symptoms from abrupt discontinuation • Worsening of depression	MAOI		No
Mirtazapine	• Remeron • Solutab	15–45 mg daily (q HS)		• Increased appetite • Hyperlipidemia • Weight gain • Constipation • Elevated transaminases		• MAOI • Clonidine • Tramadol • Fluoxetine • Fluvoxamine • Linezolid • Olanzapine • Venlafaxine	• Dosed at bedtime due to somnolence • Off-label use for appetite stimulation	Yes

Storage and Administration Pearls

- Store at room temperature in a dry place that is protected from light.

PATIENT EDUCATION PEARLS

- It may take several weeks for medication to demonstrate maximal efficacy. Allow adequate trial before determining if medication is ineffective.
- Patients should not abruptly discontinue their medication. They should consult with a healthcare professional to determine appropriate tapering procedures.
- Patients on MAOIs should avoid excessive caffeine intake, chocolate, and foods containing high levels of tyramine, including red wine, aged cheeses, avocado, eggplant, figs, and soy-based foods.

ANXIETY

Definition

Anxiety disorders consist of a number of disorders, including generalized anxiety disorder (GAD) and panic disorder. This chapter focuses on these two most common subtypes of anxiety disorders. The pathophysiology of anxiety is poorly understood but is theoretically linked to abnormal function of several neurotransmitters, including GABA, serotonin, and norepinephrine.

Diagnosis

GAD diagnosis is based on the presence of anxiety or excessive worry (1) that has been present on most days over at least 6 months, and (2) over which the patient feels a lack of control. Three or more subjective symptoms must be present in order to make the diagnosis.

Panic disorder is a complex disorder characterized by panic attacks. During a panic attack, at least four psychic and somatic symptoms will be present. In order to be diagnosed with panic disorder, a patient must have a history of recurrent panic attacks

Signs and Symptoms

- Subjective symptoms of GAD include restlessness, feeling easily fatigued, difficulty concentrating, irritability, muscle tension, and sleep difficulties.
- Psychic symptoms of panic disorder include depersonalization, fear of dying, derealization, fear of losing control, and fear of going "crazy."
- Somatic symptoms of panic disorder include sweating, trembling, shaking, choking, chest pain, nausea, abdominal pain, palpitations, tachycardia, shortness of breath, dizziness, light-headedness, chills, and hot flashes.

Summary of Treatment Recommendations

- Goals of therapy include improvement in overall functionality and quality of life through reduction of symptom frequency and intensity. Complete remission of illness is the long-term treatment goal.
- Treatment options are detailed in the medication charts and no consensus exists as to the preferred initial therapy or order of options thereafter.
- Many clinicians prefer the SSRIs as initial therapy due to their favorable side-effect profile as compared to other therapies. Subsequently, other antidepressants such as venlafaxine or tricyclics can be utilized. Benzodiazepines are commonly used, especially in acute situations. Although efficacious, these agents lend themselves to issues related to dependence, increased fall risk in the elderly, and potential for negative cognitive effects in general. Buspirone is a unique treatment option that is effective but requires 2 to 3 weeks to reach efficacy; thus, it is not useful in acute situations.
- Benzodiazepine selection should take into account varying pharmacokinetic profiles of agents. In elderly patients, preference is given to those agents that are shorter-acting (less accumulation) and those metabolized by glucoronidation (e.g., lorazepam, oxazepam) versus oxidation (e.g., alprazolam, diazepam). Agents with a rapid onset have a greater potential for dependence.

Anxiolytics

Mechanism of action – benzodiazepines bind to GABA receptors, causing an influx of chloride which results in hyperpolarization and a less excitable state; metabolized by CYP450, benzodiazepines have a potential interaction with all CYP450 inhibitors and inducers

Generic	Brand	Dose & Max mg (frequency)	Contra-indications	Primary Side Effects	Key Monitoring Parameters	Pertinent Drug Interactions	Med Pearls	Top 200
Alprazolam	• Xanax • Xanax XR • Nirazax ODT • Alprazolam • Intensol	• Immediate release (IR) 0.25–2 mg (q day–TID) • Extended release (ER) 0.5–3 mg (q day) • Max: 4 mg/day	• Hypersensitive • Narrow-angle glaucoma	• Somnolence • Ataxia • Dizziness • Changes in appetite • Decreased libido • Confusion • Constipation • Blurred vision	• Orthostasis • Excessive sedation • Signs of withdrawal • Periodic basic metabolic panel (BMP) • Liver function tests (LFTs) and complete blood count (CBC) in chronic therapy	• Ketoconazole • Itraconazole • Alcohol • Central nervous system (CNS) depressants • Digoxin • Fluoxetine • Propoxyphene • Nefazodone	• Schedule C-IV • Pregnancy category D • Smoking decreases concentration up to 50% • Pediatric dosing • Rapid onset, short-acting	Yes
Chlordiazepoxide	Librium	5–25 mg (TID–QID)				• Alcohol • CNS depressants • Ketoconazole	• CrCl <10% give 50% of recommended dose • IV injection available • Avoid in elderly • Schedule C-IV • Pregnancy category D • Slower-onset, long-acting	No
Clonazepam	• Klonopin, • Klonopin Wafers	• 0.5–2 mg (BID) • Orally disintegrating tablet (ODT) 0.125–2 mg (BID)					• Decrease dose by 50% in elderly and hepatic disease • Pregnancy category D • Schedule C-IV • Rapid-onset, long-acting	Yes
Clorazepate	• Gen-XENE • Tranxene T-Tab • Tranxene-SD • Tranxene	• IR: 3.75–15 mg (BID–QID) • ER: 11.25–22.5 mg (q day)					• Avoid in elderly • Schedule C-IV • Pregnancy category D • Rapid-onset, long-acting	No
Diazepam	• Valium • Diazepam Intensol	2–10 mg (BID–QID)					• IV and liquid dosage forms available • Schedule C-IV • Pregnancy category D • Rapid-onset, long-acting	Yes

Anxiolytics *(cont'd)*

Generic	Brand	Dose & Max mg (frequency)	Contra-indications	Primary Side Effects	Key Monitoring Parameters	Pertinent Drug Interactions	Med Pearls	Top 200
Lorazepam	• Ativan • Lorazepam • Intensol	• 0.5–2 mg (BID–TID) • Max: 10 mg/day					• Available in IV and liquid form • Schedule C-IV • Pregnancy category D • Medium-onset, short-acting	Yes
Oxazepam	• Alepam, Medopam, Murelax, Noripam, Oxpam, Purata, Serax, and Serepax	10–30 mg (TID–QID)					• Schedule C-IV • Pregnancy category C • Medium-onset, short-acting	No

Mechanism of action — SSRIs: selectively inhibit the reuptake of serotonin by presynaptic neuronal membranes with little to no effect on norepinephrine or dopamine reuptake

Generic	Brand	Dose & Max mg (frequency)	Contra-indications	Primary Side Effects	Key Monitoring Parameters	Pertinent Drug Interactions	Med Pearls	Top 200
Citalopram	Celexa	Details above in antidepressants table			Unlabeled use for panic disorder, GAD, posttraumatic stress disorder (PTSD), and obsessive-compulsive disorder (OCD)			Yes
Escitalopram	Lexapro				Indicated for GAD			Yes
Fluoxetine	• Prozac • Sarafem				Indicated for OCD, panic disorder			Yes
Paroxetine	Paxil, Paxil CR				Indicated for panic disorder, PTSD, GAD, OCD, social anxiety disorder (SAD)			Yes
Sertraline	Zoloft				Indicated for OCD, panic disorder, SAD, PTSD			Yes
Fluvoxamine	Luvox				Indicated for OCD			No

Anxiolytics *(cont'd)*

Generic	Brand	Dose & Max mg (frequency)	Contra-indications	Primary Side Effects	Key Monitoring Parameters	Pertinent Drug Interactions	Med Pearls	Top 200
Mechanism of action — nonselective beta-adrenergic blocker which competitively blocks response to beta1- and beta2-adrenergic stimulation in the heart muscle, vascular smooth muscle, and bronchial muscles								
Propranolol (nonselective BB)	• Inderal, Inderal LA • InnoPran XL • Propranolol • Intensol	10–80 mg 1 hr prior to anxiogenic event	• Hypersensitivity • Severe bradycardia • Heart block • Uncompensated congestive heart failure (CHF) • Severe chronic obstructive pulmonary disease (COPD) or asthma	• Dizziness • Fatigue • Gastrointesinal (GI) upset • Hypotension	• Heart rate • BP	Inhibitors/inducers of CYP450 major CYP1A2), non-dihydropyridine calcium channel blockers (CCBs)	Unlabeled for situational anxiety, acute panic	Yes
Mechanism of action — exact mechanism is unknown; high affinity for 5-HT$_{1A}$ and 5-HT$_2$ receptors, mild affinity for dopamine D$_2$ receptors								
Buspirone	BuSpar	• 5–30 mg (BID–TID) • Max 60 mg/day		• Headache • Dizziness • Nausea • Hostility • Confusion • Drowsiness	• Mental status • Symptoms of anxiety • Pseudo-parkinsonism	• MAOIs • Nondihydropyridine CCBs • Inhibitors/inducers of CYP450 • Macrolides • SSRIs	• Pregnancy category B • Avoid use in renal and hepatic impairment • Pediatric dosing for 6 yrs and older • Takes 2–3 wks to reach efficacy	Yes
Mechanism of action — selective norepinephrine reuptake inhibitor (SNRI): inhibits reuptake of neuronal serotonin and norepinephrine; may have weak inhibitory effect on reuptake of dopamine								
Venlafaxine	• Effexor • Effexor XR	• 25–100 mg (q day) • ER: 37.5–150 mg (q day) • Max: 225 mg/day	• Hypersensitivity • Concurrent use of MAOI	• Drowsiness • Dizziness • Insomnia • Xerostomia • Weakness (generalized) • Changes in appetite	• BP • Mental status • Symptoms/signs of serotonin syndrome	• Alcohol • CNS depressants—SSRIs • TCAs • MAOIs • Buspirone • Tramadol • Lithium • Haloperido • Clozapine • Nefazodone • Trazodone	• Labeled for GAD, panic disorder, SAD • Pregnancy category C • Use with caution in renal impairment	Yes

Anxiolytics *(cont'd)*

Generic	Brand	Dose & Max mg (frequency)	Contra-indications	Primary Side Effects	Key Monitoring Parameters	Pertinent Drug Interactions	Med Pearls	Top 200
Mechanism of action – inhibits neuronal reuptake of serotonin and norepinephrine; also blocks 5-HT$_2$ and alpha1 receptors								
Nefazodone	Serzone	• 50–250 mg (q day–BID) • Max: 600 mg/day	• Hypersensitivity • Acute liver disease • Elevated LFTs • Concurrent use of carbamazepine • Cisapride • Pimozide	• Headache • Drowsiness • Insomnia • Dizziness • Xerostomia • Nausea • Constipation • Hypotension • Edema	• LFTs: discontinue at 3x upper limit of normal (ULN) and do not reintroduce • mental status	• Triazolam • Alprazolam • Lovastatin • Simvastatin • Other statins to lesser extent • Digoxin • Alcohol • CNS depressants • Inhibitors/inducers of CYP3A4	• Does not inhibit REM sleep • Unlabeled use in GAD, panic disorder PTSD, SAD • Black box warning for suicidal ideation • Pregnancy category C	No
Mechanism of action – competes with histamine for H$_1$-receptor sites on effector cells in GI, blood vessels, and respiratory tract								
Hydroxyzine	Vistaril	10–100 mg (QID)	• Hypersensitivity • Early pregnancy	• Dizziness • Drowsiness • Fatigue • Xerostomia • Blurry vision • Urinary retention	• BP • Mental status • Blood urea nitrogen (BUN) serum creatinine (SCr) with chronic use	• Antihistamines • MAOIs • CNS depressants	• Use with caution in benign prostatic hyperplasia (BPH), respiratory disease, glaucoma • Pregnancy category C • Avoid in elderly • Avoid in renal impairment	Yes
Mechanism of action – appears to affect the thalamus and limbic system; also appears to inhibit multineuronal spinal reflexes								
Meprobamate	Miltown	• 200–400 mg (TID–QID) • Max: 2,400 mg/day	• Hypersensitivity to carbamates • Porphyria	• Drowsiness • Ataxia • Nausea, vomiting, diarrhea • Anorexia • Hypotension	• Signs/symptoms of withdrawal • Mental status • LFTs with chronic use	• Alcohol • CNS depressants	• Schedule C-IV • Pregnancy category D • Dose adjustment in hepatic and renal insufficiency	No

STORAGE AND ADMINISTRATION PEARLS

- Tablets and capsules should all be stored at room temperature, in dry area out of direct sunlight.
- Keep liquid preparations from freezing or overheating. Do not expose to temperatures >77°F (25°C).

PATIENT EDUCATION PEARLS

- Take as directed by physician.
- Patients should *not* abruptly discontinue any anxiety medication.
- SSRIs, SNRIs, MAOIs may take up to several weeks (2–4 weeks) to see effect
- Patients should avoid alcohol when taking any of these medications.
- Patients should avoid driving or operating heavy machinery while taking benzodiazepines until they know how they respond to the medication.

BIPOLAR DISORDER

Definition

Bipolar disorder is an episodic, lifelong illness with symptoms of depression alternating with symptoms of mania or hypomania. Bipolar disorder is classified on the basis of the frequency of alternating symptoms and the subtype of manic symptoms demonstrated. Bipolar I disorder is defined as one or more manic episodes plus one or more major depressive episodes. Bipolar II disorder is defined as one or more episodes of major depression and one or more hypomanic episodes with no history of a full manic or mixed episode.

Diagnosis

The diagnosis of bipolar disorder is based on the DSM IV criteria for each of the subtype mood disorders (mania, hypomania, depression, mixed episode). Bipolar disorder diagnosis requires that a patient exhibits diagnosed episodes of both major depression plus manic, hypomanic, or mixed episodes. Acute manic symptoms are hallmarks of the disorder and consist of elevated, expansive, or irritable mood lasting for at least 1 week or requiring hospitalization. Hypomania is defined as symptoms of mania that do not meet the criteria for manic episode and last for at least 4 days. Mixed episode is one that meets criteria for major depression and a manic episode for at least 1 week.

Signs and Symptoms

Acute mania requires that three of the following symptoms must be present: flight of ideas or racing thoughts, decreased need for sleep, inflated self-esteem or grandiosity, more talkative than usual or pressured speech, distractibility, psychomotor agitation, and excessive involvement in pleasurable activities with high potential for negative consequences.

Major depressive symptoms are detailed in the depression section of this chapter.

GUIDELINES

Texas Implementation of Medication Algorithms: update to the algorithms for the treatment of bipolar disorder. *J Clin Psychiatry*, no. 66 (2005): 870–86.

GUIDELINES SUMMARY

- First-line treatment options for patient with acute manic episodes include lithium, valproate, aripiprazole, quetiapine, risperidone, ziprasidone, olanzapine, or carbamazepine. Antipsychotic medications are detailed in medication charts later in this chapter.
- First-line treatment options for acute depressive episodes include lamotrigine monotherapy or lamotrigine in combination with antimania therapy.
- Maintenance therapy generally consists of continuation of therapy used in acute phases. Lithium and valproate have long history of clinical success in maintenance therapy.

Mood Stabilizers

Generic	Brand	Dose & Max mg (frequency)	Contra-indications	Primary Side Effects	Key Monitoring Parameters	Med Pearls	Top 200
Mechanism of action – lithium: altered sodium transport leads to a shift toward intraneuronal metabolism of catecholamines; the specific mechanism in mania is not fully understood							
Lithium	• Tablets • Lithobid extended-release tablets	• 300–1,200 mg daily (TID) • 300–1,200 mg daily (BID)	• Significant renal or cardiovascular disease • Dehydration	• Diarrhea • Vomiting • Drowsiness • Muscle weakness • Lack of coordination • Ataxia • Blurred vision • Tinnitus	Serum drug concentration 0.6–1.5 mEq/L	Significant drug interactions with angiotensin converting enzyme (ACE) inhibitors and diuretics which decrease lithium clearance and increase toxicity	No
Mechanism of action – valproic acid: not fully understood; thought to increase gamma amino butyric acid (GABA) concentrations in the brain							
Valproic acid (divalproex sodium)	• Depakote • Depakote ER • Depakene • Depacon	10–60 mg/kg/day	• Hepatic dysfunction • Hypersensitivity • Urea cycle disorders	• Hepatic impairment • Thrombocytopenia • Hyperammonemia • Weight gain • Pancreatitis	• Serum drug concentration: (50–100 mcg/mL) • LFTs at baseline and periodically • Periodic CBC and serum ammonia levels	• Highly teratogenic • Available in oral capsules, tablets, ER tablets, sprinkle caps, oral syrup, and IV solution • Drug interactions detailed in neurological disorders chapter	Yes
Mechanism of action – oxcarbazepine: blocks voltage-sensitive sodium channels, resulting in stabilization of hyperexcitable neuronal membranes							
Oxcarbazepine	Trileptal tablets and oral suspension	600–2,400 mg daily (BID)	Hypersensitivity	• Sedation • Dizziness • Ataxia • Nausea • Rash (Stevens-Johnson possible) • Hyponatremia	Periodic Na, renal function; serum concentrations 12–30 mcg/mL	• CrCl <30 mL/min requires half of initial dose • Drug interactions detailed in neurological disorders chapter	Yes
Mechanism of action – lamotrigine: affects sodium channels stabilizing neuronal membranes; the exact mechanism in bipolar disorder is unknown							
Lamotrigine	• Lamictal • Oral tablets, chewable tablets	25–700 mg daily (once to BID)	• Hypersensitivity • History of Stevens-Johnson rash	• Stevens-Johnson rash • Other rash • Diplopia • Dizziness • Headache	• Response to therapy • Presence of side effects	• Risk of rash increased when combined with valproate • Slow dose titration necessary • Drug interactions detailed in neurological disorders chapter	Yes

Storage and Administration Pearls

- All medications should be stored at room temperature in a dry area away from direct sunlight.
- Patient may take medications with food if GI upset occurs.

Patient Education Pearls

- It is important that medications be continued once the symptoms have resolved.
- Patients should discuss any new medications with a healthcare professional prior to use due to risk of drug interactions.

SCHIZOPHRENIA

Definition

Schizophrenia is a psychiatric disorder that manifests as symptoms including hallucinations or delusions, and has a dramatic impact on the affected individual's functionality and quality of life. The pathophysiology is not fully understood, but theories suggest an excessive firing of dopamine and potential activity of additional neurotransmitters such as norepinephrine, serotonin, and glutamate.

Diagnosis

Persistent disturbances in social, occupational, and self-care functioning must be present for at least 6 months, with 1 month of symptoms including at least two of the following: hallucinations, delusions, disorganized speech, disorganized behavior, or negative symptoms.

SIGNS AND SYMPTOMS

There are multiple subtypes of schizophrenia and symptoms vary widely between them, ranging from catalepsy or stupor to disorganized speech. Potential symptoms include auditory or visual hallucinations, delusions, disorganized speech or behavior, flat or inappropriate affect, and catatonic behavior.

GUIDELINES

American Psychiatric Association. Practice guideline for the treatment of patients with schizophrenia. 2nd Ed. Arlington, VA. American Psychiatric Association, no. 114 (2004): 1–114.

GUIDELINES SUMMARY

For many years, atypical antipsychotics were considered the obvious first-line choice because of significantly reduced incidence of extrapyramidal side effects. Recently, considerable controversy has surfaced, because of the ability of these medications to increase the risk of the metabolic syndrome. At this time, choice of either class is appropriate as first-line therapy. It should be considered, however, that atypical agents have better efficacy in treating negative symptoms.

- Goals of therapy include: Reduce or eliminate symptoms, minimize adverse effects of pharmacological treatment, and prevent relapse.
- Atypical and typical antipsychotics have similar efficacy profiles. Decision on first-line therapy is based on consideration of side-effect profiles, adherence issues, history of response, and cost.

Typical Antipsychotics

Generic	Brand	Dose & Max mg (frequency)	Contra-indications	Primary Side Effects	Key Monitoring Parameters	Pertinent Drug Interactions	Med Pearls	Top 200
Mechanism of action – phenothiazines: block postsynaptic mesolimbic dopaminergic receptors in the brain								
Chlorpromazine	Thorazine	• 10–200 mg (BID–QID) • Max: 2,000 mg/day	• Hypersensitivity • Severe CNS depression • Coma	• Orthostatic hypotension • Drowsiness • Xerostomia • Constipation • Nausea	• Vital signs • Mental status • Lipid profile • Fasting blood glucose • Severity of EPS	• Alcohol • CNS depressants • Lithium • Warfarin • Other phenothiazine	• Available in IV • May produce false-positive phenylketonuria (PKU) test results and pregnancy • Pregnancy category C	No
Fluphenazine	Prolixin	• 1–10 mg (TID–QID) • Max: 40 mg/day	• Hypersensitivity • Severe CNS depression • Coma • Subcortical brain damage • Blood dyscrasias • Hepatic disease	• Urinary retention • Blurred vision • Photosensitivity • Extrapyramidal symptoms (EPS)	• LFTs • Involuntary movement • Neuroleptic malignant syndrome (NMS) • CBCs	• Propranolol • Pindolol • Valproic acid • Phenytoin • Atropine	• Available as elixir and injection • Pregnancy category C	No
Perphenazine	Trilafon (only generic available)	• 2–16 mg (BID–QID) • Max: 64 mg/day					Pregnancy category C	No
Trifluoperazine	Stelazine (only generic available)	• 1–10 mg (q day–BID) • Max: 40 mg/day					• Pregnancy category C • False-positives on PKU and pregnancy tests	No
Prochlorperazine	• Compazine • Compro (suppository)	• 5–15 mg (TID–QID) • 2.5–25 mg (BID) • Max: 150 mg/day					False-positives on PKU and pregnancy tests	No
Thioridazine	Mellaril (only generic available)	• 10–200 mg (BID–QID) • Max: 800 mg/day				• Alcohol • CNS depressants • Propranolol • Pindolol • Drugs that prolong QT interval	• Pregnancy category C • Black box warning for altered cardiac conduction • Use with caution in respiratory disease and hepatic disease	No

Typical Antipsychotics *(cont'd)*

Generic	Brand	Dose & Max mg (frequency)	Contra-indications	Primary Side Effects	Key Monitoring Parameters	Pertinent Drug Interactions	Med Pearls	Top 200
Mechanism of action – haloperidol: not well established; thought to block postsynaptic mesolimbic dopaminergic D$_2$ receptors in the brain								
Haloperidol	• Haldol • Haldol Deconade (Injection)	• 0.5–20 mg (BID-TID) • 50–100 mg/mL (q day) • Max: 100 mg/day	• Hypersensitivity • Parkinson's disease • Severe CNS depression • Bone marrow suppression • Severe cardiac or hepatic disease • Coma	• Xerostomia • Drowsiness • Constipation • Nausea • Urinary retention • Blurred vision • EPS • Dyspepsia • Priapism • QT prolongation	• Vital signs • CBCs • Mental status • ECG at baseline • EPS • Involuntary movement	• Alcohol • CNS depressants • Antiparkinson medication • Lithium • Inhibitors/ inducers of CYP450	• Available in IV and liquid dosage form • Pregnancy category C • IV form uses sesame oil	No
Mechanism of action – Pimozide: a potent, centrally acting dopamine-receptor antagonist								
Pimozide	Orap	• 1–2 mg (q day) • Max: 0.2 mg/kg or 10 mg, whichever is less	• Severe CNS depression • Coma • History of dysrhythmia • Prolonged QT syndrome • Hypokalemia, hypomagnesemia • Drugs that are inhibitors of CYP3A4 (azole antifungals, fluvoxamine, macrolide antibiotics)	• Somnolence • Drowsiness • Rash • Xerostomia • Constipation • Diarrhea • Increased appetite • Taste disturbance • Impotence • Weakness • Visual disturbance • Speech disorder • Hypotension	• Vital signs • CBCs • Mental status • ECG at baseline • EPS • Involuntary movement	• Alcohol • CNS depressants • Anticonvulsants • Propranolol • macrolide antibiotics • Lithium • Sertraline • TCAs • CYP3A4 inhibitors	• FDA-labeled for Tourette's disorder • Pregnancy category C	No

Typical Antipsychotics *(cont'd)*

Generic	Brand	Dose & Max mg (frequency)	Contra-indications	Primary Side Effects	Key Monitoring Parameters	Pertinent Drug Interactions	Med Pearls	Top 200
Mechanism of action – loxapine: blocks postsynaptic mesolimbic D_1 and D_2 receptors in the brain, and also possesses serotonin 5-HT$_2$ blocking activity								
Loxapine	Loxitane	• 5–50 mg (BID–QID) • Max: 250 mg/day	• Hypersensitivity • Severe CNS depression • Coma	• Hypotension • Nausea • Constipation • Vomiting • Xerostomia • Weakness • Sexual disturbance • Dizziness	• Vital signs • Mental status • EPS • CBCs • Thyroid function tests • Involuntary movement	• Lorazepam • Alcohol • CNS depressants • TCAs • Anticonvulsants • Lithium	• Use with extreme caution in patients with thyroid disease • False-positive PKU test • Pregnancy category C	No
Mechanism of action – molindone: exerts effect on the ascending reticular activating system								
Molindone	Moban	• 5–50 mg (TID–QID) • Max: 225 mg/day	• Severe cardiovascular disorders • Hypersensitivity	• Drowsiness • Xerostomia • Constipation • Hypotension • Tachycardia	• Vital signs • Mental status • EPS • CBCs	• Phenytoin • Tetracycline • Alcohol • CNS depressants	Pregnancy category C	No
Mechanism of action – thiothixene: blocks postsynaptic dopamine receptors, resulting in inhibition of dopamine-mediated effects; also has alpha-adrenergic blocking activity.								
Thiothixene	Navane	• 1–20 mg (TID) • Max: 60 mg/day	• Hypersensitivity • Severe CNS depression • Circulatory collapse • Blood dyscrasias • Coma	• Hypotension • Dizziness • GI upset • Constipation • Libido changes • Tachycardia • Insomnia	• Vital signs • CBCs • Thyroid function tests • EPS	• Alcohol • CNS depressants	May cause false-positive pregnancy tests	No

Typical Antipsychotics

Mechanism of action — mixed and varied (per agent) D_2/5-HT_2 antagonist activity

Generic	Brand	Dose & Max mg (frequency)	Contra-indications	Primary Side Effects	Key Monitoring Parameters	Pertinent Drug Interactions	Med Pearls	Top 200
Aripiprazole	• Abilify • Abilify Discmelt; Oral tablet, disintegrating tablet, solution, immediate IM injection	• 10–30 mg PO daily (q day) • 9.75 IM (q 2 hours up to 30 mg/day)	Hypersensitivity	• Weight gain • Constipation • Nausea • Vomiting • Akathisia • Dizziness • Hyperglycemia • Hyperlipidemia • Anxiety • Restlessness • Sedation • Prolonged QT interval • Hyperprolactinemia (rare) • EPS (rare) • Tardive dyskinesia (rare) • Tachycardia	• Blood sugar • Fasting lipid panel, BP, and heart rate • Weight/body mass index • Symptoms of psychosis or EPS • ECG	• Ranolazine • Carbamazepine • Quinidine • Ketoconazole • Medications that prolong QT interval • Metoclopramide	Among the lowest risk of metabolic syndrome	Yes
Olanzapine	• Zyprexa • Oral tablets; oral disintegrating tablets; immediate IM injection	• 10–20 mg IM daily (q day) • 10–30 mg IM daily					Higher degree of weight gain than some other atypicals	Yes
Paliperidone	Invega	• 6–12 mg daily (q day)					• Major active metabolite of risperidone • Newest med in this class, least clinical evidence	No
Quetiapine	• Seroquel • Oral tablets, ER tablets	• IR: 50–750 mg daily (BID–TID) • ER: 300–800 mg daily (q day)					Dosed at bed time due to somnolence	Yes
Iloperidone	Fanapt	Initial: 1 mg BID recommended dosage range: 6–12 mg BID (max: 24 mg/day) Recommended titration schedule: increase in 2 mg increments every 24 hours on days 2–7					Lower risk of weight gain than many atypical, low risk of somnolence; may improve cognitive function	No
Asenapine	Saphris	• Schizophrenia: 5 mg BID • Bipolar disorder: 10 mg BID					Very low incidence of EPS	No

Atypical Antipsychotics *(cont'd)*

Generic	Brand	Dose & Max mg (frequency)	Contra-indications	Primary Side Effects	Key Monitoring Parameters	Pertinent Drug Interactions	Med Pearls	Top 200
Risperidone	• Risperdal • Risperdal Consta • Risperdal M–Tab • Tablet, liquid, disintegrating tablet, long-acting injection	• 2–16 mg PO daily (q day–BID) • 25–50 mg IM q 2 wks	(same as above)	(same as above)	(same as above)	(same as above)	Sedation often leads to bedtime dosing	Yes
Ziprasidone	Geodon	40–160 mg daily (BID)	• History of cardiac arrhythmias • Uncompensated heart failure • Hypersensitivity • Acute or recent MI • QT prolongation history • Drugs that cause QT prolongation				Lower risk of metabolic syndrome when compared to other atypicals	Yes
Lurasidone	Latuda	40–80 mg PO once daily	Hypersensitivity; concomitant use with CYP3A4 inhibitors or inducers			• Potent inducers (rifampin) and inhibitors (ketoconazole) of CYP3A4, diltiazem • Metoclopramide (increased risk of EPS)	Metabolized by CYP3A4	No

Atypical Antipsychotics *(cont'd)*

Generic	Brand	Dose & Max mg (frequency)	Contra-indications	Primary Side Effects	Key Monitoring Parameters	Pertinent Drug Interactions	Med Pearls	Top 200
Clozapine	• Clozaril • FazaClo	12.5–900 mg daily (q day–TID)	• History of clozapine-induced agranulocytosis or severe granulocytopenia • Myelo-proliferative disorder • Paralytic ileus • CNS depression or comatose states • Other agents that cause agranulocytosis	• Hypotension • Tachyarrhythmia • Rash • Weight gain • Agranulocytosis • Neuroleptic malignant syndrome (rare)	• WBC and absolute neutrophil count (ANC) wkly for 6 mo, q 2 wks for 6 mo, and then q 4 wks • S/S of psychotic behavior • Blood sugar, fasting lipid panel • Symptoms of neuroleptic malignant syndrome • BP and heart rate • Orthostatic hypotension • ECG	• Droperidol • Buspirone • Carbamazepine • Lithium • Tramadol • Zotepine	• Used less frequently than other atypicals due to requirement for frequent monitoring • Effective in treatment of refractory cases and in patients at high risk for suicide	Yes

Storage and Administration Pearls

- All medications should be stored at room temperature in a dry area away from direct sunlight.
- Patient may take medications with food if GI upset occurs.

Patient Education Pearls

- Grapefruit Juice should be avoided when taking these medications.
- Alcohol should be avoided due to excessive CNS depression.
- Driving or operating heavy machinery should be avoided until patients know how they respond to medication.
- All medications can take up to several weeks (2–4 weeks) to see full effect.
- Medications should *not* be abruptly discontinued.
- Patients should not self-adjust dose.
- Patients should report to a physician any side effects that disrupt their daily life (i.e., EPS).

LEARNING POINTS

- The most commonly used antidepressants are the SSRIs. These agents may take several weeks to reach maximal efficacy.
- Bupropion is the antidepressant of choice in patients with sexual side effects resulting from other classes of antidepressants.
- The treatment of anxiety and panic disorder may include acute therapies such as benzodiazepines but may also include chronic prophylactic therapies with antidepressants.
- Mood stabilizer therapy is the mainstay of treatment for bipolar disorder. Lithium has a narrow therapeutic window and requires therapeutic serum monitoring.
- While atypical antipsychotic medications exhibit fewer extrapyramidal side effects than typical agents, they do carry a greater risk of metabolic side effects such as weight gain, hyperglycemia, and hyperlipidemia. Atypical antipsychotics are more effective in treating the negative symptoms of schizophrenia.

ALZHEIMER'S DISEASE

Definition

Alzheimer's disease (AD) is a dementia of progressive nature that affects, in the early stages, primarily cognition and in later stages behavior and functional status. The pathophysiology is not fully understood but is known to involve destruction of neurons and synapses and cortical atrophy.

Diagnosis

The *Diagnostic and Statistical Manual of Mental Disorders, Fourth Edition* (DSM IV) criteria describe an insidious onset of memory impairment plus one additional cognitive defect. The diagnosis is based upon evidence of progressive cognitive decline from baseline that has reached the point of impacting social or occupational functioning along with the ruling out of reversible causes such as thyroid abnormalities, vitamin deficiencies, medication side effects, and infections.

Signs & Symptoms

Problems with memory, difficulty performing familiar tasks, forgetting information that was recently acquired, poor judgment, difficulty with abstract concepts, mood changes, and loss of interest in usual activities include some of the most common elements of the clinical presentation. The Folstein Mini-Mental State Examination (MMSE) is often used to provide staging and clinical guidance. MMSE scores of 20 or greater are considered mild AD, scores of 10–19 indicated moderate disease, and scores less than 10 indicate severe cases.

Guidelines

American College of Physicians/American Academy of Family Physicians (ACP/AAFP). Current pharmacologic treatment of dementia: a clinical practice guideline from the American College of Physicians and the American Academy of Family Physicians. Ann Intern Med 2008 Mar 4;148(5):370–8.

Guidelines Summary:

- Goals of treatment include preservation of function and symptomatic slowing of cognitive decline. A commonly used benchmark is the change in MMSE within one year. Without therapy, MMSE would be expected to decrease approximately two to four points per year. Therapeutic efficacy is often determined if MMSE decreases by two or fewer points per year. None of the available therapies has an impact on halting disease progression or reversing pathophysiology.

- Cholinesterase inhibitors are the treatment of choice in mild to moderate AD. Although slight differences exist in the mechanisms of these agents, there is no evidence to indicate greater efficacy with one agent over another. Agent selection is typically made based upon patient preference, cost, and potential for drug interactions. There is insufficient evidence to support a dose-response relationship within this class. It is currently recommended that patients be started on the lowest dose and titrated slowly to the typical maintenance dose.

- Memantine is the only currently available NMDA receptor agonist and has been studied and approved in moderate to severe AD as either monotherapy or an adjunct to a cholinesterase inhibitor.

- The most widely accepted approach to treatment is to initiate a low-dose cholinesterase inhibitor at the time of diagnosis with slow titration to typical maintenance dose. After 6 months to one year, efficacy is assessed. If this therapy is not efficacious, the patient can be switched to an alternate cholinesterase inhibitor, dose can be increased, or memantine can be added (in moderate to severe disease).

Cholinesterase Inhibitors

Generic	Brand	Dose & Max	Contraindications	Primary Side Effects	Key Monitoring Parameters	Pertinent Drug Interactions	Med Pearls	Top 200
Mechanism of action – inhibits the activity of cholinesterase enzyme, thereby allowing greater acetylcholine activity								
Donepezil	• Aricept • Tablets and orally disintegrating tablets	• 5 mg daily, titrated to 10 mg daily after 4–6 weeks • Max of 23 mg daily in moderate–severe AD	Hypersensitivity	• Nausea • Vomiting • Diarrhea • Urinary incontinence • Dizziness • Headache • Syncope • Salivation • Sweating • Bradycardia • Hypertension	• Presence of side effects • Heart rate, blood pressure, MMSE at 6–12 month intervals	• Succinylcholine: prolonged neuromuscular blockade (AVOID) • Oxybutynin/tolterodine: decrease efficacy of donepezil • Ramelteon, ketoconazole, bethanechol, quinidine	• Slow titration can increase tolerability • Donepezil and galantamine available as generic	Yes
Galantamine	• Razadyne: oral solution, tablet • Razadyne ER: extended release capsule	• 4–12 mg PO BID • 8–24 mg PO once daily				• Oxybutynin/tolterodine: decrease efficacy of galantamine • Quinidine, ketoconazole, paroxetine, fluoxetine, fluvoxamine: increased galantamine concentrations		No
Rivastigmine	Exelon: transdermal patch	4.6–9.5 mg/24 hours				• Metoclopramide: increased risk of EPS (contraindicated) • Oxybutynin/tolterodine: decrease efficacy of rivastigmine		No

NMDA Receptor Antagonists

Generic	Brand	Dose & Max	Contraindications	Primary Side Effects	Key Monitoring Parameters	Pertinent Drug Interactions	Med Pearls	Top 200
Mechanism of action – NMDA receptor antagonist								
Memantine	• Namenda • Namenda XR	• 5–10 mg PO BID • 7–28 mg PO daily	Hypersensitivity	• Confusion • Constipation • Dizziness • Headache • Diarrhea • Vomiting • Hypertension	• Presence of side effects • Blood pressure, MMSE at 6–12 month intervals	• Carbonic anhydrase inhibitors • Nicotine polacrilex • Quinidine • Ranitidine • Sodium bicarbonate • Cimetidine • Hydrochlorothiazide	Indicated for moderate–severe AD as monotherapy or in combination with cholinesterase inhibitor	No

Storage and Administration Pearls

- Donepezil: Should be taken in evening prior to bed with or without food. Oral disintegrating tablets should be allowed to dissolve on tongue and then followed with glass of water.

- Galantamine: Ensure adequate fluid intake while on therapy, and take with food. Do not crush, break, or chew extended-release capsules.

- Rivastigmine: Apply patch to a dry, hairless area of skin (preferably upper back) and rotate site of application daily.

Patient Education Pearls

- The most common side effects are nausea, vomiting, diarrhea, and dizziness.

- Abrupt discontinuation of therapy may cause worsening of symptoms.

- The expected outcome is that the medications will slow progression. Significant improvement is not likely to be observed.

PRACTICE QUESTIONS

1. Which of the following is first-line in the treatment of acute depressive episode in a patient with bipolar disorder?

    (A) Lithium
    (B) Valproic acid
    (C) Oxcarbazepine
    (D) Lamictal
    (E) Carbamazepine

2. Which of the following medications can be used in the treatment of anxiety?

    I.   Clonazepam
    II. Venlafaxine
    III. Hydroxyzine

    (A) I only
    (B) III only
    (C) I and II only
    (D) II and III only
    (E) I, II, III

ANSWERS

1. **D**

According to the guidelines, first-line treatment options for acute depression episodes include lamotrigine as monotherapy or in combination with antimania agents. Lithium (A) and valproic acid (B) are used as first-line treatment options for acute manic episodes. Oxcarbazepine (C) and carbamazepine (E) would also be used as first-line treatment options of acute manic episodes. Maintenance therapy may consist of a combination of medications for both depression and manic episodes.

2. **E**

All of the named medications can be used in the treatment of anxiety. Clonazepam (I) is a benzodiazepine, which is commonly used for the acute treatment of anxiety. Venlafaxine (II) is generic Effexor, which is labeled for GAD, PD, and SAD. Hydroxyzine (III) competes with histamine and can also be used in the treatment of anxiety.

Bone and Joint Disorders

9

This chapter covers the following disease states:

- **Osteoarthritis**
- **Rheumatoid arthritis**
- **Osteoporosis**
- **Gout**

 Suggested Study Time: **45 minutes**

OSTEOARTHRITIS

Definition

Osteoarthritis (OA) is a disease of the cartilage resulting from an imbalance between cartilage destruction and formation with subsequent bony proliferation within the joint, which results in pain, potentially decreased range of motion, and local inflammation.

Diagnosis

The diagnosis of OA is based on history, physical exam, and radiographs. History and physical exam will reveal symptoms and signs consistent with OA (detailed below) and should be used to rule out other potential conditions such as rheumatoid arthritis. Radiologic changes may include joint space narrowing, osteophytes, or subchondral bone sclerosis.

Signs and Symptoms

- Osteoarthritis signs: Physical exam may reveal tenderness, crepitus, and/or enlargement of the affected joints. Radiologic evaluation is necessary to identify presence of OA and disease progression. Radiographic changes may not be easily identifiable in early, mild disease but with disease progression may include narrowing of the joint spaces, presence of osteophytes, subchondral bony sclerosis, and eventual subluxation and deformity.

- Osteoarthritis symptoms: Patients with OA present with pain, stiffness, and instability of joints that can be unilateral or bilateral. The pain is often worsened with weight-bearing activity and is described as deep and aching. Stiffness may resolve with motion but may limit physical activity. Commonly affected joints include the hands, knees, and hips.

Guidelines

American College of Rheumatology Subcommittee on Osteoarthritis Guidelines: Recommendations for medical management of osteoarthritis of the hip and knee. *Arthntis Rheum* no. 43(9) (2000): 1905–15. www.rheumatology.org/publications/guidelines/oa-mgmt/oa-mgmt.asp.

Guidelines Summary

The goals of therapy are to decrease pain and stiffness, maintain/improve joint mobility and limit functional impairment, and increase the quality of life.

- Nonpharmacological therapy: Rest, physical therapy, and weight loss
- Pharmacological therapy:
  - First-line: Scheduled acetaminophen up to a maximum daily dose of 4 g
  - Second-line: Nonsteroidal anti-inflammatory drugs (NSAIDs); specific agent chosen based on cost, prior response, and gastrointestinal risk factors
  - Third-line: Narcotic analgesics or hyaluronate injections
  - Adjunctive therapy: Topical capsaicin cream, glucosamine sulfate

Drugs for Osteoarthritis

Generic	Brand	Dose & Max mg (frequency)	Contraindications	Primary Side Effects	Key Monitoring Parameters	Pertinent Drug Interactions	Med Pearls	Top 200
Mechanism of action – decreases pain through inhibition of central cyclo-oxygenase, which in turn inhibits prostaglandin synthesis							
Acetaminophen	Tylenol	• 325–1,000 • TID–QID • Max dose = 4 g/day	• Hepatic disease • Alcoholism	Very few	Pain relief	Alcohol	• Over-the-counter (OTC) • Best if taken on scheduled basis vs. as needed (PRN)	No, OTC
Tramadol	• Ultram • Ultram ER	• Immediate release (IR) 25–400 daily (q 4–6 hrs) • Extended release (ER) 100–300 daily	Hypersensitivity	Confusion, sedation, rash, stomach upset, orthostatic hypotension	Pain relief, renal and hepatic function periodically	• Alcohol • Opioids • Selective serotonin reuptake inhibitors (SSRIs) • Monoamine oxidase inhibitors (MAOIs) • Warfarin	Renal dose adjustment for CrCl <30 mL/min	Yes
Mechanism of action – induces the release of substance P, the principle chemomediator of pain impulses from the periphery							
Capsaicin cream	Various	0.025–0.1% applied 3–4x daily	Do not apply to wounds or damaged skin	Localized stinging	Pain relief	None	• OTC • Must be used regularly for 2 wks or more for maximal efficacy	No
Mechanism of action – nonsteroidal anti-inflammatory drugs (NSAIDs): decrease pain and inflammation by inhibition of prostaglandin synthesis through inhibition of cyclooxygenase enzymes.							
Aspirin	Various	• IR 325–3,600 daily (q 4–6 hrs) • XR product 650–1,300 TID	• Allergy • Fever in children • Active bleeding	• Gastrointestinal (GI) (upset stomach, bleeding) • Rash	Pain relief, GI symptoms	• Warfarin • Other NSAIDs • Angiotensin-converting enzyme (ACE) inhibitors • Antiplatelets	• OTC • Anti-inflammatory only at high doses (>3 g/day)	No, OTC
Nonacetylated salicylates							
Salsalate	Various	500–3,000 daily (BID–TID)	Hypersensitivity	• GI (upset stomach, bleeding) • Rash • Diminished renal function • Edema	Pain relief, GI symptoms	• Other salicylates • Warfarin • ACE inhibitors	• Monitor serum salicylate levels with chronic use or very high doses • Desired range 10–30 mg/100 mL	No
Diflunisal	None	500–1,500 daily (BID)					Administer with food	No

Drugs for Osteoarthritis *(cont'd)*

Generic	Brand	Dose & Max mg (frequency)	Contraindications	Primary Side Effects	Key Monitoring Parameters	Pertinent Drug Interactions	Med Pearls	Top 200
Acetic acids								
Etodolac	None	200–1,200 daily (Q 6–8 hrs)	Hypersensitivity	• GI (upset stomach, bleeding) • Rash • Diminished renal function • ↑ Blood pressure (BP) • Edema	• Pain relief • GI symptoms • Renal function • Blood pressure	• Other salicylates • Warfarin • Lithium • ACE inhibitors	Administer with food	Yes
Diclofenac	• Cataflam • Voltaren	50–150 daily (BID–TID)						Yes
Indomethacin	• Indocin • Indocin SR	• IR 25–200 daily (BID–TID) • Sustained release (SR) 75–150 1x daily		• GI (upset stomach, bleeding) • Rash • Diminished renal function • ↑ BP • Edema • Central nervous system (CNS) disturbances			• Most commonly used for treatment of gout • Fat-soluble, crosses blood brain barrier • Administer with food	No
Ketorolac	Toradol	30 mg IM or 15 mg IV initial; 10 mg PO q 4–6 hrs up to 40 mg daily	• Active peptic ulcer disease (PUD) or bleeding • History of GI bleeding • Severe renal impairment • Labor and delivery	• GI (upset stomach, bleeding) • Rash • Diminished renal function • ↑BP • Edema			• Only approved for moderate-severe pain for ≤5 days duration • Available IM and IV as well	No
Nabumetone	Relafen	500–2,000 daily (q day–BID)	Hypersensitivity				Administer with food	Yes

Drugs for Osteoarthritis *(cont'd)*

Generic	Brand	Dose & Max mg (frequency)	Contraindications	Primary Side Effects	Key Monitoring Parameters	Pertinent Drug Interactions	Med Pearls	Top 200
Propionic acids								
Fenoprofen	Nalfon	200–3,200 daily (TID–QID)	Hypersensitivity	• GI (upset stomach, bleeding) • Rash • Diminished renal function • Increase BP • Edema	• Pain relief • GI symptoms • Renal function • BP	• Other salicylates • Warfarin • ACE inhibitors • Lithium	Administer with food	No
Flurbiprofen	Ansaid	50–300 daily (BID–QID)						No
Ibuprofen	• Motrin • Advil	200–3,200 daily (TID–QID)					• Available OTC and Rx (400–800 mg tabs) • Administer with food • Available in pediatric preparations	Yes
Ketoprofen	• Orudis • Oruvail • Rhodis • Apo-Keto-E	• IR: 50–300 daily (TID–QID) • SR: 75–200 daily						No
Naproxen	• Naprosyn • Naprosyn • Naprelan	• IR: 250–1,500 daily (BID) • EC: 375–1,500 daily (BID) • Controlled release (CR): 375–1,500 daily (BID)					• Available OTC and Rx • Administer with food	Yes
Naproxen sodium	Anaprox	275–1,650 daily (BID)						Yes
Oxaprozin	Daypro	600–1800 daily (1x daily)					Administer with food	No

Drugs for Osteoarthritis *(cont'd)*

Generic	Brand	Dose & Max mg (frequency)	Contraindications	Primary Side Effects	Key Monitoring Parameters	Pertinent Drug Interactions	Med Pearls	Top 200
Fenamates								
Meclofenamate	None available	50–400 mg daily (q 4–6 hrs)	Hypersensitivity	GI (upset stomach, bleeding); rash; diminished renal function; ↑ BP; edema	Pain relief, GI symptoms, renal function, BP	Other salicylates, warfarin, ACE inhibitors, lithium	Administer with food	No
Oxicams								
Piroxicam	Feldene	10–20 mg daily (1x daily)	Hypersensitivity	GI (upset stomach, bleeding); rash; diminished renal function; ↑ BP; edema	Pain relief, GI symptoms, renal function, BP	Other salicylates, warfarin, ACE inhibitors, lithium	More COX-2 selectivity than traditional NSAIDs; slightly less GI symptoms	No
Meloxicam	Mobic	7.5–15 mg daily (1x daily)						Yes
Selective COX-2 inhibitors								
Celecoxib	Celebrex	50–200 mg daily (q day–BID)	Hypersensitivity	GI (upset stomach, bleeding—less than other NSAIDs); rash; diminished renal function; ↑ BP; edema	Pain relief, GI symptoms, renal function, BP	Other salicylates (including aspirin), warfarin, ACE inhibitors, lithium	• Lower incidence of GI toxicity than with nonselective NSAIDs • Concern about cardiovascular adverse effects prompted withdrawal of similar drug from market (rofecoxib)	Yes
Narcotic analgesics – stimulate opioid receptors in the brain								
Hydrocodone/ APAP	• Various • Lortab • Vicodin	• 5–60 mg hydrocodone daily (q4–6 hrs)	• Hypersensitivity • Severe hepatic impairment • Alcoholism	• Constipation • CNS depression • Confusion • Sedation • Respiratory depression • Hypotension • Bradycardia	• Presence of side effects (constipation, confusion) • Pain relief • Respiratory rate • BP • Heart rate	• Alcohol • Other CNS depressants	• Take with food • Often need laxative in addition • High abuse potential	Yes
APAP/Codeine	• Various • Tylenol #3	7.5–360 mg codeine daily (q4–6 hrs)						Yes

Drugs for Osteoarthritis *(cont'd)*

Generic	Brand	Dose & Max mg (frequency)	Contraindications	Primary Side Effects	Key Monitoring Parameters	Pertinent Drug Interactions	Med Pearls	Top 200
Morphine	Various	See chapter on pain management						Yes
Oxycodone/ APAP	• Various • Percocet • Roxicet	5–40 mg daily oxycodone (q6 hrs PRN)						Yes
Adjunctive therapies/nutritional supplements								
Glucosamine Sulfate	Various	500–1,500 daily (q day–BID)	Unknown	• Itching • GI upset	• Pain relief • Presence of side effects	Unknown	• Nutritional supplement • Available OTC • Conflicting clinical trial data	No
Intra-articular injections								
Mechanism of action – serves as a lubricant for joint tissue								
Hyaluronate and derivates	• Synvisc • Synvisc-One	• Inject 16 mg (2 mL) once weekly for 3 wks (total of 3 injections) • Inject 48 mg (6 mL) once per knee	Hypersensitivity	• Injection site reaction • Bruising • Erythema • Lumps • Pain • Swelling • Pruritus • Skin discoloration • Arthralgia • Infection	• Intraocular pressure • Signs and symptoms of inflammation or infection	No known significant drug interactions	None	No

Storage and Administration Pearls

- NSAIDs should be administered with food to decrease the risk of gastrointestinal side effects.
- Capsaicin cream may take several weeks for maximal efficacy to be demonstrated. Regular daily use, 2–4 times daily for 4 weeks, is considered an adequate trial.

Patient Education Pearls

- Take NSAIDs with food to avoid stomach upset.
- Avoid alcohol when taking acetaminophen or narcotic analgesics due to the risk of liver damage.
- Avoid driving or operating heavy machinery while taking narcotics.
- Capsaicin cream may take 2–4 weeks to become effective. Allow an adequate trial before determining efficacy.
- Wash your hands very thoroughly after capsaicin application.

RHEUMATOID ARTHRITIS

Definition

Rheumatoid arthritis (RA) is an autoimmune disease characterized by chronic inflammation of the synovial tissue lining the joint capsule. The erosive synovitis is generally symmetrical and extra-articular involvement may also occur, including rheumatoid nodules, cardiopulmonary disease, lymphadenopathy, splenomegaly, and neurological dysfunction.

Diagnosis

RA diagnosis is based on history and physical, laboratory evidence, and radiographic evaluation. History and physical will reveal consistent signs and symptoms of RA. Laboratory evidence will demonstrate rheumatoid factor presence in 60–70% of affected patients, elevated erythrocyte sedimentation rate and c-reactive protein, and radiographic evidence of joint space narrowing or erosions.

Signs and Symptoms

- Symmetrical symptoms of joint pain and stiffness (especially in the morning) for more than 6 weeks' duration
- Joint tenderness, erythema, swelling, and, potentially, rheumatoid nodules

Guidelines

American College of Rheumatology 2008 recommendations for the use of nonbiologic and biologic disease-modifying antirheumatic drugs in rheumatoid arthritis. At: http://www.rheumatology.org/practice/clinical/guidelines/recommendations.pdf.

Guidelines Summary

- Disease modifying antirheumatic drug (DMARD) should be initiated within 3 months of diagnosis to retard disease progression.
- Leflunomide, sulfasalazine, hydroxychloroquine, and methotrexate are first-line DMARD options.
- In patients with moderate to severe disease activity or those with features of poor prognosis (functional limitation, extra-articular disease, rheumatoid factor positivity, bony erosions) at the time of diagnosis, combination therapy may be considered initially.
- NSAIDs are useful for symptomatic relief during onset of DMARD and PRN otherwise. NSAIDs do not alter disease progression in RA.
- Corticosteroids are used as adjunctive therapy in patient with refractory symptoms.
- Biologic agents are used when initial DMARD has been demonstrated to be ineffective as monotherapy. Additional DMARDs may be tried prior to use of biologics.
- Biologic therapies increase the risk of serious infections and should not be initiated in a patient with an active infection.

Drugs for Rheumatoid Arthritis

Generic	Brand	Dose & Max mg (frequency)	Contraindications	Primary Side Effects	Key Monitoring Parameters	Pertinent Drug Interactions	Med Pearls	Top 200
Mechanism of action – corticosteroids: exert anti-inflammatory and immunosuppressive effects by inhibiting prostaglandins and leukotrienes, which results in decreased inflammation, decreased pain, and a potential decrease in joint destruction								
Prednisone	Various	5–60 mg daily initially; individualized	• Systemic fungal infection • Hypersensitivity	• High blood sugar • High BP • Reduced bone mineral density • Fluid retention • Impaired wound healing	Blood sugar, BP, bone mineral density, presence of edema/weight	Warfarin	Side effects generally present with chronic and/or long-term use	Yes
Disease-modifying antirheumatic drugs (DMARDs)								
Mechanism of action – inhibits cytokine production, inhibits purine biosynthesis, thereby decreasing inflammation in affected joints								
Methotrexate	• Rheumatrex • Trexall	7.5 mg 1x wkly	• Hypersensitivity • Alcoholism • Severe hepatic impairment • Immuno-deficiency • Significant blood dyscrasias/anemias • Pregnancy • CrCl <40 mL/min	• GI upset (nausea, diarrhea, abdominal pain) • Stomatitis • Thrombocytopenia • Leukopenia • ↑ liver enzymes • Malaise • Fatigue • Fever/chills • Infections	• Pain relief • Liver function tests (LFTs) • Periodic complete blood count (CBC) • Folate	Salicylates, sulfonamides, phenytoin	• May supplement folic acid to decrease adverse effects and prevent folate deficiency • Myelosuppression is biggest concern • Should be taken with food	Yes
Mechanism of action – not fully understood; thought to be related to immunosuppressant properties								
Hydroxy-chloroquine	Plaquenil	200–600 mg daily (1x daily)	• Hypersensitivity • Retinal changes with agent in past	Macular damage, corneal deposits, retinopathy; rash; nausea, diarrhea	• Ocular exams q 3 mo • Periodic CBC	Cyclosporine, digoxin	Older drug without risk of myelosuppression but ocular risk	No

Drugs for Rheumatoid Arthritis *(cont'd)*

Generic	Brand	Dose & Max mg (frequency)	Contraindications	Primary Side Effects	Key Monitoring Parameters	Pertinent Drug Interactions	Med Pearls	Top 200
Mechanism of action – leflunomide: inhibits pyrimidine synthesis, thereby decreasing lymphocyte proliferation and inflammation								
Leflunomide	Arava	Load 100 mg daily for 3 days; 20 mg daily maintenance	• Hepatic disease • Pregnancy • Immuno-deficiency	• Diarrhea • Elevated liver enzymes • Alopecia • Rash	Alanine transaminase (ALT) monthly x 6 mo, then periodically	Cholestyramine, rifampin	• Oral DMARD with low risk of bone marrow toxicity • Appropriate contraception should be used • Highly teratogenic	No
Mechanism of action – not fully understood; related to anti-inflammatory properties								
Sulfasalazine	Azulfidine	250–2,000 mg daily (BID)	Hypersensitivity to any sulfa-containing drug	• Frequent diarrhea, nausea, vomiting • Rash • Urticaria • Photosensitivity • Leukopenia • Alopecia • Stomatitis • Elevated liver enzymes	• Response to therapy • Presence of adverse effects • CBC • Liver enzymes	Warfarin, methotrexate, cyclosporine, digoxin, thiopurines	• Warfarin interaction very clinically significant • Monitor international normalized ratio (INR) closely	No
Biologics								
Mechanism of action – binds to and inhibits the cytokine tumor necrosis factor (TNF), thereby inhibiting the subsequent inflammatory cascade								
Etanercept	Enbrel	50 mg SC 1x wk	• Sepsis • Active infection • Hypersensitivity	• Local injection site reactions • Infections	Response to therapy	Anakinra; cyclophosphamide; live vaccines	• Refrigerate prior to use • Discontinue temporarily if infection occurs • Can be self-administered • Can be used alone or in combination with methotrexate (MTX)	No

Drugs for Rheumatoid Arthritis (cont'd)

Generic	Brand	Dose & Max mg (frequency)	Contraindications	Primary Side Effects	Key Monitoring Parameters	Pertinent Drug Interactions	Med Pearls	Top 200
Mechanism of action – monoclonal antibody that binds to TNF and prevents interaction with TNF receptors on inflammatory cells								
Infliximab	Remicade	3–10 mg/kg IV infusion at initiation; wks 2 and 6 and q8 wks thereafter	• Active infection • Hypersensitivity	• Infections (upper respiratory common) • Acute infusion reactions (fever, chills, rash)	• Response to therapy	• Anakinra • Live vaccines	• *Always* used in combination with MTX • Dose limited to ≤5 mg/kg in patients with heart failure	No
Mechanism of action – monoclonal antibody that binds to TNF, blocking its interaction with cell surface receptors and decreasing inflammation								
Adalimumab	Humira	40 mg subcutaneously (SC) q other wk to wkly	• Active infection • Untreated latent tuberculosis (TB)	Injection-site reactions; infections	• Tuberculin skin test (PPD) prior to initiation • Ongoing monitoring for response to therapy and presence of infection • Response to therapy	• Anakinra • Live vaccines	• Caution use in patients with heart failure • Discontinue during serious infections • Used as monotherapy or in combination with MTX or other DMARDs	No
Mechanism of action – Binds to interleukin-1 (IL-1) receptors on target cells, thereby preventing release of chemotactic factors and adhesion molecules and subsequently decreasing inflammation and connective tissue damage								
Anakinra	Kineret	100 mg SC daily	• Hypersensitivity • Active infections	Injection-site reactions (inflammation, ecchymosis); infections; neutropenia	• CBC periodically • Response to therapy • Presence of adverse effects	• Etanercept, infliximab, adalimumab • Live vaccines	Used alone or in combination with DMARDs (other than TNF blockers)	No
Mechanism of action – interluekin-6 (IL-6) receptor antagonist								
Tocilizumab	Actemra	IV: Initial: 4 mg/kg every 4 weeks; may be increased to 8 mg/kg based on clinical response (maximum: 800 mg per infusion)	None	• Serious: potentially fatal infections, TB • Common: upper respiratory tract infection, nasopharyngitis, elevated aspartate aminotransferase (AST)/ alanine aminotransferase (ALT)	• Signs and symptoms of infection • TB test prior to initiation and during therapy • CBC, lipid panel, and AST/ ALT prior and every 4–8 weeks during therapy • LFT • Signs and symptoms of CNS demyelinating disorders	• May diminish the therapeutic effect of immunosuppressants • Not to be used with live vaccines	• Discontinue use if serious infection • Do not use with live vaccines • Monotherapy or in addition to MTX • Indicated for patients that have failed one or more TNF agents	No

Drugs for Rheumatoid Arthritis *(cont'd)*

Generic	Brand	Dose & Max mg (frequency)	Contraindications	Primary Side Effects	Key Monitoring Parameters	Pertinent Drug Interactions	Med Pearls	Top 200
Mechanism of action — TNFα inhibitor								
Golimumab	Simponi	50 mg SC once per month	None	• Infection • Nasopharyngitis • Injection site reaction • Elevated AST/ALT	• TB test prior to initiation and during therapy • Signs and symptoms of infection and heart failure • CBC • Hepatitis B virus (HBV) screening	• May diminish the therapeutic effect of immunosuppressants • Not to be given with live vaccines	• Once monthly SC injection may increase use due to convenience • Indicated for use in combination with MTX • Caution use in patients with heart failure • Discontinue use if serious infection • Refrigerated (not frozen)	No
Mechanism of action — Selective co-stimulation modulator; inhibits T-cell activation								
Abatacept	Orencia	IV according to body weight; repeat dose at 2 wks, 4 wks, and every 4 wks thereafter <60 kg: 500 mg 60–100 kg: 750 mg >100 kg: 1,000 mg	Hypersensitivity	• Headache • Nausea • Nasopharyngitis • Upper respiratory tract infection • Antibody formation	• TB and hepatitis test prior to initiation • Signs and symptoms of infection and infusion reaction	• May diminish the therapeutic effect of immunosuppressants • Should not be given with live vaccines • Increased risk of infection with TNF antagonists	• Not to be given with TNF antagonists or live vaccines • Discontinue use if serious infection • Infections more likely in patients with chronic obstructive pulmonary disease (COPD) • Can be used as monotherapy or in combination with MTX	No

Storage and Administration Pearls

- NSAIDs should be administered with food to decrease risk of gastrointestinal side effects.

- Oral methotrexate should be administered with food to avoid stomach upset.

- The following medications should be refrigerated to 2–8°C (36–46°F): MTX injectable, etanercept, infliximab, adalimumab, anakinra, and golimumab. These medications should *not* be frozen and should be protected from light.

- The following medications are administered through SC injection: etanercept, adalimumab, anakinra.

- Methotrexate is administered orally or through intramuscular (IM) injection.

- Infliximab, tocilizumab, and abatacept cannot be self-administered and are delivered through IV infusion.

- The following medications are available in prefilled syringes and/or pen devices: etanercept, adalimumab, anakinra, and golimumab.

Patient Education Pearls

- Promptly report any signs of infection to your physician. A temporary withdrawal of medication may be necessary during this time.

- Do not receive live vaccines while you are on biologic therapies.

- Appropriate administration of injectable therapies is as follows:
  - Visually inspect the products for particulate matter or discoloration. Do not use if either is present.
  - MTX is injected IM.
  - All other injectables are SC administration.
  - Rotate injection site.
  - Do not inject into tender, bruised, hard, or ulcerated skin.
  - Do not reuse needles or syringes.
  - Properly dispose of needles in a puncture-proof container.

OSTEOPOROSIS

Definition

Osteoporosis is a condition of low bone mass, which results in increased fragility of bone and subsequent increased risk of fracture. Potential etiologies of the characteristic decreased bone mass include age-related physiologic changes, disorders of estrogen or testosterone levels, or use of medications associated with drug-induced osteoporosis. Although more common in women, osteoporosis also occurs in men.

Normal bone physiology includes constant bone remodeling, which consists of bone formation via osteoblasts and bone resorption via osteoclasts. Bone mineral density (BMD) reflects the balance between resorption and formation. Osteoporosis occurs when there is an imbalance between formation and resorption resulting in a decreased BMD.

Diagnosis

The diagnosis of osteoporosis is most commonly based on the results of BMD measurement with dual energy x-ray absorptiometry (DXA) at the hip and spine. Results of the DXA are reported as the T score. The T score represents the number of standard deviations away from the mean BMD for a young, healthy individual. Normal BMD would be considered any T score greater than –1, while osteopenia would be a T score –1 to –2.5; a T score of less than –2.5 would be diagnostic for osteoporosis. Osteoporosis can also be diagnosed based on the occurrence of a nontraumatic fracture.

Signs and Symptoms

Typical signs of osteoporosis include kyphosis, shortened stature, and nontraumatic fractures of the vertebrae, hip, or forearm. Some patients may have symptoms of bone pain, and often vertebral fractures go undiagnosed as patients complain of chronic back pain. In a patient with risk factors for osteoporosis, radiographic investigation of back pain is warranted. Pain and physical changes associated with osteoporosis may lead to depression and lowered self-esteem.

Guidelines

American Association of Clinical Endocrinologists medical guidelines for clinical practice for the prevention and treatment of osteoporosis: 2001 Edition, with selected updates for 2003. *Endocr Pract,* no. 9(6) (2003): 544–64. www.aace.com/pub/pdf/guidelines/osteoporosis2001Revised.pdf.

Guidelines Summary

- Oral calcium and vitamin D supplementation is an important prerequisite to pharmacological therapy. Without adequate calcium and vitamin D available, other therapies will be limited in their ability to improve bone architecture.
- Bisphosphonates are the first-line therapy for the prevention and treatment of osteoporosis in patients without contraindications.
- Oral bisphosphonates are approved for prevention and treatment of osteoporosis (including glucocorticoid-induced osteoporosis) in men and women.
- Raloxifene is recommended as an alternative choice for the treatment of osteoporosis in patients with contraindications to bisphosphonates or in patients who are unable to comply with the appropriate bisphosphonate administration instructions.
- Calcitonin is reserved for third-line therapy because of a lack of compelling evidence indicating fracture reductions and lack of long-term data. Calcitonin is approved for the treatment of acute pain secondary to vertebral fractures and is well tolerated, so may have specific role in certain situations.
- Teriparatide is approved for treatment of osteoporosis and is indicated in patients with a history of fracture secondary to osteoporosis and in those with multiple risk factors for fracture who have not responded or are intolerant to bisphosphonate therapy.
- Denosumab is reserved for second-line therapy for the treatment of osteoporosis in postmenopausal females at high risk for fracture (previous osteoporotic fractures, multiple fracture risk factors, failed other therapies).

Drugs for Osteoporosis

Mechanism of action – bisphosphonates: adsorb to bone apatite and inhibit osteoclast activity

Generic	Brand	Dose & Max	Contra-indications	Primary Side Effects	Key Monitoring Parameters	Pertinent Drug Interactions	Med Pearls	Top 200
Alendronate	Fosamax	• 10 mg daily or 70 mg 1x wk (treatment) • 5 mg daily or 35 mg 1x wk (prevention)	Esophageal stricture; hypersensitivity; inability to sit upright or stand for 30 minutes; CrCl <35 mL/min; hypocalcemia	Nausea, dyspepsia, esophageal irritation, ulceration, muscle pain	BMD	NSAIDs/aspirin increase risk of GI symptoms	• Must be taken with at least 8 oz of water ≥30 minutes prior to other medications/food • Patient should remain upright for 30 min or more	Yes
Risedronate	Actonel	5 mg daily or 35 mg 1x wk						Yes
Ibandronate	Boniva	(PO) 2.5 mg daily or 150 mg 1x month						Yes
Zoledronic acid	Reclast	5 mg IV infusion 1x year	Hypersensitivity; CrCl <35 mL/min	Hypotension, agitation, confusion, fever, nausea, constipation, hypocalcemia, muscle pain	BMD	Aminoglycosides	Annual IV infusion	No

Mechanism of action – selective estrogen receptor modulators: through selective binding to estrogen receptors, decreases bone resorption and reduces biochemical markers of bone turnover

Generic	Brand	Dose & Max	Contra-indications	Primary Side Effects	Key Monitoring Parameters	Pertinent Drug Interactions	Med Pearls	Top 200
Raloxifene	Evista	60 mg 1x daily	• Hypersensitivity • History of pulmonary embolism or deep vein thrombosis • Pregnancy/lactation	Hot flushes, leg cramps, thrombo-embolism	BMD; presence of adverse effects	Cholestyramine, warfarin	• Monitor international normalized ratio (INR) closely for patients on warfarin (expect INR increase) • Lipid effects include decreased LDL with no effect on HDL/triglycerides	Yes

Drugs for Osteoporosis *(cont'd)*

Miscellaneous agents

Mechanism of action – inhibits bone resorption through inhibition of osteoclast activity, to a small decrease stimulates bone formation through stimulation of osteoblast activity

Generic	Brand	Dose & Max	Contra-indications	Primary Side Effects	Key Monitoring Parameters	Pertinent Drug Interactions	Med Pearls	Top 200
Calcitonin	• Miacalcin Nasal Spray • Injection	• 200 units (1 spray) daily intranasally • 100 units q other day (SC or IM)	Hypersensitivity	Nasal irritation and dryness, rhinitis	BMD	None	• Refrigerate • Keep nasal spray at room temp while in use (<86°F/30°C) • Discard unused nasal spray after 30 days	No

Mechanism of action – acts as a parathyroid hormone (PTH) agonist; thereby increases bone formation by the stimulation of osteoblast activity and increases renal reabsorption of calcium

Generic	Brand	Dose & Max	Contra-indications	Primary Side Effects	Key Monitoring Parameters	Pertinent Drug Interactions	Med Pearls	Top 200
Teriparatide (PTH)	Forteo	20 mcg 1x daily SC	• Hypersensitivity • Primary hyperparathyroidism • Hypercalcemia • Paget's disease	Orthostatic hypotension, dizziness, nausea, hypercalcemia	BMD	Digoxin (may predispose to digoxin toxicity)	Reduces risk of vertebral and nonvertebral fractures	No

Mechanism of action – monoclonal antibody, bone-modifying agent

Generic	Brand	Dose & Max	Contra-indications	Primary Side Effects	Key Monitoring Parameters	Pertinent Drug Interactions	Med Pearls	Top 200
Denosumab	Prolia	60 mg SC q6 months	Hypocalcemia	• Fatigue • Diarrhea • Nausea • Hyperlipidemia • Hypophosphatemia	• BMD • Serum phosphorous • Calcium • Magnesium	None	• Refrigerate • Should be clear and colorless	No

Storage and Administration Pearls

- Oral bisphosphonates should be taken on an empty stomach first thing in the morning with at least 8 oz of water. At least 30 to 60 minutes should pass prior to ingestion of any medication or food. Patient should remain upright for 30 to 60 minutes after taking dosage.
- Zoledronic acid solution for injection should be refrigerated prior to use. IV infusion administered only by healthcare professional.
- Calcitonin injection and nasal spray should be refrigerated at 2–8°C (36–46°F). Nasal spray can be kept at room temperature up 30°C to (86°F) during use.
- Nasal spray should be primed prior to use. Discard unused portion after 30 days.
- Calcitonin injection can be administered SC or IM.
- Teriparatide injection is available in a prefilled pen device and should be refrigerated at 2–8°C (36–46°F). The product should not be frozen, and any unused portion should be discarded after 28 days of use.
- Denosumab injection is available in a prefilled pen device and should be refrigerated at 2–8°C (36–46°F). The product should be brought to room temperature prior to injection (15–30 minutes) and injected by a health care professional. Once at room temperature it should be used within 14 days.

Patient Education Pearls

- Take oral bisphosphonates on an empty stomach first thing in the morning with at least 8 oz of plain water. You should then remain upright for 30–60 minutes and avoid lying down. Avoid ingestion of food, beverages (other than water), and other medications for 30–60 minutes after taking this medication.
- Calcitonin nasal spray should be primed prior to use and any unused portion should be discarded after 30 days.
- Teriparatide injection should be refrigerated at all times and should be discarded after 28 days of use.
- Denosumab injection should be refrigerated prior to use and brought to room temperature in its original container prior to injection into the upper arm, thigh, or abdomen. Once at room temperature, the prefilled syringe should be used within 14 days. Injection is typically administered by a health care professional.
- Oral bisphosphonate therapy has been associated with a low potential risk for osteonecrosis of the jaw. Use of bisphosphonate therapy should be shared with your dental health professional.

GOUT

Definition

Gout is a syndrome of acute or chronic recurrent arthritis characterized by deposits of monosodium urate crystals in synovial fluid and/or tissues and is most often associated with hyperuricemia. Hyperuricemia can result from either an overproduction or underexcretion of uric acid. Overproduction of uric acid is most common in myeloproliferative and lymphoproliferative disorders. A decrease in the renal excretion of uric acid can be the result of renal dysfunction, certain drugs, or a number of predisposing conditions, including obesity and hypothyroidism. Acute gouty attacks may be precipitated by a number of conditions including stress, trauma, and alcohol ingestion.

Diagnosis

The diagnosis of gout is based on clinical presentation along with the presence of uric acid crystals detected on joint aspiration of the synovial fluid of affected joints. Evaluation of a 24-hour urinary uric acid will allow classification of the patient as a uric acid overproducer (urinary uric acid excretion ≥600 mg) or a uric acid underexcretor (urinary uric acid >600 mg), which will assist in pharmacotherapeutic decisions.

Signs and Symptoms

Patients presenting with acute gouty arthritis complain of a quick onset of excruciating pain, inflammation, and swelling that most commonly affects the first metatarsophalangeal (MTP) joint and can also affect the feet, ankles, heels, knees, wrists, fingers, and elbows. Severe cases of gout can result in uric acid nephrolithiasis, nephropathy, or urate deposits (tophi) in affected joints.

Summary of Treatment Recommendations

Treatment of Acute Gouty Arthropathy

- Asymptomatic hyperuricemia does not require therapy.
- First-line treatment for gout includes the use of an NSAID. The majority of acute gout attacks will respond to an NSAID within 72 hours of therapy. Indomethacin is the most common NSAID used in the treatment of gout, but other NSAIDs are also appropriate. Please see the medication chart in the osteoarthritis section of this chapter for more specific NSAID information.
- If patients have a contraindication to the use of an NSAID, evaluation of the time course of symptoms is necessary.
  - If gout symptoms have been present for less than 48 hours, colchicine is recommended for acute treatment.

- • If gout symptoms have been present for more than 48 hours, use of a corticosteroid is recommended.
- ▪ If the patient demonstrates an inadequate response to either NSAIDs or colchicine, corticosteroids should be considered.
- ▪ The use of oral (preferred) or parenteral corticosteroids is recommended for multijoint involvement, while an intraarticular corticosteroid can be used to target one specific symptomatic joint.
- ▪ Allopurinol or febuxostat should never be used in the treatment of acute gout. This agent is reserved for chronic prophylactic therapy in patients with multiple gout exacerbations each year.
  - • If these agents are used in the treatment of an acute gout exacerbation, the symptoms may be worsened due to the mobilization of uric acid stores.

Prophylaxis of Gout

- ▪ Colchicine maintenance therapy is indicated for prophylaxis in patients with only slightly elevated serum uric acid levels.
- ▪ Allopurinol is indicated for prophylaxis of gout exacerbations in patients with a moderately elevated serum uric acid level and a history of nephrolithiasis, tophi, serum creatinine >2.0 g/dL, or urinary uric acid excretion indicative of overproduction.
- ▪ Uricosuric drugs are indicated for prophylaxis of gout exacerbations in patients who are not candidates for allopurinol therapy and have a urinary uric acid excretion indicative of underexcretion.
- ▪ When initiating prophylactic therapy in a patient with gout, colchicine should be initiated with allopurinol, febuxostat, or a uricosuric and continued for the first 3–6 months of therapy to avoid causing an exacerbation.
- ▪ Pegloticase is indicated for refractory chronic gout in patients that do not respond to or have contraindications to traditional therapy.

Drugs for Gout

Generic	Brand	Dose & Max	Contra-indications	Primary Side Effects	Key Monitoring Parameters	Pertinent Drug Interactions	Med Pearls	Top 200
Mechanism of action – colchicine: inhibits lactic acid production, decreases uric acid production, decreases uric acid deposition, reduces phagocytosis, and decreases inflammation								
Colchicine	None	1 mg followed by 0.5 mg q2 hrs until symptoms resolve, diarrhea occurs, or 8 mg taken	Hypersensitivity; serious GI, renal, hepatic or cardiac disorders	• Diarrhea, nausea, vomiting • Rare: bone marrow suppression, aplastic anemia, thrombocytopenia	• Response to therapy • Serum uric acid • GI symptoms • Periodic CBC	None significant	• Patients may be provided with a prescription to be filled on a PRN basis and used during an exacerbation • Used for treatment and prophylaxis	Yes
Mechanism of action – xanthine oxidase inhibitor: by inhibition of xanthine oxidase, impairs the conversion of xanthine to uric acid, thereby decreasing the production of uric acid								
Allopurinol	Zyloprim	100–800 mg daily (renal dose adjustment necessary)	Hypersensitivity	Skin rash, leukopenia, GI upset	Response to therapy, serum uric acid, renal function	Mercaptopurine, azathioprine	Renal dose adjustment	Yes
Febuxostat	Uloric	40–80 mg PO daily	Concurrent use with azathioprine, mercaptopurine, or theophylline	Rash, liver abnormalities, arthralgia	• LFTs 2 and 4 months after initiation and periodically thereafter • Serum uric acid levels	Azathioprine, mercaptopurine, theophylline, didanosine	• No renal dose adjustment necessary • Not to be used during acute gout flares	No
Mechanism of action – uricosuric agents: increase the renal clearance of uric acid by inhibiting tubular reabsorption								
Sulfinpyrazone	Anturane	50–800 mg daily (BID)	• Hypersensitivity • CrCl <50 mL/min • History of renal calculi • Overproducers of uric acid • PUD	GI upset, rash, stone formation	• Response to treatment • Serum uric acid • Renal function	Warfarin (↑ INR), salicylates	May precipitate acute gouty attacks; avoid use during acute gouty arthritis	No
Probenecid	None	250–2,000 mg daily (BID)	• Hypersensitivity • CrCl <50 mL/min • History of renal calculi • Overproducers of uric acid • PUD	GI upset, rash, stone formation	• Response to treatment • Serum uric acid • Renal function	Methotrexate (↓ MTX levels), salicylates, penicillins	May precipitate acute gouty attacks; avoid use during acute gouty arthritis	No

Drugs for Gout *(cont'd)*

Generic	Brand	Dose & Max	Contra-indications	Primary Side Effects	Key Monitoring Parameters	Pertinent Drug Interactions	Med Pearls	Top 200
Mechanism of action – catalyzes oxidation of uric acid to allantoin, thereby decreasing serum uric acid								
Pegloticase	Krystexxa	8 mg IV infusion (over 2 or more hours) q2 weeks	• Glucose-6-phosphate-dehydrogenase deficiency • Risk of hemolysis • Methemoglobinemia	Acute gout exacerbation, infusion reactions	• Serum uric acid • Signs/symptoms of anaphylaxis/infusion reactions 1 hour after infusion • Symptoms of congestive heart failure after infusion	None	• Indicated only for refractory cases • Patient should receive pretreatment with antihistamines and corticosteroids • Gout flare prophylaxis with colchicine or NSAID one week prior to administration is recommended	No

Storage and Administration Pearls

- Medications should be stored in a dry place and protected from light.

Patient Education Pearls

- Patient should drink plenty of water (6–8 eight-oz glasses) while taking sulfinpyrazone or probenecid to avoid formation of kidney stones.

LEARNING POINTS

- First-line therapy for mild to moderate osteoarthritis is acetaminophen.
- NSAIDs and other pain medication should be administered with food to minimize stomach upset.
- Biologic therapies for RA suppress immunity and therefore cannot be initiated during infection and may be temporarily withdrawn during active infection.
- Biologic therapy for RA requires parenteral administration.
- First-line therapy for osteoporosis is the bisphosphonate class. Frequency of administration varies greatly from once daily to once annually. Oral formulations require very specific adherence to administration instructions to avoid esophageal side effects.
- Allopurinol and febuxostat are used for gout prophylaxis only and should be avoided during acute attacks because of their ability to exacerbate acute gout arthropathy by mobilizing uric acid stores.

PRACTICE QUESTIONS

1. Pharmacists dispensing narcotic analgesics to patients with severe osteoarthritis should inform the patients that

    (A)   medication will work better on an empty stomach.
    (B)   if taken as directed, there is little potential for addiction.
    (C)   it is okay to consume small amounts of alcohol with the medication.
    (D)   they may need to take a stool softener or laxative with the medication.
    (E)   they may need to take acetaminophen between doses.

2. Which of the following is NOT correctly matched with its trade name?

    (A)   Methotrexate – Rheumatrex
    (B)   Hydroxychloroquine – Azulfidine
    (C)   Leflunomide – Arava
    (D)   Etanercept – Enbrel
    (E)   Infliximab – Remicade

ANSWERS

1. **D**

Narcotic analgesics may cause constipation and often require the need for a laxative or stool softener. Narcotics may cause stomach upset and should be taken with food (A). Narcotics are controlled substances and have the potential for addiction and abuse even if taken correctly (B). Narcotics may cause CNS depression and should not be used with any amount of alcohol (C). Many narcotics are formulated in combination with acetaminophen, so recommending extra acetaminophen between dosing intervals may provide over the daily recommendation of acetaminophen (E) and should not be advised.

2. **B**

Hydroxychloroquine is generic for Plaquenil. Azulfidine is the brand name for sulfasalazine. The other answer choices are correctly matched with their trade names. Methotrexate (A) is generic for Rheumatrex or Trexall.

Pain Management

 10

This chapter covers the following drug classes:

- **Nonsteroidal anti-inflammatory drugs (NSAIDs)**
- **Nonopioid pain management**
- **Opioid pain management**

The text also provides an overview of basic treatment and management of pain.

Suggested Study Time: **30 minutes**

PAIN MANAGEMENT

Definitions

Pain management can be a very complicated and a very involved condition because pain is subjective and therapy must be individualized. Such objective measures as tachycardia are not reliable. There are five main types of pain: Acute, chronic, chronic cancer, breakthrough, and neuropathic pain. Pain can also be classified as somatic, visceral, nociceptive, neuropathic, psychologically based pain syndromes, and mixed or undetermined pathophysiology. Acute pain usually requires only temporary therapy for less than 30 days. Chronic pain is persistent and adversely affects the function or well-being of the patient for longer than 6 months. Somatic and visceral pain are treated like acute pain. Nociceptive, neuropathic, psychologically based pain syndromes, and mixed or undetermined pathophysiologic pain, however, are chronic pain types. Nonnarcotic preparations should be used when possible; however, patients are at greater risk for potential addiction and dependences. Often, chronic pain will intensify, requiring more complex regimens and combination therapy with narcotics and nonnarcotics. Chronic cancer pain occurs in 60–90% of patients with cancer. It is similar to chronic nonmalignant pain. Breakthrough pain is intermittent and occurs at a greater intensity over baseline chronic pain. Neuropathic pain is characterized by a burning or tingling feeling, and can often be treated using anticonvulsants and antidepressants (also known as co-analgesics) with great success.

Diagnosis

Because pain is identified principally through self-reports and is very much subjective, it is challenging for a clinician to accurately assess and is virtually impossible to diagnose.

- Pain is always subjective.
- No neurophysiological or laboratory test can measure pain.
- The clinician must accept the patient's report of pain.

Signs and Symptoms

- Objective observations such as grimacing, limping, or tachycardia may be helpful in assessing patients, but theses signs are often absent in patients with chronic pain caused by structural lesions.
- Pain intensity scales help patients communicate the signs and symptoms and pain intensity. This assessment can help guide treatments.
- Most adults and children above the age of 7 can score their pain intensity on a verbal numerical rating scale: 0 = no pain; 10 = the worst pain imaginable.

Guidelines

- Healthcare Association of New Jersey, July 2006. Pain management. www.hcanj.org.
- Institute for Clinical Systems Improvement, March 2007. Assessment and Management of Chronic Pain. www.icsi.org/pain_chronic_assessment_and_management_of_14399/pain_chronic_assessment_and_management_of_guideline_.html.

Guidelines Summary

- Drug therapy is the mainstay of management for acute pain and cancer pain in all age groups, including neonates, infants, children, and adults. The drugs discussed in this review are classified into three categories: Nonopioid analgesics, including acetaminophen and nonsteroidal anti-inflammatory drugs (NSAIDs); opioid pain management; and co-analgesics. The drug classes can be used in monotherapy and combination for pain.
- As the pain increases, so does the dose of medications, the migration to stronger medications, and the use of combinations of medications with different mechanisms of actions.

- Acetaminophen and NSAIDs are useful for acute and chronic pain arising from a variety of causes, including surgery, trauma, arthritis, and cancer.
- NSAIDs are indicated for pain involving inflammation because acetaminophen lacks clinically effective anti-inflammatory agents.
- NSAIDs differ from opioid analgesic by the following mechanisms:
  - NSAIDs are both analgesics and inflammatory in nature.
  - There is a dose ceiling of affect in relationship with adverse affects.
  - NSAIDs do not produce physical or psychological dependence.
  - NSAIDs are antipyretic.
- Initiation of opioid analgesics should be based on a pain-directed history and physical that includes repeated pain assessment.
  - Opioid analgesics should be added to nonopioids to manage acute pain and cancer-related pain that does not respond to nonopioids alone.
  - There is enormous variability in doses of opioids required to provide pain relief, even among opioid-naïve patients.
  - It is important to give each analgesic an adequate trial. As a result, a clinician will increase the opioid dose until unacceptable side effects appear before changing to another opioid.
  - It is recommended to administer analgesics on a regular schedule if pain is present most of the day. This allows the patient to stay ahead of the pain.
    - » For chronic pain, consider having a scheduled long-acting agent on board and a short-acting agent for times of breakthrough pain.
- Patient-controlled intravenous opioid administration (PCA) for acute pain is a commonly used technique for pain control.
  - PCA is used with a microprocessor-controlled infusion pump.
  - PCA is most often used for the intravenous (IV) administration of opioids for acute pain.
  - PCA allows patients considerable control over the experience of pain.
  - PCA is not recommended in situations in which oral opioids could readily manage pain.

Nonnarcotic Oral and Nonsteroidal Anti-inflammatory Drugs (NSAIDs)

Generic	Brand	Dose & Max mg (frequency)	Contraindications	Primary Side Effects	Key Monitoring Parameters	Pertinent Drug Interactions	Med Pearls	Top 200
Mechanism of action – decreases pain through inhibition of central cyclooxygenase, which in turn inhibits prostaglandin synthesis								
Acetaminophen	Tylenol	• 325–1,000 mg TID–QID • Max: 4,000 mg	• Hepatic disease • Alcoholism	Very few	Pain relief	Alcohol	• Over-the-counter (OTC) • Best if taken on scheduled basis vs. as needed (PRN)	No
Mechanism of action – NSAIDs: decrease pain and inflammation by inhibition of prostaglandin synthesis through inhibition of cyclooxygenase enzymes								
Aspirin	Various	• Immediate release (IR): 325–3,600 mg daily (q4–6 hrs) • Extended release (ER) product 650–1,300 mg TID • Max: 5.4 g/day	• Allergy • Fever in children • Active bleeding	Gastrointestinal (GI) (upset stomach, bleeding); rash	Pain relief, GI symptoms	• Warfarin • Other NSAIDs • Angiotensin-converting enzyme (ACE) inhibitors	• OTC • Anti-inflammatory only at high doses (>3 g/day)	No
Nonacetylated salicylates								
Salsalate	Various	• 500–3,000 mg daily (BID–TID) • Max: 3 g/day	Hypersensitivity	• GI (upset stomach, bleeding) • Rash • Diminished renal function • Edema	Pain relief, GI symptoms	• Other salicylates • Warfarin • ACE inhibitors	• Monitor serum salicylate levels with chronic use or very high doses • Desired range 10–30 mg/100 mL	No
Diflunisal	None	500–1,500 mg daily (BID)	Hypersensitivity				Administer with food	No

Nonnarcotic Oral and Nonsteroidal Anti-inflammatory Drugs (NSAIDs) *(cont'd)*

Generic	Brand	Dose & Max mg (frequency)	Contraindications	Primary Side Effects	Key Monitoring Parameters	Pertinent Drug Interactions	Med Pearls	Top 200
Acetic acids								
Etodolac	None	200–1,200 mg daily (q6–8 hrs)	Hypersensitivity	• GI (upset stomach, bleeding) • Rash • Diminished renal function • ↑ blood pressure • Edema	• Pain relief • GI symptoms • Renal function • Blood pressure	• Other salicylates • Warfarin • Lithium • ACE inhibitors	Administer with food	Yes
Diclofenac	• Cataflam • Voltaren • Zipsor • Flector	50–150 mg daily (BID–TID)	Hypersensitivity	• GI (upset stomach, bleeding) • Rash • Diminished renal function • ↑ blood pressure • Edema	• Pain relief • GI symptoms • Renal function • Blood pressure	• Other salicylates • Warfarin • Lithium • ACE inhibitors	Administer with food	Yes
Indomethacin	• Indocin • Indocin SR	IR: 25–200 mg daily (BID–TID) • Suspended release (SR) 75–150 mg 1x daily • Max: 200 mg/day	Hypersensitivity	• GI (upset stomach, bleeding) • Rash • Diminished renal function • ↑ blood pressure • Edema • Central nervous system (CNS) disturbances	• Pain relief • GI symptoms • Renal function • Blood pressure	• Other salicylates • Warfarin • Lithium • ACE inhibitors	• Most commonly used for treatment of gout • Fat-soluble, crosses blood-brain barrier • Administer with food	No
Ketorolac	Toradol	30 mg intramuscular (IM) or 15 mg IV initial; 10 mg PO q4–6 hrs up to 40 mg daily	• Active peptic ulcer disease (PUD) or bleeding • History of GI bleeding • Severe renal impairment • Labor and delivery	• GI (upset stomach, bleeding) • Rash • Diminished renal function • ↑ blood pressure	• Pain relief • GI symptoms • Renal function • Blood pressure	• Other salicylates • Warfarin • Lithium • ACE inhibitors	Only approved for moderate–severe pain for ≤5 days' duration, due to risk of renal and GI dysfunction	No
Nabumetone	Relafen	500–2,000 mg daily (q day–BID)	Hypersensitivity				Administer with food	No

Nonnarcotic Oral and Nonsteroidal Anti-inflammatory Drugs (NSAIDs) *(cont'd)*

Generic	Brand	Dose & Max mg (frequency)	Contraindications	Primary Side Effects	Key Monitoring Parameters	Pertinent Drug Interactions	Med Pearls	Top 200
Propionic acids								
Fenoprofen	Nalfon	200–3,200 mg daily (TID–QID)	Hypersensitivity	• GI (upset stomach, bleeding) • Rash • Diminished renal function • ↑ blood pressure	• Pain relief • GI symptoms • Renal function • Blood pressure	• Other salicylates • Warfarin • Lithium • ACE inhibitors	• Administer with food	No
Flurbiprofen	Ansaid	50–300 mg daily (BID–QID)	Hypersensitivity				• Administer with food	No
Ibuprofen	• Motrin • Advil • Caldolor	• 200–3,200 mg daily (TID–QID) • Max: 3.2 g/day	Hypersensitivity				• Available OTC and Rx (400–800 mg tabs) • Administer with food • Available in pediatric preparations	Yes
Ketoprofen	• Orudis • Oruvail • Rhodis	• IR: 50–300 mg daily (TID–QID) • SR: 75–200 mg daily	Hypersensitivity				• Available OTC and Rx • Administer with food	No
Naproxen	• Naprosyn • EC Naprosyn • Naprelan	• IR: 250–1,500 mg daily (BID) • Enteric coated (EC) 375–1,500 mg daily (BID) • Controlled release (CR) 375–1,500 mg daily (BID)	Hypersensitivity				• Available OTC and Rx • Administer with food	Yes
Naproxen sodium	Anaprox	275–1,650 mg daily (BID)	Hypersensitivity				• Available OTC and Rx • Administer with food	Yes
Oxaprozin	Daypro	600–1,800 mg daily (1x daily)	Hypersensitivity				• Administer with food	No

Nonnarcotic Oral and Nonsteroidal Anti-inflammatory Drugs (NSAIDs) *(cont'd)*

Generic	Brand	Dose & Max mg (frequency)	Contraindications	Primary Side Effects	Key Monitoring Parameters	Pertinent Drug Interactions	Med Pearls	Top 200
Fenamates								
Meclofenamate	Meclomen	50–400 mg daily (q 4–6 hrs)	Hypersensitivity	• GI (upset stomach, bleeding) • Rash • Diminished renal function • ↑ blood pressure	• Pain relief • GI symptoms • Renal function • Blood pressure	• Other salicylates • Warfarin • Lithium • ACE inhibitors	administer with food	No
Oxicams								
Piroxicam	Feldene	10–20 mg daily (1x daily)	Hypersensitivity	• GI (upset stomach, bleeding) • Rash • Diminished renal function • ↑ blood pressure	• Pain relief • GI symptoms • Renal function • Blood pressure	• Other salicylates • Warfarin • Lithium • ACE inhibitors	• More COX-2 selectivity than traditional NSAIDs • Slightly less GI symptoms	No
Meloxicam	Mobic	7.5–15 mg daily (1x daily)	Hypersensitivity					No
Selective COX-2 inhibitors								
Celecoxib	Celebrex	50–200 mg daily (q day–BID)	Hypersensitivity	• GI (upset stomach, bleeding—less than other NSAIDs) • Rash • Diminished renal function • ↑ blood pressure; edema	• Pain relief • GI symptoms • Renal function • Blood pressure	• Other salicylates (including aspirin) • Warfarin • Lithium • ACE inhibitors	• Lower incidence of GI toxicity than with NSAIDs • Concern about cardiovascular adverse effects prompted withdrawal of similar drug from market (rofecoxib)	Yes

Narcotic Analgesics

Narcotic analgesics: stimulate opioid receptors in the brain

Generic	Brand	Dose & Max mg (frequency)	Contraindications	Primary Side Effects	Key Monitoring Parameters	Pertinent Drug Interactions	Med Pearls	Top 200
Hydrocodone/APAP	• Various • Lortab • Vicodin	5–60 mg hydrocodone daily (q4–6 hrs)	Hypersensitivity, severe hepatic impairment, alcoholism	• Constipation • CNS depression • Confusion • Sedation • Respiratory depression • Hypotension • Bradycardia	• Presence of side effects (constipation, confusion) • Pain relief • Respiratory rate • Blood pressure • Heart rate	• Alcohol • Other CNS depressants	• Take with food • Often need laxative in addition • High abuse potential	Yes
APAP/Codeine	• Various • Tylenol #3	7.5–360 mg codeine daily (q4–6 hrs)		• Constipation • CNS depression • Confusion • Sedation • Respiratory depression • Hypotension • Bradycardia	• Presence of side effects (constipation, confusion) • Pain relief • Respiratory rate • Blood pressure • Heart rate			Yes
Morphine	• Various • Roxanol • Oxycontin • Kadian	No max					• Take with food • Often need laxative in addition • High abuse potential • Initiate IR and switch to CR/ER	Yes
Morphine sulfate and naltrexone hydrochloride	Embeda ER	20 mg/0.8–100 mg/4 mg daily or BID	Hypersensitivity to morphine, respiratory depression, acute or severe bronchial asthma or hypercarbia, or paralytic ileus	• Constipation • Nausea • Somnolence	• Comprehensive metabolic panel (CMP) • Liver function test (LFT) • Thyroid-stimulating hormone (TSH)			Yes

Narcotic Analgesics *(cont'd)*

Generic	Brand	Dose & Max mg (frequency)	Contraindications	Primary Side Effects	Key Monitoring Parameters	Pertinent Drug Interactions	Med Pearls	Top 200
Morphine sulfate extended release capsules	Avinza	30–120 mg/day		• Constipation • CNS depression • Confusion • Sedation • Respiratory depression • Hypotension • Bradycardia	• Presence of side effects (constipation, confusion) • Pain relief • Respiratory rate • Blood pressure • Heart rate	• CNS depressants • Alcohol • Cimetidine • MAOIs	Do not crush or chew, must be swallowed whole	Yes
Morphine sulfate extended release capsules	Kadian	10–200 mg/day or BID	Hypersensitivity to morphine or any of its components, respiratory depression with no resuscitative equipment, acute or severe bronchial asthma, and paralytic ileus	• Constipation • CNS depression • Confusion • Sedation • Respiratory depression • Hypotension • Bradycardia	• Presence of side effects (constipation, confusion) • Pain relief • Respiratory rate • Blood pressure • Heart rate	• CNS depressants • Alcohol • Cimetidine • Diuretics • MAOIs	• 100 mg and 200 mg doses are for opioid-tolerant patients only • Pellets may be sprinkled over applesauce but must not be chewed, crushed, or dissolved	
Oxycodone/APAP	• Various • Percocet • Roxicet	5–40 mg daily oxycodone (q6 hrs PRN)		• Constipation • CNS depression • Confusion • Sedation • Respiratory depression • Hypotension • Bradycardia	• Presence of side effects (constipation, confusion) • Pain relief • Respiratory rate • Blood pressure • Heart rate	• Alcohol • Other CNS depressants	• Take with food • Often need laxative in addition • High abuse potential	Yes

Narcotic Analgesics *(cont'd)*

Generic	Brand	Dose & Max mg (frequency)	Contraindications	Primary Side Effects	Key Monitoring Parameters	Pertinent Drug Interactions	Med Pearls	Top 200
Fentanyl	• Duragesic • Actiq • Fentora • Onsolis	• Infusion, injection, lozenge, tab, transdermal patch • No max • Dosages different for each delivery system • Buccal soluble film				CYP450 and CYP3A4	• Patch takes 24 hrs to begin working • Fentanyl remains in patch at 72 hrs; fold in half to avoid diversion	Yes
Hydromorphone	• Dilaudid • Dilaudid –HP	• 3, 6, 12, 18, 24, 30 mg • No max	Hypersensitivity, asthma, respiratory depression, CNS depression			None	• Tolerance can develop • High potential for abuse • Dilaudid-HP is highly concentrated	Yes
Meperidine	Demerol	Injection, PCA pump, tablet 25–100 mg	• Avoid in renal failure • Avoid hepatic disease		Same as above; add seizure due to potential metabolite-normeperidine	• CYP450 • CYP2B6, CYP2C19, CYP3A4	• Not recommended as an analgesic • Use less than 48 hrs and in doses less than 600 mg/day	No
Methadone	Dolophine	• Initial opioid naïve: 2.5–10 mg q8–12 hrs • No max	Same as above but add concurrent use of selegiline		Pain relief, mental status, blood pressure	• CYP450 Inhibits: CYP2D6, CYP3A4	Long half-life and difficult to titrate	Yes
Tapentadol	Nucynta	• 50–100 mg q4–6 hours • Max dose is 600 mg/day	Impaired pulmonary function, paralytic ileus, or use of MAOIs	• Nausea • Dizziness • Vomiting • Somnolence • Along with the other side effects of the drugs in this class	Pain relief and signs of abuse	• Centrally acting • Alcohol • MAOIs		No

Analgesic Adjuncts

Generic	Brand	Dose & Max mg (frequency)	Contraindications	Primary Side Effects	Key Monitoring Parameters	Pertinent Drug Interactions	Med Pearls	Top 200
Mechanism of action – increases synaptic concentration of norepinephrine, desensitization of adenyl cyclase, downregulation of serotonin receptors								
Desipramine	Norpramin	• Initial: 75–150 mg • Max: 300 mg	Use of MAOI past 14 days; acute recovery phase following a myocardial infarction	• Orthostatic hypotension • Tachycardia • Anticholinergic	• Blood pressure • Suicidal ideation	CYP450 inhibits CYP1A2, CYP2C9, CYP2D6, CYP2E1	• Increased suicidal behavior in young adults age 18–25 yrs • Chronic pain is an unlabeled indication	No
Amitriptyline	Elavil	• Initial: 50–150 mg/day • Max: 400 mg						Yes
Mechanism of action – induces the release of substance P, the principle chemomediator of pain impulses from the periphery								
Gabapentin	Neurontin	• Initial 300 mg TID • Max: 3,600	None	• Somnolence • Dizziness • Peripheral edema	Pain scale	Sedative effects: CNS depressants, alcohol, opiates	Chronic pain is not an official indication	Yes
Pregabalin	Lyrica	• Initial: 75 mg BID • Max: 450 mg/day					• Controlled substance (C5) • Has official FDA indication for neuropathic pain associated with diabetes	Yes
Mechanism of action – binds to μ-opiate receptors in the CNS, causing inhibition of ascending pain pathways								
Tramadol	• Ultram • Ultram ER • Ryzolt	• IR: 25–400 daily (q4–6 hrs) • ER: 100–300 daily	Hypersensitivity	• Confusion • Sedation • Rash • Stomach upset • Orthostatic hypotension	• Pain relief • Renal and hepatic function periodically	• Alcohol • Opioids • SSRIs • MAOIs • Warfarin	• Renal dose adjustment for CrCl <30 mL/min • Not a controlled substance	Yes
Mechanism of action – induces the release of substance P, the principal chemomediator of pain impulses from the periphery								
Capsaicin Cream	Various	0.025–0.1% applied 3–4x daily	Do not apply to wounds or damaged skin	Localized stinging	Pain relief	None	• OTC • Must be used regularly for 2 wks or more for maximal efficacy	No

STORAGE AND ADMINISTRATION PEARLS

- Do not freeze acetaminophen suppositories.
- Hydrolysis of aspirin occurs upon exposure to water or moist air, resulting in salicylate and acetate, which possess a vinegar-like odor. Do not use if a strong odor is present.
- Ibuprofen, indomethacin, ketoprofen, and ketoralac must be protected from light.
- With codeine, protect injection from light.
- Amitriptyline, oxycodone, fentanyl, hydromorphone, meperidine, and methadone all need to be protected from light.

PATIENT EDUCATION PEARLS

- The patient should always take exactly what is prescribed. Never increase the dose without discussing with the prescriber
- The narcotic medications may cause physical and psychological dependence.
- While using pain medications, it is recommended not to use alcohol or other prescription or OTC medications.

LEARNING POINTS

- NSAIDs are both analgesics and inflammatory in nature.
- No NSAID is any more effective than any other in the general population.
- Symptoms of overdose for narcotic medications include: CNS depression, bradycardia, hypotension, respiratory depression, miosis, apnea, pulmonary edema, and convulsions.
- Onset of action of most pain medication occurs within 45 minutes, with peak drug effect in 1 to 2 hours after oral administration for most immediate-release medications.
- PCA provides the important advantage of medication that is rapidly administered when needed, delaying pain exacerbation.
- In chronic pain, continuous opioid administration is recommended with controlled release medication, transdermal patch, or infusion. Short-acting medications should be available for breakthrough pain.

PRACTICE QUESTIONS

1. Which of the following is NOT a muscle relaxer?

    (A) Baclofen
    (B) Relafen
    (C) Robaxin
    (D) Parafon Forte
    (E) Zanaflex

2. Which of the following drugs is/are contraindicated for a patient with a history of a gastrointestional bleed?

    I.   Aspirin
    II. Warfarin
    III. Toradol

    (A) I only
    (B) III only
    (C) I and II only
    (D) II and III only
    (E) I, II, and III

ANSWERS

1. **B**

Relafen (nabumetone) is an NSAID, so (B) is correct. The other choices are all muscle relaxer: Baclofen (Lioresal), Robaxin (methocarbamol), Parafon Forte (chlorzoxazone), and Zanaflex (tizanidine).

2. **E**

Aspirin, warfarin, and Toradol are all contraindicated for someone who has had a GI bleed, so (E) is correct. Aspirin and Toradol inhibit prostaglandins, which protect the lining of the stomach. Warfarin and aspirin both increase the bleeding time.

Ophthalmologic Disorders

This chapter covers the following disorder:

- **Glaucoma**

Suggested Study Time: 20 minutes

GLAUCOMA

Definitions

Glaucoma is a group of eye disorders caused by damage to an area of the optic nerve (optic disk), which results in loss of visual sensitivity and field. The two types of glaucoma include open-angle and closed-angle glaucoma. Open-angle glaucoma is the most common form of this disorder and can be due to either genetic causes (most prevalent is primary open-angle glaucoma [POAG]) or other factors such as trauma, surgery, or medications (secondary open-angle glaucoma). Although it was previously believed that increased intraocular pressure (IOP) was solely responsible for the damage to the optic disk, it appears that factors such as ischemia, changes in blood flow, and autoimmune factors may also play a role.

Given that up to 70% of all cases of glaucoma in the United States are characterized as POAG, the discussion in this chapter focuses only on this form of the ocular disorder.

Diagnosis

The diagnosis of POAG is based on the presence of characteristic changes to the optic disk and visual field loss with or without an increased IOP. An increased IOP does not need to be present to confirm the diagnosis of POAG. In general, an IOP greater than 21 mmHg is considered to be elevated.

Signs and Symptoms

Symptoms for glaucoma usually do not develop until significant damage to the optic disk and significant visual field loss has already occurred. Patients may complain of blind spots, reduced peripheral vision, and changes in color perception.

Guidelines

American Academy of Ophthalmology. http://one.aao.org/CE/PracticeGuidelines/default.aspx.

Overview of Treatment

Because the above guidelines do not specify which drugs should be used as first-line or second-line therapy, this section should not be considered as a "Guidelines Summary" but rather as a general overview of the pharmacologic treatment of glaucoma.

The initial goal is to achieve at least a 20% reduction in the IOP. Additional lowering may be necessary based upon the baseline IOP, the extent of damage to the optic disk, and the extent of visual field loss.

- β-blockers or prostaglandin analogs are considered first-line therapy for POAG. Prostaglandin analogs are often used as initial therapy. These agents can be used as monotherapy or in combination with each other.
  - If a patient does not tolerate or does not respond at all (no reduction in IOP) to an agent, an alternative drug should be used.
  - If a patient partially responds to an agent (some reduction in IOP, but not at goal), addition of another drug should be considered.
- α_2 agonists or topical carbonic anhydrase inhibitors can be considered if the patient does not respond to or tolerate one of the above first-line agents.
- Cholinergic agonist are usually considered as last-line drug therapies because of their increased risk of side effects.
- Laser or surgical procedures may also be considered during the course of therapy.

β-Blockers

Mechanism of action — ↓ IOP by ↓ production of aqueous humor

Generic	Brand	Dose	Contra-indications	Primary Side Effects	Key Monitoring	Pertinent Drug Interactions	MedPearl	Top 200
Betaxolol (β₁-selective)	• Betoptic • Betoptic-S	• Solution: 1–2 drops 2x daily • Suspension: 1 drop 2x daily	• Sinus bradycardia • ≥2nd-degree heart block (in absence of pacemaker) • Decompensated heart failure • Severe chronic obstructive pulmonary disease/asthma	Local effects • Burning • Stinging • Tearing • Blurred vision • Dry eyes Systemic effects • Bradycardia • Heart block • Hypotension • Heart failure exacerbation • Bronchospasm • Fatigue	IOP every 2–4 wks until target achieved, then every 6 mo	• ↑ risk of systemic side effects with oral β-blockers • ↑ risk of bradycardia or heart block with digoxin, verapamil, diltiazem, or clonidine	• All have similar efficacy in ↓ IOP • Tachyphylaxis may occur with long-term use • Effect on IOP may be lessened in patients receiving oral β-blockers	No
Carteolol (nonselective, ISA properties)	Only available generically	1 drop 2x daily						No
Levobunolol (nonselective)	• AKBeta • Betagan	1 drop 1–2x daily						No
Metipranolol (nonselective)	OptiPranolol	1 drop 2x daily						No
Timolol (nonselective)	• Solution: Timoptic, Betimol, Istalol • Gel-forming solution: Timoptic-XE	• Solution: 1 drop 1–2x daily • Gel-forming solution: 1 drop 1x daily						No

Prostaglandin Analogs

Mechanism of action – ↓ IOP by ↑ outflow of aqueous humor

Generic	Brand	Dose	Contraindications	Primary Side Effects	Key Monitoring	Pertinent Drug Interactions	Med Pearl	Top 200
Bimatoprost	Lumigan	1 drop 1x daily in evening	Hypersensitivity	• Change in iris, eyelash, and eyelid pigmentation (become darker) • Growth of eyelashes • Eyelid edema • Itching, redness, blurred vision, dry eyes	IOP every 2–4 wks until target achieved, then every 6 mo	No significant interactions	• Do not exceed 1x daily dosing (may worsen IOP) • Iris discoloration is not reversible (highest incidence with latanoprost) • Eyelid discoloration and eyelash changes may be reversible • Travatan Z does not contain benzalkonium chloride • Most effective in ↓ IOP • Bimatoprost also available as Latisse → to ↑ eyelash growth	Yes
Latanoprost	Xalatan	1 drop 1x daily in evening						Yes
Tafluprost	Zioptan	1 drop 1x daily in evening						No
Travoprost	Travatan Z	1 drop 1x daily in evening						Yes

α₂-Agonists

Mechanism of action – ↓ IOP by ↓ production of aqueous humor (brimonidine may also ↑ outflow of aqueous humor)

Generic	Brand	Dose	Contraindications	Primary Side Effects	Key Monitoring	Pertinent Drug Interactions	Med Pearl	Top 200
Apraclonidine	Iopidine	1 drop 3x daily	Concurrent or recent use (within 14 days) of monoamine oxidase inhibitors	Local effects • Eyelid edema • Itching, redness, burning Systemic effects • Dizziness • Fatigue • Dry mouth • Headache • Hypotension • Bradycardia	IOP every 2–4 wks until target achieved, then every 6 mo	↑ risk of systemic side effects with central nervous system depressants (e.g., alcohol, opiates, sedatives, barbiturates)	• Structurally similar to clonidine • Apraclonidine primarily used to control postoperative ↑ IOP	No
Brimonidine	Alphagan P	1 drop 3x daily						Yes

Carbonic Anhydrase Inhibitors

Mechanism of action – ↓ IOP by ↓ production of aqueous humor

Generic	Brand	Dose	Contra-indications	Primary Side Effects	Key Monitoring	Pertinent Drug Interactions	Med Pearl	Top 200
Brinzolamide	Azopt	1 drop 3x daily	Sulfa allergy (risk of cross-sensitivity)	• Eyelid reactions • Burning, stinging, tearing, blurred vision	IOP every 2–4 wks until target achieved, then every 6 mo	No significant interactions	• Topical therapy rarely associated with systemic side effects • Oral carbonic anhydrase inhibitor therapy (e.g., acetazolamide) may be used in patients refractory to maximal doses of topical therapy; associated with higher risk of side effects	No
Dorzolamide	Trusopt	1 drop 3x daily		• Bitter taste in mouth				No

Cholinergic Agonists (Direct-Acting)

Mechanism of action – ↓ IOP by ↑ outflow of aqueous humor

Generic	Brand	Dose	Contra-indications	Primary Side Effects	Key Monitoring	Pertinent Drug Interactions	Med Pearl	Top 200
Carbachol	Isopto Carbachol	1–2 drops 2–3x daily	Ocular inflammatory condition (may worsen condition)	• Impaired night vision • Headache • Eyelid twitching • Stinging, burning, tearing	IOP every 2–4 wks until target achieved, then every 6 mo	No significant interactions	• Patients with darker eyes may require higher concentrations of pilocarpine to ↓ IOP • Pilocarpine concentrations >4% may be associated with ↑ risk of systemic side effects (e.g., ↑ urinary frequency, sweating, vomiting, salivation, bronchospasm, bradycardia)	No
Pilocarpine	• Solution: Isopto Carpine • Gel: Pilopine HS	• 1–2 drops 3–4x daily • At bedtime						No

Combination Drugs

Generic	Brand
Timolol/brimonidine	Combigan
Timolol/dorzolamide	Cosopt

STORAGE AND ADMINISTRATION PEARLS

- Most ophthalmic preparations (gels, solutions, suspensions) should be stored at room temperature.
  - Latanoprost should be refrigerated until opened; once opened, the bottle can be stored at room temperature.
- Ophthalmic suspensions should be shaken well prior to using.

PATIENT EDUCATION PEARLS

- Patient should be educated on the appropriate administration of ophthalmic preparations:
  - Wash and dry hands.
  - If suspension is being used, shake the bottle well.
  - Contact lenses should be removed prior to administration.
  - Tilt head back and look at the ceiling.
  - Pull down the lower eyelid to form a pocket into which the medication will be instilled.
  - Place the dropper over the eye, look up, and then place a single drop in the eye.
  - To avoid contamination, the tip of the dropper should not touch any part of the eye.
  - Close the eyes for several minutes. Do not rub the eyes.
- If the patient is using more than one ophthalmic drug, administration of these drugs should be separated by at least 10 minutes to prevent loss of the initially administered drug.
- Patient should be educated on use of nasolacrimal occlusion when administering eye drops to minimize the development of systemic side effects and to enhance drug efficacy.
  - Once the eye drop is instilled, instruct patient to close eye and place index finger over nasolacrimal drainage system in the inner corner of the eye for 1–3 minutes.

LEARNING POINTS

- Know examples of ophthalmic β-blockers, prostaglandin analogs, and α₂ agonists.
- β-blocker eye drops can cause systemic adverse effects. Use caution in patients also receiving oral β-blocker therapy.
- Prostaglandin analogs can cause pigmentation changes in the iris, eyelid, and eyelashes.
- Carbonic anhydrase inhibitors should not be used in patients with sulfa allergies.
- Know combination drug products.

PRACTICE QUESTIONS

1. Which of the following medications is likely to cause a darkening of the iris of the eye?

   (A) Apraclonidine
   (B) Carbachol
   (C) Dorzolamide
   (D) Latanoprost
   (E) Timolol

2. Lumigan belongs to which of the following classes of drugs?

   (A) α_2 agonist
   (B) Antihistamine
   (C) β-blocker
   (D) Cholinergic agonist
   (E) Prostaglandin analog

ANSWERS

1. D

Latanoprost, an ophthalmic prostaglandin analog, is likely to cause darkening of the iris, so choice (D) is correct. This class of drugs may also cause increased pigmentation of the eyelid and eyelashes.

2. E

Lumigan, the brand name for bimatoprost, is a prostaglandin analog, so choice (E) is correct.

Hematologic Disorders

12

This chapter covers the following diseases:

- **Iron deficiency anemia**
- **Anemia of chronic kidney disease and dialysis**
- **Pernicious anemia**

 Suggested Study Time: **45 minutes**

IRON DEFICIENCY ANEMIA

Definitions

Iron deficiency anemia (IDA) is a common disorder worldwide. In the United States, most cases are caused by menstrual blood loss, GI blood loss, and increased iron requirements of pregnancy. Decreased iron absorption or increased iron requirements may also lead to iron deficiency.

Diagnosis

- Evidence of a source of blood loss should be sought.
- Iron deficiency anemia is classically described as a microcytic anemia (MCV <80).
- The differential diagnosis includes thalassemia, sideroblastic anemias, some types of anemia of chronic disease, and lead poisoning.
- Cells start out normochromic but become more hypochromic as the anemia progresses.
- Serum ferritin is the preferred initial diagnostic test. Total iron-binding capacity, transferrin saturation, serum iron, and serum transferrin receptor levels may be

helpful if the ferritin level is between 46 and 99 ng/mL (46 and 99 mcg/L); bone marrow biopsy may be necessary in these patients for a definitive diagnosis.

- Laboratory tests:
  - Low serum Fe
  - Low ferritin (main lab indicator)
  - Increased TIBC
  - Hgb and Hct decrease in later stages
  - Decreased MCV, MCH, MCHC
  - Decreased transferrin saturation

Signs and Symptoms

There are many symptoms of IDA. Different patients will experience different combinations of symptoms; and, if the anemia is mild, the symptoms may not be noticeable. Some of the symptoms are: Pale skin color, fatigue, irritability, dizziness, weakness, shortness of breath, sore tongue, brittle nails, decreased appetite (especially in children), and frontal headaches.

Guidelines

American Family Physicians, *Am Fam Physician*, no. 75 (2007): 671–8. www.aafp.org/afp/20070301/671.pdf.

Guidelines Summary

Routine iron supplementation is recommended for high-risk infants 6 to 12 months of age. In children, adolescents, and women of reproductive age, a trial of iron is a reasonable approach if the review of symptoms, history, and physical examination are negative; however, the hemoglobin should be checked at 1 month. If there is not a 1–2 g/dL increase in the hemoglobin level in that time, possibilities include malabsorption of oral iron, lack of compliance, continued bleeding, or presence of an unknown lesion.

Transfusion should be considered for patients of any age with IDA who are complaining of symptoms such as fatigue or dyspnea on exertion. Transfusion should also be considered for asymptomatic cardiac patients with hemoglobin less than 10 g/dL (100 g/L). However, oral iron therapy is usually the first-line therapy for patients with IDA. As noted in the etiology section, iron absorption varies widely based on type of diet and other factors.

- Bone marrow response to iron is limited to 20 mg/day of elemental iron.
- An increase in the hemoglobin level of 1 g/dL (10 g/L) should occur every 2 to 4 weeks on iron therapy.

- It may take up to 4 months for the iron stores to return to normal after the hemoglobin has corrected. Iron sulfate in a dose of 300 mg provides 60 mg of elemental iron, whereas 325 mg of iron gluconate provides 36 mg of elemental iron.

- Sustained-release formulations of iron are not recommended as initial therapy because they reduce the amount of iron that is presented for absorption to the duodenal villi.

- Gastrointestinal (GI) absorption of elemental iron is enhanced in the presence of an acidic gastric environment.

- This can be accomplished through simultaneous intake of ascorbic acid (i.e., vitamin C).

- Patients should be counseled to take iron 2 hours before or 4 hours after antacids.

- Although iron absorption occurs more readily when taken on an empty stomach, this increases the likelihood of stomach upset because of iron therapy. Increased patient adherence should be weighed against the inferior absorption.

- Laxatives, stool softeners, and adequate intake of liquids can alleviate the constipating effects of oral iron therapy.

- Indications for the use of intravenous (IV) iron include:
  - Chronic uncorrectable bleeding
  - Intestinal malabsorption
  - Intolerance to oral iron: Often results in nonadherence by the patient
  - Hemoglobin levels less than 6 g/dL (60 g/L) with signs of poor perfusion in patients who would otherwise receive transfusion (e.g., those who have religious objections).

Drugs for Iron Deficiency Anemia

Generic	Brand	Dose	Contraindications	Primary Side Effects	Key Monitoring	Pertinent Drug Interactions	Med Pearl	Top 200
Mechanism of action – replaces iron found in hemoglobin, myoglobin; allows the transportation of oxygen via hemoglobin								
Ferrous sulfate, gluconate, fumarate	• Sulfate: Feosol, Fer-In-Sol, Fer-Iron, Slow-FE • Gluconate	• Sulfate: treatment: 300 mg BID • Gluconate/ fumarate: 60 mg BID prophylaxis 1x daily	Hypersensitivity to iron salts, hemochromatosis (GI absorbs excess iron), hemolytic anemia	• GI irritation • Epigastric pain • Nausea • Dark stools • Vomiting • Stomach cramping • Constipation	• Serum iron • Total iron-binding capacity • Reticulocyte count • Hemoglobin	• Absorption: tetracyclines, fluoroquinolones, levodopa, methyldopa, penicillamine • Proton pump inhibitors (PPIs) and H$_2$ blockers can affect iron absorption	• The advantage of iron dextran is the ability to administer large doses (200 to 500 mg) at one time • One major drawback of iron dextran is the risk of anaphylactic reactions that can be fatal	No
Mechanism of action – release iron from the plasma; eventually replenishes the depleted iron stores in the bone marrow								
Dextran 40, 70	Dexferrum	IV: 500–1,000 mL at 20–40 mL/min for 5 days	• Hypersensitivity to dextran • Thrombocytopenia • Hypofibrinogenemia	• Mild hypotension • Tightness in the chest • Wheezing	• Circulatory overload • Anaphylactoid reaction • Hemoglobin	Enhance the anticoagulant effect of abciximab	• Rifabutin often will be used with drug interaction to prevent the use of rifampin • Test dose is required	No
Sodium ferric gluconate	Ferrlecit	IV: 125 mg/10 mL infused approximately 8x	Use in any anemia not caused by iron deficiency	• Angina, bradycardia • Hypotension • Agitation • Chills, dizziness, fatigue	• Hematocrit • Electrolytes • Vital signs	Decrease the absorption of oral iron	• A safer form of parenteral iron compared to dextran • No test dose is required	No
Mechanism of action – iron sucrose is dissociated by the reticuloendothelial system into iron and sucrose; increases serum iron levels								
Iron sucrose	Venofer	IV: 100 mg administered 1–3x/ wk during dialysis	• Evidence of iron overload • Anemia not caused by iron deficiency	• Hypotension • Peripheral edema • Headache and nausea	• Circulatory overload • Anaphylactoid reaction • Hemoglobin • Hematocrit • Electrolytes • Vital signs	Decrease the absorption of oral iron	Safety profiles are similar to sodium ferric gluconate	No

Storage and Administration Pearls

- Sodium ferric gluconate and iron sucrose should not be frozen.
- Iron is a leading cause of fatal poisoning in children. Store out of children's reach and in child-resistant containers.

Patient Education Pearls

- If taking rifampin, report any tingling or numbness in hands of feet.
- If taking streptomycin, maintain adequate hydration.

ANEMIA OF CHRONIC KIDNEY DISEASE AND DIALYSIS

Definitions

Anemia of chronic kidney disease is a hypoproliferative disorder associated with certain infectious or inflammatory processes, tissue injury, or conditions that release proinflammatory cytokines. It is attributed primarily to decrease endogenous erythropoietin (EPO) production and may occur as the creatinine clearance declines below approximately 50 mL/min. Eventually, the patient may require dialysis to filtrate metabolic waste. There are several types of dialysis, including:

- Hemodialysis, which diffuses small molecular-weight solutes across a semipermeable membrane
- Peritoneal dialysis, which uses the peritoneum as a dialysis membrane
- Ultrafiltration and hemofiltration, which removes large volumes of fluid with minimal removal of metabolic wastes

Diagnosis

- There is currently no definitive test for anemia of chronic kidney disease. It is a diagnosis of exclusion.
- May coexist with iron deficiency and folate deficiency
- Low serum iron
- Normal or increased ferritin
- Decreased TIBC
- Normal MCV
- Normochromic red blood cells on peripheral smear

Signs and Symptoms

There are many symptoms of anemia of kidney disease. Different patients will experience different combinations of symptoms; and, if the anemia is mild, the symptoms may not be noticeable. Some of the symptoms are: Pale skin color, fatigue, irritability, dizziness, weakness, shortness of breath, sore tongue, brittle nails, decreased appetite (especially in children), and frontal headaches.

Guidelines

National Kidney Foundation. KDOQI Clinical Practice Guidelines and Clinical Practice Recommendations for Anemia in Chronic Kidney Disease. Am J Kidney Dis. 2006;47(5).

Guidelines Summary

- Treatment guidelines for stress treatment are based on hemoglobin (Hb).
- Hb should be between 11–12 mg/dL.
- Hb targets are not intended to apply to the treatment of iron deficiency in patients receiving iron therapy without the use of erythropoiesis-stimulating agents (ESAs).
- ESAs are the drug of choice.
- In dialysis and nondialysis patients with chronic kidney disease (CKD) receiving ESA therapy, the Hb target should not be greater than 13.0 g/dL.
  - Hb should not be greater than 13.0 g/dL due to the all-cause mortality and adverse cardiovascular event in patients with CKD and Hb greater than 13.0 g/dL.

Drugs for Anemia of Chronic Renal Disease and Dialysis

Mechanism of action – induces erythropoiesis by stimulating the division and differentiation of committed erythroid progenitor cells; induces the release of reticulocytes from the bone marrow into the bloodstream

Generic	Brand	Dose	Contraindications	Primary Side Effects	Key Monitoring	Pertinent Drug Interactions	Med Pearl
Epoetin alfa	Procrit	IV, subcutaneous (SC) initial: 50–100 units/kg 3x wk	• Hb >12 g/dL • Hb increase >1 g/dL per 2-wk time period	• Hypertension • Hypotension • Peripheral edema • Dizziness • Diarrhea • Infection	• Hb 1–2x wk until maintenance dose established and after dosage changes • Iron stores • Blood pressure	None	Indicated for IDA, sickle-cell disease, autoimmune hemolytic anemia, bleeding, chronic renal failure (CRF)
Darbepoetin alfa	Aranesp	IV, SC initial: 0.45 mcg/kg 1x wkly	• Uncontrolled hypertension				Only indicated for patients with CRF and nonmyeloid malignancies whose anemia is a result of chemotherapy

Storage and Administration Pearls

- Refrigerate vial between 36–46°F.
- Do not freeze or shake.
- Multidose vials, with preservative, are stable for 1 week at room temperature.

Patient Education Pearls

- These medications can be administered only by infusion or injection.
- Frequent blood tests will be needed to determine appropriate dosages.
- Avoid alcohol and do not make significant changes in dietary iron without consulting prescriber.
- Check blood pressure frequently.

PERNICIOUS ANEMIA

Definitions

Pernicious anemia is a type of megaloblastic anemia. Pernicious anemia is a decrease in red blood cells that occurs when the body cannot properly absorb vitamin B12 (cyanocobalamin) from the GI tract. Vitamin B12 is necessary for the formation of RBCs. Megaloblastic anemia is a blood disorder characterized by RBCs that are larger than normal due to deficiency in folate or cyanocobalamin.

Diagnosis

- Detecting antibodies to intrinsic factor is specific for the diagnosis of pernicious anemia.
- A Schilling test is used to detect antibodies to intrinsic factor.
- Serum vitamin B12 should be measured.
- Serum methylmalonic acid and homocysteine are elevated in pernicious anemia.
- Homocysteine is elevated only in folic acid deficiency.

Signs and Symptoms

- Symptoms similar to IDA
- May find glossitis, jaundice, and splenomegaly
- Ataxia, paresthesias, confusion, and dementia
- Folate acid deficiency: does not result in neurologic disease

Treatment Summary

- No major guidelines have been recently published on the treatment of pernicious anemia.
- Treatment is directed toward replacing the deficient factor.
- Blood transfusions are rarely required.
- Pernicious anemia is treated with vitamin B12.
- Treatment should always be initiated with intramuscular injections before moving to oral formulations.
- With therapy the reticulocytosis should begin within 1 week, followed by a rising Hb over 6–8 weeks.
- Coexisting iron deficiency is present in one-third of patients and is a common cause of incomplete response to therapy.

Drugs for Pernicious Anemia

Mechanism of action – coenzyme for various metabolic functions, cell replication, and hematopoiesis

Generic	Brand	Dose	Contraindications	Primary Side Effects	Key Monitoring	Pertinent Drug Interactions	Med Pearl	Top 200
Cyanocobalamin (B12)	• Nascobal • Vitamin B12	• Initial: 1,000 mcg IM daily for 1 week, then 1,000 mcg IM monthly for 6 months • Maintenance: 1,000 mcg IM monthly • Oral: 1 mg/day • Intranasal: 500 mcg in one nostril weekly	Hypersensitivity to cobalt	• Anxiety • Itching • Diarrhea	• Vitamin B12 • HCT • Reticulocyte count • Folate • Iron	• May decrease the effect of chloramphenicol • Long-term treatment with metformin may decrease the absorption of vitamin B12	• Oral neomycin or aminosalicylic acid may significantly reduce B12 absorption • Hydroxycobalamin is a longer-acting form of vitamin B12	No

Mechanism of action – coenzyme in many metabolic systems, particularly for purine and pyrimidine synthesis

Generic	Brand	Dose	Contraindications	Primary Side Effects	Key Monitoring	Pertinent Drug Interactions	Med Pearl	Top 200
Folic acid (folate)	Apo-Folic	• Oral: 0.4 mg/day • Prevention of neural tube: 0.4–0.8mg/day	Hypersensitivity to folic acid	• Allergic reaction • Bronchospasm • Flushing • Malaise • Pruritus • Rash	• HCT • Reticulocyte count • Folate • Iron	Folic acid administration may decrease serum levels of phenytoin	• Phenytoin and other anticonvulsant may inhibit folic acid absorption • Products containing more than 0.8 mg of folic acid are Rx-only	Yes

Storage and Administration Pearls

- Cyanocobalamin injection is clear pink-to-red solution, stable at room temperature.
- Cyanocobalamin must be protected from light.
- Intranasal spray must be stored in the refrigerator and not frozen.

Patient Education Pearls

- Pernicious anemia may require treatment for life.
- Report rashes on extremities or acute persistent diarrhea.

LEARNING POINTS

- Coexisting iron deficiency is present in many forms of anemia and should always be assessed.
- When treating with ESA, Hb should not be greater than 13.0 g/dL due to the all-cause mortality and adverse cardiovascular event in patients with CKD and Hb greater than 13.0 g/dL.
- Iron absorption is enhanced through simultaneous intake of ascorbic acid (i.e., vitamin C).
- Laxatives, stool softeners, and adequate intake of liquids should be regularly recommended to patients taking iron therapy, to alleviate the medication's constipating effects.
- Long-term metformin therapy can decrease the absorption of vitamin B12.

PRACTICE QUESTIONS

1. Which of the following drugs need to be protected from light?

        I. Lasix
       II. Epoetin alfa
      III. Enalaprilat

    (A) I only
    (B) III only
    (C) I and II only
    (D) II and III only
    (E) I, II, and III

2. Which of the following is NOT a characteristic of pernicious anemia?

    (A) Weakness
    (B) Forgetfulness
    (C) Pica
    (D) Tendency to fall easily
    (E) Treatment includes B12 replacement

3. Which of the following is NOT a treatment for anemia of chronic renal failure?

    (A) Darbepoetin alfa
    (B) Ferrous sulfate
    (C) Cyanocobalamin
    (D) Erythropoietin
    (E) All of the above

ANSWERS

1. **A**

Lasix (furosemide) is the only drug on this list that needs to be protected from light. Epoetin alfa (II) should not be frozen or shaken. Enalaprilat (III) is the only IV angiotensin-converting enzyme inhibitor; however, it does not require an amber bag to protect it from light.

2. **C**

Pica, or the craving to eat nonfood substances such as ice or dirt, is characteristic of iron deficiency anemia but not pernicious anemia. Weakness, forgetfulness, and the tendency to fall easily are all commonly seen symptoms associated with pernicious, or B12 deficiency, anemia. And because pernicious anemia is caused by a decrease in vitamin B12, a common treatment is B12 replacement (E).

3. **C**

Cyanocobalamin is the correct choice. Cyanocobalamin, or B12, is a treatment option in pernicious anemia. In anemia of chronic renal failure, the kidneys are not able to adequately produce red blood cells, so treatment options include drugs that stimulate red blood cell production. Darbepoetin alfa (A) and erythropoietin (D) are drugs that stimulate red blood cell production. In addition to the need for red blood cells, these patients also require iron supplementation during erythropoietin therapy, hence the need for ferrous sulfate (B).

Dermatologic Disorders

13

This chapter covers the following disease states:

- **Acne**
- **Psoriasis**

 Suggested Study Time: **20 minutes**

ACNE

Definitions

Acne vulgaris is an inflammatory skin disorder that results in comedones, papules, pustules, nodules, or cysts on the face, back, or chest. The disorder occurs most commonly in teenagers at or near puberty but can occur at any age.

Diagnosis

Although no strict diagnostic criteria exist, the presence of five or more lesions (of any type) is generally considered sufficient for diagnosis.

Signs and Symptoms

Acne vulgaris lesions appear most commonly on the face but also on the back and chest. The severity of acne vulgaris varies and is based on the types of lesions present. Type I acne is the mildest form and is associated with a mostly noninflammatory presentation of open and closed comedones. Type II acne is a more moderate form with multiple papules present. Type III acne is associated with a more severe form of acne consisting of an inflammatory condition with multiple pustules. Type IV is the most severe form, consisting of inflammatory nodules and cysts that lead to scarring.

Guidelines

Guidelines of care for acne vulgaris management. *J Am Acad Dermatol*, no. 56 (4) (April 2007): 651–63.

www.guideline.gov/summary/summary.aspx?doc_id=10797&nbr=005625&string= acne+AND+vulgaris.

Guideline Summary

- Topical benzoyl peroxide is the first-line therapy recommendation for most mild to moderate forms of acne vulgaris (type I).

- Topical antibiotics and topical retinoids are considered first-line for moderate acne vulgaris (type II) and second-line for mild-moderate (type I).

- Moderate-severe, inflammatory acne (type III) should be treated with topical therapy (benzoyl peroxide, retinoids, or antibiotics) plus oral antibiotics.

- Severe, inflammatory acne (type IV) can be treated with the combination of oral antibiotics and topical therapy but often requires the use of oral isotretinoin therapy.

- Oral isotretinoin is an effective therapy option for the treatment of severe, inflammatory acne, or more moderate forms that have been refractory to other treatment options.

- All females of child-bearing age that have been prescribed isotretinoin must agree to use two forms of contraception during isotretinoin use. Because of the known teratogenic risk associated with isotretinoin therapy, all patients, pharmacies, physicians, and wholesalers must register with the iPLEDGE program. This is an FDA program designed to monitor and decrease the risk of fetal exposure to isotretinoin.

Drugs for Acne

Generic	Brand	Dose & Max	Contraindications	Primary Side Effects	Key Monitoring Parameters	Pertinent Drug Interactions	Med Pearls	Top 200
Topical								
Nonprescription								
Benzoyl peroxide	Many	2.5–10% cream, lotion, gel, wash	Hypersensitivity	Excessive drying, photo sensitivity, peeling, erythema	Presence of adverse effects, efficacy	Retinoids: combination causes significant irritation	Over-the-counter (OTC)	No
Sulfur	SAStid	3–8% soap				Other topical agents: additive drying		No
Salicylic acid	Many	0.5–2% wash						No
Antimicrobials								
Clindamycin	Cleocin T	1% gel, lotion apply BID	Hypersensitivity, ulcerative colitis	Burning, itching, dryness, irritation	Presence of adverse effects, efficacy	Neuromuscular blocking agents		Yes
Erythromycin	• Theramycin Z • Benzamycin • Emgel	2% gel, liquid, ointment, pledgets	Hypersensitivity			None		No
Retinoids								
Tretinoin	• Retin-A • Renova • Avita	0.015–0.1% gel, cream, lotion	Hypersensitivity	Photosensitivity, burning, dryness, erythema, irritation	Presence of adverse effects	Other topical drying agents – additive drying Other photosensitizing medications	Apply after freshly washed face is completely dry	Yes
Adapalene	Differin	0.1% gel, cream, and lotion						Yes
Tazarotene	Tazorac	0.05–0.1% gel						No
Alitretinoin	Panretin	0.1% gel						No
Other								
Azelaic acid	Azelex, Finevin	• 15% cream, 20% gel • Apply BID	Hypersensitivity	Burning, stinging, tingling, pruritus, photosensitivity	Presence of adverse effects	None		No

Drugs for Acne *(cont'd)*

Generic	Brand	Dose & Max	Contraindications	Primary Side Effects	Key Monitoring Parameters	Pertinent Drug Interactions	Med Pearls	Top 200
Oral								
Antimicrobials								
Tetracycline	• Achromycin • Sumycin	250–3,000 mg daily (divided BID–QID)	Hypersensitivity	Rash, photosensitivity, gastrointestinal (GI) upset	Presence of adverse effects	Antacids, penicillin, oral contraceptives, anticoagulants	Take 2 hrs before or after meals, avoid calcium containing foods (dairy)	Yes
Doxycycline	Vibramycin	50–200 mg daily (divided BID)						Yes
Minocycline	Minocin	50–200 mg daily (divided BID)				As above, and isotretinoin		Yes
Erythromycin	• E.E.S. • Erythrocin	250–3,000 mg daily (divided BID)	Hypersensitivity; use of terfenadine, astemizole, cisapride	GI upset, diarrhea, nausea, vomiting, abdominal pain	Presence of adverse effects	Terfenadine, astemizole, cisapride: combination of these agents with erythromycin increases the risk of fetal arrhythmia; anticoagulants, lovastatin, digoxin	Significant drug interactions and GI side effects limit use	Yes
Isotretinoin								
Isotretinoin	Accutane	0.5–2 mg/kg/day (divided BID)	Pregnancy, hypersensitivity	Cheilitis, dry mouth, dry skin, pruritus, erythema, GI upset, headaches, hyperlipidemia, depression (rare)	Periodic lipid panel, presence of adverse effects	Isotretinoin increases concentrations of corticosteroids, phenytoin; and has additive toxicity with vitamin A	• Females must agree to at least two forms of contraception during therapy • Must register in iPLEDGE program	No

Storage and Administration Pearls

- Apply topical acne products only after washing the face and then waiting for the skin to dry completely (approximately 30 minutes).
- Protect tetracycline from light. Tetracycline, doxycycline, and minocycline should be taken 2 hours before or after a meal, and interact with calcium-containing products such as dairy items.

Patient Education Pearls

- Topical agents and antimicrobials increase risk of excessive burning from the sun. Apply sunscreen prior to sun exposure.

PSORIASIS

Definitions

Psoriasis is a chronic inflammatory skin disease associated with silvery scalelike lesions. There are two primary types of psoriasis identified: Type I is diagnosed early in life in patients with a family history, while type II develops later in life and generally has no family history present.

Diagnosis

Diagnosis is based on thorough history and physical and depends primarily on the observation of lesions.

Signs and Symptoms

Sharp, demarcated, erythematous papules and plaques covered with silvery scales is a sign. Affected areas may include the scalp, trunk, back, arms, legs, palms, soles, face, and/or genitalia. Psoriatic arthritis refers to secondary joint inflammation that occurs in patients with psoriasis. The most commonly affected joints are the elbows, wrists, ankles, and knees.

Guidelines

Guidelines of care for the management of psoriasis and psoriatic arthritis: Section 4. Guidelines of care for the management and treatment of psoriasis with traditional systemic agents. *J Am Acad Dermatol* 2009 Sep;61(3):451–85.

Summary of Treatment Recommendations

- The goal of therapy is complete resolution of lesions.
- There is significant interpatient variability in response to the available medications. Options for initial treatment include topical agents such as emollients and keratolytics (salicylic acid or sulfur), coal tar, anthralin, calcipotriene, or retinoids.
- Systemic treatment is considered as initial therapy in very severe cases or as second-line therapy in patients that do not respond to topical options. Systemic options include antimetabolite therapy (methotrexate, cyclosporine, tacrolimus), oral corticosteroids, psoralens, immunosuppressants, or retinoids.

Drugs for Psoriasis

Generic	Brand	Dose & Max	Contraindications	Primary Side Effects	Key Monitoring Parameters	Pertinent Drug Interactions	Med Pearls	Top 200
Coal Tar								
Coal tar	• Medotar • Fototar	1–25% ointment, cream, lotion apply 1–4x daily	Hypersensitivity	Photosensitivity	Presence of adverse effects	Other photosensi-tizing agents	OTC	No
Retinoids								
Tretinoin	• Retin-A • Renova • Avita	0.015–0.1% gel, cream, lotion	See details above					
Adapalene	Differin	0.1% gel						
Tazarotene	Tazorac	0.05–0.1% gel						
Alitretinoin	Panretin	0.1% gel						
Anthralin								
Dithranol	• Anthralin • Psoriatec	0.5–1% cream, apply 1x daily	Hypersensitivity, inflamed eruptions	Discoloration of skin, hair, fabrics, irritation	Presence of adverse effects	Topical steroids	Staining of fabric can be permanent	No
Calcipotriene								
Calcipotriene	Dovonex	0.005% cream, ointment, solution; apply 1–2x daily	Hypersensitivity, hypercalcemia	Burning, itching, skin irritation, drying	Presence of adverse effects	Other topical agents: additive drying		No
Topical Vitamin D Analog								
Calcitriol	Vectical	Apply 2 x (max 200 g/week)	Do not apply to face or eyes	Pruritis, erythema, blisters, skin discomfort, dermatitis, photosensitivity	Response to therapy	Concomitant use with vitamin D or calcium supplements, or calcium- or magnesium-containing antacids may increase likelihood of clinically significant increases in serum levels	Topical product unlikely to cause drug interactions or serum abnormalities due to limited systemic absorption	No

Drugs for Psoriasis *(cont'd)*

Generic	Brand	Dose & Max	Contraindications	Primary Side Effects	Key Monitoring Parameters	Pertinent Drug Interactions	Med Pearls	Top 200
Systemic								
Antimetabolites								
Methotrexate (MTX)	None	7.5 mg PO 1x wkly	Hypersensitivity, alcoholic liver disease, pre-existing blood dyscrasias	Leukopenia, nausea, fatigue, chills, fever, hepatotoxicity, photosensitivity	Periodic complete blood count (CBC), liver enzymes	Nonsteroidal anti-inflammatory drugs (NSAIDs), salicylates, probenecid, phenytoin, sulfonamides increase MTX levels	Necessary to use contraception in female patients (pregnancy category X)	Yes
Immunosuppressants								
Alefacept	Amevive	15 mg IM wkly	CD4 count <250 cells/mcL, HIV	Lymphopenia, headache, chills, dizziness, myalgias	Periodic white blood cell (WBC) count, CD4 count prior to first dose and wkly during 12 wks of therapy	Other immuno-suppressants; live or attenuated vaccines	Alefacept pregnancy registry program for female patients who become pregnant	No
Etanercept	Enbrel	50 mg SC 2x wkly	Hypersensitivity	Injection site reactions, infections, headache, rash, nausea, neutropenia	Periodic WBC	Risk of blood dyscrasias and infection when combined with anakinra or other immuno-suppressants	Available in prefilled syringes; pregnancy registry for pregnant females on medication	No
Efalizumab	Raptiva	0.7–1 mg/kg SC wkly	Hypersensitivity	Headache, chills, fever, increased risk of infection, myalgia, thrombocytopenia	Presence of side effects, signs and symptoms of infection, periodic platelet counts	Other immuno-suppressants; live or live-attenuated vaccines	Efalizumab pregnancy registry for females who become pregnant	No
Ustekinumab	Stelara	45–90 mg SC every 12 weeks	Hypersensitivity	Nasopharyngitis, upper respiratory tract infection, headache, and fatigue	PPD prior to initiation of therapy, response to therapy, presence of infection	Not to be given with live vaccines or other immuno-suppressants	Indicated for moderate to severe plaque	No
Retinoids								
Acitretin	Soriatane	25–50 mg PO daily	Hypersensitivity, impaired hepatic or renal function, use with MTX	Dry skin, alopecia, rash, chelitis, peeling, pruritus	Presence of adverse effects	• MTX: increased risk of hepatitis • Tetracyclines: increased intra-cranial pressure	Law requires medication guide be given to the patient each time acitretin is dispensed; pregnancy category X	No

Storage and Administration Pearls

- Store out of reach of children.
- Avoid application of topical agents near the eyes.
- Alefacept and ustekinumab should be stored in a refrigerator between 2–8°C (36–46°F), protected from light, and retained in drug/diluent pack until time of use.
- Efalizumab (lyophilized powder) must be refrigerated at 2–8°C (36–46°F). Protect the vial from exposure to light. Store in original carton until time of use.
- Etanercept solution must be refrigerated at 2–8°C (36–46°F) and should not be frozen.

Patient Education Pearls

- Wash hands thoroughly after application of topical agents.
- Keep topical agents away from eyes.

LEARNING POINTS

- First-line therapy for mild to moderate acne vulgaris is topical benzoyl peroxide.
- Topical retinoids should not be combined with other topical acne agents due to risk of excessive drying and photosensitivity.
- Oral isotretinoin is reserved for refractory or severe cases of acne vulgaris. Patients, pharmacists, and physicians must register with the FDA iPLEDGE program to use this medication.
- Oral isotretinoin is associated with significant teratogenicity. Females on isotretinoin therapy must agree to use two forms of contraception during the course of therapy.
- Significant interpatient variability exists in the response to psoriasis treatments. Initial therapy generally consists of topic agents such as keratolytics, coal tar, or anthralin.
- Antimetabolite and immunosuppressant therapy carries significantly greater adverse effect risk and therefore should be reserved for severe or refractory cases.

PRACTICE QUESTIONS

1. Which of the following is appropriate initial treatment for type III acne?

   (A) Topical antibiotics and topical retinoids
   (B) Topical antibiotics + oral antibiotics
   (C) Topical benzoyl peroxide
   (D) Oral antibiotics
   (E) Isotretinoins

2. Which of the following psoriasis medications is NOT pregnancy category X?

      I. Dovonex
     II. Methotrexate
    III. Soriatane

   (A) I only
   (B) III only
   (C) I and II only
   (D) II and III only
   (E) I, II, III

ANSWERS

1. B

First-line therapy for type III acne is topical therapy (benzoyl peroxide, retinoids, or antibiotics) plus oral antibiotics. First-line therapy for type I acne is topical benzoyl peroxide (C). First-line therapy for type II acne is topical antibiotics and topical retinoids (A). Oral antibiotics are not used alone (D) without topical agents. Isotretinoins (E) are usually reserved for type IV or other types that are refractory to other treatment options.

2. A

Methotrexate (II) is pregnancy category X and requires the use of contraception when used by females of child-bearing age. This rules out choices (C), (D), and (E). Soriatane (III) is a retinoid that is also pregnancy category X and requires a medication guide dispensed with each medication, thus eliminating choice (B). Dovonex (I) is calcipotriene and is one of the first-line therapy options for psoriasis. It is not pregnancy category X (it is pregnancy category C). Therefore, (A) is the answer.

Antidotes

14

The following chapter addresses drugs that are used as antagonist drugs to do one of the following:

- **Reverse the effect of one drug**
- **Prevent toxicity**
- **Treat toxicity**

🕐 Suggested Study Time: **15 minutes**

ANTIDOTES

Definitions

The drugs included in this chapter act in a variety of ways to counter the toxic effects of exogenous and endogenous substances in the body. Therefore, they are used in the management of poisoning and overdosage. Many antidotes are used to protect against the toxicity of drugs such as antineoplastics, and in the management of metabolic disorders such as Wilson's disease, where toxic substances accumulate.

Accidental and deliberate drug overdosage is a common problem seen by ambulance staff and emergency workers. The majority of these episodes of poisoning are dealt with along similar lines with general supportive care, but some require more specific action.

Some antagonists, such as the opioid antagonist naloxone, compete with the poison for receptor sites. Other antagonists, such as atropine, block substances that mediate the effects of the toxin. This may reduce absorption of the toxin from the gastrointestinal tract, inactivate or reduce the activity of the toxin, or increase the toxin's elimination via drugs that affect the metabolism of the toxin.

Some antidotes, such as fomepizole in methyl alcohol poisoning, act by reducing the rate of metabolism to a toxic metabolite. Others, such as methionine and glutathione, promote the formation of inactive metabolites. Acetylcysteine also acts by bypassing the effect of the toxin. On the NAPLEX, antidotes questions can be an easy way to earn points if you learn the correct antidote for the toxicity.

ACUTE POISONING

In the management of suspected acute poisoning, it is often impossible to determine with any certainty the identity of the poison or the size of the dose received. As a result, a common procedure needs to be in place:

- First, call the poison control center: (800) 222-1222.
- Next, take a history of the event and drug, or substance, involved.
  - What mode of poisoning has occurred (i.e., ingestion or inhalation)?
  - When did it happen?
  - Has any treatment occurred yet (i.e., induced vomiting)?

Few poisons have specific antidotes or methods of elimination, and the mainstay of treatment for patients with suspected acute poisoning is therefore supportive and symptomatic therapy; in many cases, nothing further is required. Clinicians should assess the ABCDs: airway, breathing, circulation, dextrose, decontamination. Symptoms of acute poisoning are frequently nonspecific, particularly in the early stages. Maintenance of the airway and ventilation is the most important initial measure; other treatment—for example, for cardiovascular or neurological symptoms—may be added as appropriate.

Some centers also recommend the routine administration of dextrose to all unconscious patients since hypoglycemia may be a cause of unconsciousness, although blood glucose measurements should be obtained first where facilities are immediately available.

Specific antidotes are available for a number of poisons and are the primary treatment where there is a severe poisoning with a known toxin. These antidotes may be lifesaving in such cases but their use is not without hazard and, in many situations, they are not necessary. These agents are discussed in greater detail in the chart below.

Measures to reduce or prevent the absorption of the poison are widely advocated. For inhalational poisoning, the victim is removed from the source of poisoning. Some toxins, particularly pesticides, may be absorbed through the skin, and clothing should be removed and the skin thoroughly washed to avoid continued absorption. Caustic substances are removed from the skin or eyes with copious irrigation. However, for orally ingested poisons the best method of gastrointestinal (GI) decontamination remains controversial; this is addressed in the following sections.

GENERAL ANTIDOTES

Activated Charcoal

Activated charcoal absorbs a wide range of toxins and is often given to reduce absorption within the GI tract. A single dose is generally effective, particularly if it is given within 1 hour of ingestion. Delayed use, however, may be beneficial for modified-release preparations or for drugs that slow GI transit time, such as those with antimuscarinic properties. Charcoal is generally well tolerated, although vomiting is common, and there is a risk of aspiration if the airway is not adequately protected. Repeated doses may be useful in eliminating some substances even after systemic absorption has occurred.

Active removal of poisons from the stomach by induction of emesis or gastric lavage has been widely used, but there is little evidence to support its role. Emesis should not be induced if the poison is corrosive or petroleum-based, or if the poison is removable by treatment with activated charcoal.

Ipecac

When used appropriately, ipecac is a safe emetic. However, its efficacy in preventing deaths has never been proven, and the routine use of ipecac at home has been questioned.

A recent survey found that increased home use of ipecac was not associated with referral to an emergency department. Additionally, there was no difference in adverse outcome rate between the poison centers that more commonly recommended ipecac compared with those centers that did not. The authors concluded that although their data cannot exclude a benefit of ipecac in a very limited set of poisonings, any benefit remains to be proven.

There are a number of drawbacks to using ipecac. Adverse effects include lethargy, diarrhea, and persistent vomiting. Persistent vomiting can be especially troublesome because it may reduce the efficacy of other orally administered treatments for poisoning, such as activated charcoal, N-acetylcysteine, or agents used for whole-bowel irrigation. Second, ipecac is sometimes given, either without medical advice or based on inappropriate medical advice, when it is not needed (i.e., in the case of ingestion of a nontoxic agent) or when it is contraindicated. Examples of contraindications to ipecac include the following:

- Lack of a gag reflex
- Lethargy
- Seizures
- Following the ingestion of caustic agents, corrosive agents, ammonia, or bleach
- Chronic misuse: May lead to cardiomyopathy

Gastric lavage may occasionally be indicated for ingestion of noncaustic poisons that are not absorbed by activated charcoal, but only if less than 1 hour has elapsed since ingestion. Gastric lavage should not be attempted if the airway is not adequately protected.

Whole-bowel irrigation using a nonabsorbable osmotic agent such as a macrogol has also been used, particularly for substances that pass beyond the stomach before being absorbed (such as iron preparations or enteric-coated or modified-release formulations), but its role is not established.

Antidotes

Toxic Agent	Generic	Brand	Dose	Contraindications	Primary Side Effects	Key Monitoring	Med Pearl	Top 200
Mechanism of action – pure opioid antagonist that competes and displaces narcotics at opioid receptor sites								
Opioids	Naloxone	Narcan	Intravenous (IV), intramuscular (IM), subcutaneous (SC) 0.4 mg q2–3 min as needed; repeat dose q20–60 min	Hypersensitivity	• Tachycardia • Ventricular arrhythmia • Anxiety • Diaphoresis	• Respiratory rate • Heart rate • Blood pressure	Adverse effects can occur secondarily to reversal (withdrawal)	No
Mechanism of action – acts as a competitive antagonist at opioid receptor sites								
Opioids	Nalmefene	Revex	IV: 0.25 mcg/kg followed by 0.25 mcg/kg at 2–5 minute intervals	Hypersensitivity	• Nausea • Tachycardia • Vomiting • Agitation	• Respiratory rate • Sedation • Blood pressure	6-Methylene analog of naltrexone	No
Mechanism of action – acts as a competitive antagonist at opioid receptor sites								
Opioids	Naltrexone	Trexan	• Alcohol dependence • Opioid antidote	• Acute opioid withdrawal • Failure to pass Narcan challenge • Positive urine drug screen	• Syncope • Headache • Arthralgia • Diarrhea	• Narcotic withdrawal • Liver function test (LFT)	• Do not give until patient is opioid-free for 7–10 days • Alcohol and opioid dependence • Highest affinity for mu receptors	No
Mechanism of action – competitively inhibits the activity at the benzodiazepine recognition site on the GABA/benzo complex								

Benzodiazepines	Flumazenil	Romazicon	IV: 0.2 mg over 15 sec; repeat until conscious	Patients showing signs of serious cyclic antidepressant overdosage	• Palpitations
					• Hot flashes
					• Tremor
					• Abnormal vision
						Benzo reversal may result in seizures in some patients	• If patient has not responded 5 min after receiving a cumulative dose of 5 mg, the sedation is likely not due to benzodiazepines
							• Reversal affects of nonbenzodiazepines
							  · Zaleplon (Sonata)
							  · Zolpidem (Ambien)
								No

Antidotes *(cont'd)*

Toxic Agent	Generic	Brand	Dose	Contraindications	Primary Side Effects	Key Monitoring	Med Pearl	Top 200
Mechanism of action – competitively inhibits alcohol dehydrogenase, an enzyme that catalyzes the metabolism of ethanol, methanol, and ethylene glycol								
• Ethanol • Methanol • Ethylene glycol	Fomepizole	Antizol	IV: loading dose 15 mg/kg, followed by 10 mg/kg q12 hrs x 4 doses	Hypersensitivity	• Headache • Nausea • Metallic taste	• Fomepizole plasma levels should be monitored • Urinary ethylene glycol or methanol levels • Renal function		No
Mechanism of action – inhibits destruction of acetylcholine by acetylcholinesterase which prolongs effects of acetylcholine (anticholinergic drug overdose)								
Anticholinergic drugs	Physostigmine	Eserine	IV, IM, SC: 0.5–2 mg to start; repeat q2 min until response	• GI or genitourinary (GU) obstruction • Asthma, gangrene, severe cardiovascular disease	• Palpitation • Bradycardia • Restlessness • Seizure	• Heart rate • Respiratory rate		No
Mechanism of action – antigen–binding fragments (Fab) are specific for the treatment of digitalis intoxication								
Digoxin	Digoxin Immune Fab	Digibind	40 mg will bind to 0.5 mcg/mL of digoxin or digitoxin	Sheep products	• Exacerbation of heart failure • Rapid ventricular response	Serum potassium levels	Digoxin levels will greatly increase with digoxin Fab use and are not an accurate determination of body stores	No
Mechanism of action – supplies a free thiol group which binds to and inactivates acrolein, the urotoxic metabolite of ifosfamide and cyclophosphamide								
• Isophosphamide • Cyclophosphamide	Mesna	Mesnex	IV: 60–80% of ifosfamide dose given TID to QID	Thiol compounds	• Bad taste • Vomiting secondary to bad taste • Platelet-count decrease	Urinalysis	Orphan drug: used for the prevention of hemorrhagic cystitis induced by ifosfamide	No

Antidotes (cont'd)

Toxic Agent	Generic	Brand	Dose	Contraindications	Primary Side Effects	Key Monitoring	Med Pearl	Top 200
Mechanism of action – cardioprotective by converting intracellularly to a ring-opened chelating agent that interferes with iron-mediated oxygen free radical generation								
Doxorubicin	Dexrazoxane	Zinecard	IV: 10:1 ratio of dexrazoxane: doxorubicin	Hypersensitivity	• Most adverse affects thought to be attributed to chemotherapy	• Adds to myelosuppressive effects • LFTs		No
Mechanism of action – free thiol metabolite is available to bind to and detoxify reactive metabolites of cisplatin								
Cisplatin	Amifostine	Ethyol	IV	Hypersensitivity to amifostine or aminothiol	• Hypotension • Nausea/vomiting	• Blood pressure should be monitored every 5 min during the infusion • Serum calcium levels	Antiemetic medication is recommend prior to and in conjunction with amifostine	No
Mechanism of action – combines with strongly acidic heparin to form a stable complex (salt) neutralizing the anticoagulant activity of both drugs								
Heparin	Protamine	Protamine	Protamine dosage is determined by the dosages of heparin; 1 mg; 90 USP units heparin; max: 50 mg	Hypersensitivity	• Hypotension • Flushing • Dyspnea	• Activated partial thromboplastin time (aPTT) • Blood pressure		No
Mechanism of action – promotes liver synthesis of clotting factors (II, VII, IX, X) which counteracts the mechanism of warfarin								
Warfarin	Vitamin K (phytonadione)	Mephyton	• Depends on international normalized ratio (INR) and bleeding risk factors; i.e., >9 INR: no significant bleeding: hold warfarin, give vitamin K 5–10 mg, expect INR to be reduced within 24–48 hrs • Hypersensitivity		• Cyanosis • Dizziness	• Prothrombin time (PT) • INR	IM route should be avoided due to hematoma formation	No
Mechanism of action – reduced form of folic acid: supplies the necessary cofactor blocked by methotrexate								
Methotrexate	Leucovorin	Leucovorin	2–15 mg/day for 3 days or until blood counts are normal	• Pernicious anemia • B12-deficient megaloblastic anemias	• Rash • Anaphylactoid reactions	Plasma methotrexate concentration	• Continue leucovorin until plasma methotrexate level <0.05 mmol/L • Decreased efficacy of cotrimoxazole against Pneumocystis carinii pneumonitis	No

Antidotes (cont'd)

Toxic Agent	Generic	Brand	Dose	Contraindications	Primary Side Effects	Key Monitoring	Med Pearl	Top 200
Mechanism of action – absorbs toxic substances or irritants, thus inhibiting GI absorption								
Activated charcoal	Activated charcoal	Actidose	25–100 g/dose	• Non-intact GI tract • GI perforation	• Hypernatremia • Hypokalemia	• Constipation • Diarrhea	Sorbitol accelerates bowel evacuation	
Mechanism of action – bind toxic agents in the biliary; forms a nonabsorbable complex with bile acids in the intestine; inhibits enterohepatic reuptake								
Leflunomide	Cholestyramine resin	• Questran • Questran Light	4 g–24 g/day administered up to 6x day	• Complete biliary obstruction • Bowel obstruction	• Constipation • Nausea • Stomach pain • Gallstones • Bloating	Serum levels of poison	Arava (leflunomide) 8 g cholestyramine TID for 1 to 3 days; plasma level should reach <0.02 mg/L	No
Mechanism of action – exact mechanism of acetaminophen toxicity is unknown								
Acetaminophen	Acetylcysteine	• Acetadote • Mucomyst	140 mg/kg followed by 17 doses of 70 mg/kg q4 hrs	Hypersensitivity	• Drowsiness • Chills • Fever	• Aspartate aminotransferase (AST), alanine aminotransferase (ALT) • Bilirubin • PT • Serum creatinine	• Therapy should continue until acetaminophen levels are undetectable and there is no evidence of hepatotoxicity • Activated charcoal • 5–10 g:g acetaminophen	No
Mechanism of action – blocks the action of acetylcholine at parasympathetic sites in the smooth muscle, secretary glands, and the central nervous system (CNS)								
Cholinergics	Atropine	AtroPen	• Dose for adults is 2–3 mg • Dose for children is 0.02–0.05 mg/kg q60–20 minutes until effects are observed	No absolute contraindications in life-threatening poisoning	• Anaphylaxis • Nausea • Vomiting • Fatigue • Insomnia • Weakness • Cardiovascular changes	• Electrocardiogram (ECG) • Respiratory status • Metabolic panels	Dose until symptoms subside	No

Antidotes *(cont'd)*

Toxic Agent	Generic	Brand	Dose	Contraindications	Primary Side Effects	Key Monitoring	MedPearl	Top 200
Mechanism of action – stimulates adrenergic receptors resulting in relaxation of smooth muscle of the bronchial tree, cardiac stimulation and dilation of skeletal musculature								
Hypersensitivity reactions	Epinephrine	• Adrenalin • EpiPen • Twinject	0.2–0.5 mg IM or subQ every 5–15 minutes until improvement	No absolute CI in life-threatening situation	• Angina • Anxiety • Flushing	• Pulmonary function • Heart rate • Blood pressure	IM administration in the anterolateral aspect of the middle third of the thigh is preferred	Yes
Mechanism of action – stimulates adenylate cyclase to produce increased cyclic AMP, which promotes hepatic glycogenolysis and gluconeogenesis								
Hypoglycemia	Glucagon	GlucaGen	IV, IM, or subQ: 1 mg, may repeat in 20 minutes as needed	• Hypersensitivity • Insulinoma	• Hypotension • Nausea	• Blood pressure • Blood glucose • ECG • Heart rate	IV dextrose should be given as soon as available	No

Storage and Administration Pearls

- Protamine: Refrigerate, stable for 2 weeks at room temperature.
- Fomepizole: If solution becomes solid in the vial, warm carefully by running warm water over the vial.
- Naltrexone: Should be stored in the refrigerator. May be kept at room temperature for <7 days prior to use.
- Digoxin immune Fab: Should be refrigerated.
- Activated charcoal: Absorbs gas from air; store in closed container.

Patient Education Pearls

- Patient should stay calm and call the poison control center.
- If patient currently has ipecac in their home, it is better to dispose of it, according to the research.
- Most drugs do not have antidotes, so it is important to take medication as prescribed.

LEARNING POINTS

- It is important to memorize the phone number for the poison control center. The number should also be pasted on every telephone in your pharmacy.
- Storing ipecac in the home in case of acute poisoning is no longer recommended because of limited data suggesting any benefit. It is better to call the poison control center or 911 for advice.
- Few poisons have specific antidotes or methods of elimination; therefore, the mainstay of treatment for patients with suspected acute poisoning is supportive and symptomatic therapy.
- Flumazenil is the antidote for benzodiazepines and is commonly used in the hospital setting.
- Do not confuse Fomepizole and flumazenil. At first glance they may seem similar, but they have completely different uses.
- Protamine is the antidote for heparin, and vitamin K is the antidote for warfarin. Protamine and vitamin K are not interchangeable and have different mechanisms of action. These two antidotes are used for both inpatient and outpatient treatment.

PRACTICE QUESTIONS

1. Which drug is used to decrease toxicities associated with cisplatin?

   (A) Amifostine
   (B) Physostigmine
   (C) Nalmefene
   (D) Fomepizole
   (E) Leucovorin

2. How many doses of activated charcoal are typically effective?

   (A) 1
   (B) 2
   (C) 3
   (D) 4
   (E) 5

ANSWERS

1. **A**

Amifostine is used to prevent cisplatin toxicities associated with renal toxicity. Physostigmine (B) is used primarily to reverse toxic CNS effects caused by anticholinergic drugs. Nalmefene (C) is used as a partial reversal of opioid drug effects. Fomepizole (D) is used for methanol and ethylene glycol poisoning, and leucovorin (E) is used as an antidote for folic acid antagonist.

2. **A**

Activated charcoal typically requires only a single dose to be effective, particularly if it is given within 1 hour of toxin ingestion.

Gynecologic, Obstetric, and Urologic Disorders

15

This chapter covers the following topics:

- **Contraception**
- **Hormone replacement therapy**
- **Erectile dysfunction**
- **Urinary incontinence**

 Suggested Study Time: **45 minutes**

CONTRACEPTION

Definition

Contraception refers to the prevention of pregnancy and is accomplished pharmacologically through two general mechanisms: (*1*) inhibition of contact between sperm and egg, and (*2*) prevention of implantation of the fertilized egg in the endometrium. Available products most commonly contain estrogen, progestin, or both. The estrogen component suppresses follicle-stimulating hormone (FSH) and prevents the development of a viable follicle. The progestin component contributes to the production of thick cervical mucus and the involution of the endometrium, and blocks ovulation.

Therapy Selection

Available Prescription Therapies

- Combination estrogen and progestin
  - Monophasic
  - Multiphasic
- Progestin only

- Implantable
- Emergency contraception
  - Start within 72 hours of unprotected intercourse
  - Approved over-the-counter (OTC) if patient is >18 years of age
  - Plan B
    » 2 tablets 0.75 mg levonorgestrel (taken q12 h x 2 doses)
  - Preven
    » 0.25 mg levonorgestrel, 0.05 mg ethinyl estradiol (taken q12 h x 2 doses)
  - Plan B One Step
    » 1 tablet by mouth, levonorgestrel 1.5 mg
  - Ella (Rx only)
    » Ulipristal acetate 30 mg by mouth within 120 hours of unprotected intercourse

Advantages and Disadvantages

Table 1.

Product type	Advantages	Disadvantages
Combination products	Long history of superior efficacy; multiple formulations allow opportunity to try multiple-dose combination of estrogen/progestin components in different dosage forms (transdermal patch, oral, multiphasic, continuous); decreased length of menses; decreased incidence of cramping; decreased risk of ectopic pregnancy	Drug interactions present; need for backup contraception with missed pills
Progestin only	Can be used in safely patients that are breastfeeding, are >35 years of age, and/or have systemic lupus erythematosus or intolerable estrogen-related side effects	Slightly less effective; requires even stricter compliance than combinations; higher incidence of breakthrough bleeding; need for backup contraception with missed pills
Implantable	Longer-term efficacy	Not readily reversible; requires insertion at medical office

Adverse Effects Associated with Hormonal Imbalance

Table 2.

Estrogen Excess	Estrogen Deficiency	Progestin Excess	Progestin Deficiency
• Breast tenderness • Cyclic weight gain • Edema • Bloating • Hypertension • Melasma • Migraine • Nausea	• Vasomotor symptoms (hot flushes) • Spotting • Breakthrough bleeding • Decreased libido • Dyspareunia	• Decreased libido • Depression • Fatigue • Weight gain • Acne • Hypomenorrhea • Vaginal candidiasis	• Heavy menstruation • Weight loss • Delayed menses • Spotting • Breakthrough bleeding

Pharmacologic Contraceptives

Hormonal Contraceptives

Oral contraceptives

Monophasic/High-dose estrogen

Generic	Brand	Dose & Max	Contra-indications	Primary Side Effects	Key Monitoring Parameters	Pertinent Drug Interactions	Med Pearls	Top 200
Ethinyl estradiol/ norgestrel	• Ovral • Ogestrel	50 mcg E. estradiol/0.5 mg norgestrel	• Pregnancy • Breast cancer • History of deep vein thrombosis (DVT) or pulmonary embolism (PE) • Lactation (<6 wks postpartum) • Smoker >35 years of age	• Breast tenderness • Increased breast size • Nausea • Edema • Bloating • Cyclic weight gain • Headaches during active pills • Thrombophlebitis (rare) *Estrogen-excess side effects most common*	• Presence of adverse effects • Pregnancy	• Effect of oral contraceptive pill (OCP): • Antibiotics (ampicillin, sulfonamides, tetracycline) • Anticonvulsants (phenytoin, topiramate, barbiturates) • Protease inhibitors • Rifampin *Need backup method of contraception during use and for at least 1 wk after; for chronic therapy with above medications use another form of contraception*	Take 1 tablet daily at the same time of day for 21 days, followed by 7 days of inactive placebo pills	No
• Ethinyl estradiol/ • Ethynodiol diacetate	• Demulen 1/50 • Zovia 1/50	50 mcg E. estradiol/1 mg E. diacetate						No
Ethinyl estradiol/ norethindrone	Ovcon 50	50 mcg E. estradiol/1 mg norethindrone						No
Mestranol/ norethindrone	• Ortho-Novum 1/50 • Necon 1/50 • Norinyl 1/50	50 mcg mestranol/ 1 mg norethindrone						No

Pharmacologic Contraceptives *(cont'd)*

Generic	Brand	Dose & Max	Contra-indications	Primary Side Effects	Key Monitoring Parameters	Pertinent Drug Interactions	Med Pearls	Top 200
Monophasic/Low-dose estrogen								
Ethinyl estradiol and levonorgestrel	• Alesse • Aviane • Lessina • Levlite	20 mcg E. estradiol, 0.1 mg levonorgestrel	• Pregnancy • Breast cancer • History of DVT or PE • Lactation (<6 wks postpartum) • Smoker >35 years of age	• Nausea • Vomiting • Breakthrough bleeding • Spotting • Melasma • Headache • Weight change • Edema • Venous thromboembolism • Side effects associated with hormonal imbalance (see Table 2) • Presence of adverse effects • Potassium with drospirenone		Effect of OCP: • Antibiotics (ampicillin, sulfonamides, tetracycline) • Anticonvulsants (phenytoin, topiramate, barbiturates) • Protease inhibitors • Rifampin *Need backup method of contraception during use and for at least 1 wk after; for chronic therapy with above medications use another form of contraception*		No
	• Levlen • Levora • Nordette • Portia • Seasonale • Lo Ovral • Low-Ogestrel	30 mcg E. estradiol, 0.15 mg levonorgestrel					Seasonale is taken continuously for 84 days with 7 placebo pills; menses only q3 mo	Yes
Ethinyl estradiol and drospirenone	• Yasmin • Yaz • Beyaz (has added folate) • Safyral (has added folate)	30 mcg E. estradiol, 3 mg drospirenone					Decreased duration of menses	Yes

Pharmacologic Contraceptives *(cont'd)*

Generic	Brand	Dose & Max	Contra-indications	Primary Side Effects	Key Monitoring Parameters	Pertinent Drug Interactions	Med Pearls	Top 200
Ethinyl estradiol and norgestrel	• Apri • Deogen • Ortho-Cept	30 mcg E. estradiol, 0.3 mg norgestrel						Yes
Ethinyl estradiol and norethindrone acetate	• Loestrin 21 1/20 • Loestrin Fe 1/20 • Microgestin Fe 1/20 • Lo Loestrin Fe	10–20 mcg E. estradiol, 1 mg n. acetate						Yes
Ethinyl estradiol and norethindrone	Ovcon 35	35 mcg E. estradiol, 0.4 mg norethindrone						No
	• Brevicon • Modicon • Neocon 0.5/35 • Nortrel 0.5/35	35 mcg E. estradiol, 0.5 mg norethindrone						Yes
	• Necon 1/35 • Norinyl 1/35 • Nortrel 1/35 • Ortho-Novum 1/35	35 mcg E. estradiol, 1 mg norethindrone						Yes
Ethinyl estradiol and desogestrel	Kariva	10–20 mcg E. estradiol, 0.15 mg desogestrel						Yes
	Mircette	10–20 mcg E. estradiol, 0.15 mg desogestrel						No
Ethinyl estradiol and norgestimate	• Ortho cyclen • Sprintec • MonoNessa • Previfem	35 mcg E. estradiol, 0.25 mg norgestimate						Yes

Pharmacologic Contraceptives *(cont'd)*

Generic	Brand	Dose & Max	Contra-indications	Primary Side Effects	Key Monitoring Parameters	Pertinent Drug Interactions	Med Pearls	Top 200
Biphasic								
Ethinyl estradiol and norethindrone	• Ortho-Novum 10/11 • Necon 10/11	35 mcg E. estradiol, 0.5–1 mg norethindrone	• Pregnancy • Breast cancer • History of DVT or PE • Lactation (<6 wks postpartum) • Smoker >35 years of age	• Nausea • Vomiting • Breakthrough bleeding • Spotting • Melasma • Headache • Weight change • Edema • Venous thromboembolism • Side effects associated with hormonal imbalance (see Table 2)	• Presence of adverse effects • Pregnancy	Effect of OCP: • Antibiotic (ampicillin, sulfonamides, tetracycline) • Anticonvulsants (phenytoin, topiramate, barbiturates) • Protease inhibitors • Rifampin *Need backup method of contraception during use and for at least 1 wk after; for chronic therapy with above medications use another form of contraception*	• Created to decrease overall hormone exposure • High incidence of breakthrough bleeding	No
Triphasic								
Ethinyl estradiol and norethindrone	• Tri-Norinyl • Necon 7/7/7 • Ortho-Novum 7/7/7 • Estrostep 21 • Estrostep Fe	35 mcg e. estradiol, 0.5–1 mg norethindrone	• Pregnancy • Breast cancer • History of DVT or PE • Lactation (<6 wks postpartum) • Smoker >35 years of age	• Nausea • Vomiting • Breakthrough bleeding • Spotting • Melasma • Headache • Weight change • Edema • Venous thrombo-embolism • Side effects associated with hormonal imbalance (see Table 2)	• Presence of adverse effects • Pregnancy	Effect of OCP (same as above)	• Many triphasics approved for treatment of acne as well • More difficult to deal with missed pills	Yes
Ethinyl estradiol and desogestrel	Cyclessa						• Decreases overall hormone exposure	No
Ethinyl estradiol and norgestimate	• Trinessa • Ortho-TriCyclen • Orth-TriCyclen Lo							Yes
Ethinyl estradiol and levonorgestrel	• Enpresse • Tri-Levlen • Triphasil • Trivora							Yes

Pharmacologic Contraceptives *(cont'd)*

Generic	Brand	Dose & Max	Contra-indications	Primary Side Effects	Key Monitoring Parameters	Pertinent Drug Interactions	Med Pearls	Top 200
Four-phasic								
Estradiol valerate and dienogest	Natazia	• Days 1–2: 3 mg estradiol valerate • Days 3–7: 2 mg estradiol valerate + 2 mg dienogest • Days 8–24: 2 mg estradiol valerate + 3 mg dienogest • Days 25–26: 1 mg estradiol valerate • Days 27–28: inactive	• Pregnancy • Lactation • Breast cancer • History of DVT or PE • Hepatic disease • Abnormal uterine bleeding • Vascular disease • Hypercoagulopathy			Effect of OCP: • Antibiotics (ampicillin, sulfonamides, tetracycline) • Anticonvulsants (phenytoin, topiramate, barbiturates) • Protease inhibitors • Rifampin *Need backup method of contraception during use and for at least 1 wk after. For chronic therapy with above medications use another form of contraception.*	• Only four-phasic option available • Demonstrated increased efficacy for heavy menstrual bleeding	No
Transdermal								
Ethinyl estradiol and norelgestromin	Ortho Evra	20 mcg E. estradiol and 0.15 mg norelgestromin	• Pregnancy • Breast cancer • History of DVT or PE • Lactation (<6 wks postpartum) • Smoker >35 years of age	• Nausea • Vomiting • Breakthrough bleeding • Spotting • Melasma • Headache • Weight change • Edema • Venous thrombo-embolism • Side effects associated with hormonal imbalance (see Table 2)	• Presence of adverse effects • Pregnancy	Same as OCP	• Safe with usual activities • Do not apply lotion to site of application • Improved compliance over oral	Yes

Pharmacologic Contraceptives *(cont'd)*

Generic	Brand	Dose & Max	Contra-indications	Primary Side Effects	Key Monitoring Parameters	Pertinent Drug Interactions	Med Pearls	Top 200
Other								
Ethinyl estradiol and etonogestrel	NuvaRing	• 0.015 mg E. estradiol and 0.12 mg etonogestrel released daily • Inserted by patient intravaginally q4 wks (active for 3 wks)	Negative pregnancy test needed for initiation	Same as OCP (systemic absorption occurs)	Same as OCP (systemic absorption occurs)	Same as OCP (systemic absorption occurs)	• May be removed before intercourse • Not to be used >4 mos after dispensed	Yes
Progestin-only contraceptives								
Oral								
Norethindrone	• Ortho Micronor • Errin • Nor-QD • Nora-BE • Camila	0.35 mg daily	Negative pregnancy test prior to initiation	• Libido depression • Fatigue • Weight gain • Acne • Hypomenorrhea	Presence of side effects	None	Can be used in breastfeeding women, those >35 who smoke, and those at risk of coronary heart disease (CHD)	No
Norgestrel	Ovrette	0.075 mg daily						No
Parenteral								
Medroxy-progesterone	Depo-Provera	150 mg/mL intramuscular (IM) q12 wks	• Must have negative pregnancy test to start therapy or to continue therapy if >14 wks since last injection • Breast cancer • Liver disease	• Weight gain • Decreased bone mineral density • Acne • Delayed return of fertility after discontinuation	Bone mineral density	None	• Supplement calcium and vitamin D due to potential bone loss • Do not use for >2 years unless unable to use other forms of contraception	Yes

Pharmacologic Contraceptives *(cont'd)*

Generic	Brand	Dose & Max	Contra-indications	Primary Side Effects	Key Monitoring Parameters	Pertinent Drug Interactions	Med Pearls	Top 200
Implantable/intrauterine								
Levonorgestrel	Norplant	• Subdermal implant in upper arm • Replace q3–5 yrs	• History or high risk of pelvic inflammatory disease (PID) or ectopic pregnancy • Breast cancer	• Spotting • Breakthrough bleeding • Amenorrhea • Mastalgia • Headache • Abdominal pain • PID	• Presence of side effects • Pregnancy	None	• Not available as new therapy, but some women may still have • Lasts 3–5 years	No
Levonorgestrel	Mirena	• 20 mcg released daily • Intrauterine	• Abnormal uterine bleeding • High risk for sexually transmitted infections (STIs) (multiple sexual partners) • Uterine or cervical cancer				Remains in place for up to 5 years	No
Progesterone	Progestasert	Intrauterine	• Acute cervicitis or vaginitis • Postpartum endometriosis				Remains in place for 1 year	No
Etonogestrel	Implanon	• 68 mg subdermal implant in upper arm • Replace q3–5 yrs	History or high risk of pelvic inflammatory disease or ectopic pregnancy	• Amenorrhea • Infrequent menses • Weight gain			Not studied in women >130% ideal body weight	No
Nonhormonal								
Copper–T380	ParaGard	Intrauterine placement for up to 10 yrs	History or high risk of PID or ectopic pregnancy	Heavy bleeding, cramping	None	None	Can remain in place for up to 8–10 yrs with efficacy	No

Storage and Administration Pearls

- Store at controlled room temperature 20–25°C (68–77°F) in a dry area, protected from direct light.
- After use, discard NuvaRing away from children or pets.

Patient Education Pearls

- Hormonal contraceptives do not prevent the transmission of STIs
- Efficacy is high with strict adherence to therapy schedule.
- Establish a regular time to take OCP, preferably as a part of daily routine, such as brushing teeth.
- Plan a backup contraceptive method.
- Smoking with OCP poses significant risks and should be avoided.
- Contact physician immediately if any of the following occur:
  - Abdominal pain
  - Chest pain (severe), shortness of breath
  - Headache (severe), dizziness, weakness, or numbness
  - Eye problems (vision loss or blurring), speech problems
  - Severe leg pain (calf or thigh)
- Specific instructions for missed doses:

Doses Missed	Instructions for Patient
1	Take missed dose immediately and next dose at regular time
2 (during first 2 wks)	Take two doses daily for the next 2 days, then resume taking
2 (during third wk)	Sunday start: Take one dose daily until Sunday, dispose of current pack, then begin next pack without placebo pills. Backup method required for 7 days. Other: Dispose of current pack and begin new pack. Backup method required for 7 days.
3 or more	

HORMONE REPLACEMENT THERAPY

Definitions

- Menopause is the cessation of menses after the loss of ovarian follicular activity.
- Perimenopause refers to the period of time immediately prior to menopause and the 1 year following menopause onset.

Diagnosis

Diagnosis is made when amenorrhea occurs for a minimum of 12 consecutive months.

Signs and Symptoms

Symptoms are related primarily to lack of estrogen and include vaginal dryness, vaginal atrophy, hot flushes, and night sweats. Other potential symptoms include arthralgia, depression, migraine, mood swings, myalgia, and insomnia.

Guidelines

Estrogen and progestogen use in peri- and postmenopausal women: March 2007 position statement of the North American Menopause Society. *Menopause*, no. 14 (2) (January 2007): 168–82. www.guideline.gov/summary/summary.aspx?doc_id=10712&nbr=005575&string=hormone+AND+replacement.

Guideline Summary

- All women should undergo careful evaluation prior to initiation of hormone replacement therapy (HRT), including comprehensive history and physical, mammography, and, potentially, bone densitometry.

- The primary indication for HRT is vasomotor symptoms of hot flushes and night sweats.

- Local vaginal therapy is recommended when vaginal symptoms are the only complaint.

- Prevention of osteoporosis with HRT should be considered only for women with a very strong risk of osteoporosis and in whom other available therapies are not options.

- In women who are receiving HRT and who have an intact uterus, progestin is indicated as a means of reducing the risk of endometrial hyperplasia and cancer that exists with unopposed estrogen use in these patients.

- There is insufficient evidence of efficacy and evidence of safety concerns with the prolonged use of HRT. Therefore, at present, HRT is not recommended for use for any of the following indications: Cardiovascular disease, stroke prevention, hyperlipidemia, or dementia prevention.

- The Women's Health Initiative (WHI) indicated increased risks of venous thromboembolism, stroke, coronary disease, and breast cancer in women who receive HRT for an extended period of time.

- The current recommendation is to use HRT at the lowest effective dose for the shortest possible duration.

Hormone Replacement Therapy

Generic	Brand	Dose & Max mg (frequency)	Contraindications	Primary Side Effects	Key Monitoring Parameters	Med Pearls	Top 200
Oral preparations							
Estrogens							
Conjugated estrogens	Premarin	0.3–2.5 mg daily	• Abnormal bleeding • Breast cancer • History of DVT or PE • Pregnancy • Estrogen-dependent tumor • Cardiovascular accident (CVA) or myocardial infarction (MI) in past year • Thromboembolic disease	• Nausea • Fluid retention • Bloating • Headaches • Mood changes • Breast tenderness • Increased risk of venous thromboembolism (VTE), stroke, MI, breast cancer	Presence of side effects (especially vaginal bleeding or symptoms of VTE, stroke, or MI)	• Most studied • No generic equivalent • Should not be abruptly discontinued; taper	Yes
Synthetic conjugated estrogen	Cenestin	0.3–1.25 mg daily				• Longer ha f-life	No
Micronized estradiol	• Estradiol • Estrace • Gynodiol	0.5–2 mg daily				• Most potent hepatic effects • Should not be abruptly discontinued; taper	Yes
Estrone sulfate	• Estropipate • Ortho-Est • Ogen	0.625–5 mg daily					No
Esterified estrogens	• Estratab • Menest	0.3–2.5 mg daily				Should not be abruptly discontinued; taper	No
Progestins							
Medroxyprogesterone	Provera	2–10 mg daily		• Decreased libido • Cramping • Mood changes • Bloating • Nausea • Depression • Headache	Presence of adverse effects		Yes
Micronized progestin	Prometrium	100–200 mg daily				Primary use in patients with adverse effects associated with synthetic estrogens	Yes

Hormone Replacement Therapy *(cont'd)*

Generic	Brand	Dose & Max mg (frequency)	Contraindications	Primary Side Effects	Key Monitoring Parameters	Med Pearls	Top 200
Combination oral preparations							
Conjugated equine estrogens and medroxyprogesterone	Prempro	0.3–0.625 mg estrogen/1.5–2.5 mg progestin	• Abnormal bleeding • Breast cancer • History of DVT or PE • Pregnancy • Estrogen-dependent tumor • CVA or MI in past year • Thromboembolic disease	• Nausea • Fluid retention • Bloating • Headaches • Mood changes • Breast tenderness • Increased risk of VTE • Stroke • MI • Breast cancer	Presence of side effects (especially vaginal bleeding or symptoms of VTE, stroke, or MI)		Yes
Conjugated equine estrogens and medroxyprogesterone	Premphase	0.625 mg/0 mg x14 days then 0.625/5 mg x14 days					No
Estradiol and drospirenone	Angelique	1/0.5 mg					No
Ethinyl estradiol and norethindrone acetate	FemHRT	2.5–5 mcg estrogen/0.5–1.0 mg progestin					No
Estradiol and norethindrone acetate	Activella	0.5–1.0 mcg estrogen/0.1–0.5 mg progestin					No
Estradiol and norgestimate	Prefest	1 mg/0 x15 days then 1/0.09 mg x15 days					No
Transdermal and topical preparations							
17β Estradiol transdermal	• Estraderm • Vivelle • Climara • Alora • Esclim	• 25–50 mcg/24 hours • Applied 1–2x wk	• Abnormal bleeding • Breast cancer • History of DVT or PE • Pregnancy • Estrogen-dependent tumor • CVA or MI in past year • Thromboembolic disease	• Skin irritation • Nausea • Fluid retention • Bloating • Headaches • Mood changes • Breast tenderness • Increased risk of VTE • Stroke • MI • Breast cancer	Presence of side effects (especially vaginal bleeding or symptoms of VTE, stroke, or MI)	• Limited hepatic effects • Useful in patients with GI disturbances • Adverse effects less common in general	Yes
17β Reservoir	Estraderm	0.025–0.1 mg (2x/wk)					No
17β Gel	• Estrogel (q day) • Elestrin (q day) • Divigel (q day)	0.2–1 mg daily					No
17β Topical emulsion	Estrasorb (2 pkt q day)	0.05 mg daily					No
17β Transdermal spray	Evamist (initial: 1 spray q day, may increase to 2–3 sprays/day)	0.021 mg/spray					No

Hormone Replacement Therapy *(cont'd)*

Generic	Brand	Dose & Max mg (frequency)	Contraindications	Primary Side Effects	Key Monitoring Parameters	Med Pearls	Top 200
Vaginal preparations							
Conjugated estrogen cream	Premarin	1.25 mg applied vaginally from 1–2x wkly to daily	• Abnormal bleeding • Breast cancer • History of DVT or PE • Pregnancy • Estrogen-dependent tumor • CVA or MI in past year • Thromboembolic disease	Systemic side effects possible but rare	• Presence of adverse effects • Efficacy	• Use in cases of vaginal symptoms only • Effective for stress incontinence	Yes
Estrone cream	Neo-estrone cream	1 mg/g					No
Estradiol ring	Estring	7.5 mcg/d x 90 days				Long-term use associated with endometrial hyperplasia	No
	Femring	5 mcg/d x 90 days					No
17β Cream	Estrace cream	2–4 g/d x 2–4 wk, 1 g/d x 1–3 wk				• Use in cases of vaginal symptoms only • Effective for stress incontinence	No
Estradiol tablet	Vagifem	2 x 25 mcg/wk					Yes

Drug Interactions

	Interacting Drug(s)	Result
Estrogen	CYP450 3A4 inducers: barbiturates, carbamazepine, rifampin, St. John's wort	↓ Effect of estrogen
	Hydantoins, thyroid hormone, anticoagulants (oral)	↓ Effect of interacting drug
	CYP450 3A4 inhibitors: azole antifungals, macrolide antibiotics, ritonavir, grapefruit juice, atorvastatin	↑ Effect of estrogen
	Corticosteroids, tricyclic antidepressants (potential increased toxicity)	↑ Effect of interacting drug
Progestin	Aminoglutethimide, rifampin	↓ Effect of progestin

Storage and Administration Pearls

- Store at controlled room temperature in a dry location.
- Dispose of patches in a safe place inaccessible to children or pets.

Patient Education Pearls

- Potential risks of HRT should be discussed thoroughly with every patient.
- Adverse effects may be decreased if a low dose is used for a short period of time.
- Contact physician promptly for any of the following: Abnormal vaginal bleeding, abdominal pain or tenderness, speech or visual disturbance, breast lumps, numbness in extremities, severe headache, vomiting, sharp pain in leg or chest, shortness of breath.

ERECTILE DYSFUNCTION

Definition

Erectile dysfunction (ED) is often referred to as impotence and is defined as the inability to achieve a penile erection suitable for sexual intercourse.

Diagnosis

Diagnostic workup of ED includes an assessment of the severity of the dysfunction, a complete history and physical, a review of medications, a physical examination, and selected laboratory tests (serum glucose, lipid profile, thyroid). Each component of the evaluation is used to rule out potential reversible causes of the ED.

Signs and Symptoms

The inability to achieve or maintain an adequate erection is the hallmark symptom; however, symptoms such as depression and anxiety are also commonly associated with ED.

Guidelines

Erectile Dysfunction Guideline Update Panel. The management of erectile dysfunction: an update. Linthicum (MD): American Urologic Association Education and Research, Inc.; 2006 May. www.guideline.gov/summary/summary.aspx?doc_id=10018&nbr=0053 32&string=erectile+AND+dysfunction.

Guidelines Summary

- Initial treatment for most patients will consist of therapy with a phosphodiesterase-5 (PDE5) inhibitor because these agents are known to be efficacious and are minimally invasive.

- PDE5 inhibitors are contraindicated in patients who are currently taking organic nitrates, due to a risk of significant, dangerous hypotension when these agents are used concomitantly.

- If a patient does not respond to therapy with a PDE5 inhibitor, alternate therapy options should be considered, including a different PDE5 inhibitor, alprostadil intra-urethral suppositories, intracavernous injection, vacuum constriction devices, and penile prostheses.

Drugs for Erectile Dysfunction

Mechanism of action – PDE5 inhibitors: enhance the activity of nitric oxide by inhibiting an enzyme (PDE5) responsible for its degradation; enhanced nitric oxide allows relaxed smooth muscles and increased vasodilation and blood flow to the penis following sexual stimulation

Generic	Brand	Dose & Max	Contra-indications	Primary Side Effects	Key Monitoring Parameters	Pertinent Drug Interactions	Med Pearls	Top 200
Oral								
Sildenafil	Viagra	• 25–100 mg as needed (PRN) 0.5–4 hrs prior to sexual activity • Max: 1x daily	• Use with nitrates (continuous or intermittent) • Hypersensitivity • Nitric oxide donors	• Hypotension • Headache • Flushing • Dyspepsia • Priapism (not common)	• Efficacy • Presence of adverse effects • Blood pressure	***Nitrates Combination results in potentially fatal hypotension. Avoid concomitant use within at least 24 hours.*** • Alpha-blockers: Potential significant reduction in blood pressure • Combination should be avoided if possible, or lowest does of each agent used with close monitoring • PDE5 inhibitors are metabolized by CYP450 3A4; therefore, inhibitors and inducers of this enzyme will affect PDE5 inhibitor levels accordingly	Erection occurs only after physical and psychological stimulation	Yes
Tadalafil	Cialis	2.5–20 mg PRN prior to sexual activity; or 2.5–5 mg PO 1x daily						Yes
Vardenafil	Levitra Staxyn (orally disintegrating tablet)	2.5–20 mg PRN ~ 1 hr prior to sexual activity						Yes
Topical								
Testosterone transdermal patch	• Testoderm • Testoderm-TTS • Androderm	2.6–6 mg patch applied daily	• Hypersensitivity • Carcinoma of the breast or prostate	• Elevated liver enzymes • Hyperlipidemia • Depression • Aggression	• Periodic liver function • Prostate-specific antigen (PSA) • Lipid panels	Increases the effects of anticoagulants and cyclosporine	Only useful in ED due to hypogonadism	No
Testosterone gel	AndroGel 1%	5–10 g daily applied to shoulders, upper arm, or abdomen						Yes

Drugs for Erectile Dysfunction *(cont'd)*

Generic	Brand	Dose & Max	Contra-indications	Primary Side Effects	Key Monitoring Parameters	Pertinent Drug Interactions	Med Pearls	Top 200
Intramuscular								
Testosterone	• Depo-testosterone (cypionate) • Delatestryl (enanthate)	200–400 mg q2–4 wks	• Hypersensitivity • Carcinoma of the breast or prostate	• Elevated liver enzymes • Hyperlipidemia • Depression • Aggression	• Periodic liver function • PSA • Lipid panels	Increases the effects of anticoagulants and cyclosporine	Only useful in ED due to hypogonadism	Yes
Intraurethral								
Alprostadil	Muse	125–1,000 mcg pellets 5–10 min before intercourse	• Hypersensitivity • Urethral stricture • Chronic urethritis	• Urethral pain • Burning • Priapism • Hypotension	• Presence of adverse effects • Efficacy • Blood pressure periodically	None	Duration of effect is 30–60 min	No
Intracavernosal								
Alprostadil	• Caverject • Edex	1–40 mcg 5–20 min before intercourse injected intracavernosal	• Hypersensitivity • Sickle-cell trait • Multiple myeloma • Leukemia	• Pain at injection site • Erythema • Priapism • Hypotension	• Presence of adverse effects • Efficacy • Blood pressure periodically	None	Self-injection training should be done in physician's office	No

Storage and Administration Pearls

- Sildenafil should be taken at least 30 minutes prior to sexual activity and can be taken, at earliest, 4 hours prior.
- Vardenafil should be taken approximately 1 hour prior to anticipated activity.
- Tadalafil can either be taken prior to activity or as a scheduled daily dose.
- Alprostadil intraurethral: Store unopened foil pouches in a refrigerator at 2–8°C (36–46°F). Do not expose alprostadil urethral suppository to temperatures above 30°C (86°F). Alprostadil urethral suppository may be kept at room temperature (below 30°C [86°F]) for up to 14 days prior to use.
- Alprostadil intracavernosal: Prepare the solution immediately before use. Do not administer unless solution is clear. Do not add any drugs or other solutions to this solution. Discard any unused solution remaining in the cartridge.

Patient Education Pearls

- Testoderm is applied to the scrotum, whereas Testoderm TTS is applied to the arm, back, abdomen, or thigh.
- Testosterone gel is applied to shoulders, arms, or abdomen.
- Males using testosterone products should not allow direct contact between the testosterone product and a pregnant female, as teratogenic effects are possible.

URINARY INCONTINENCE

Definitions

This is a condition associated with the involuntary loss of urine. There are multiple subtypes of urinary incontinence differentiated by etiology. The major classifications are: (1) urethral underactivity (stress incontinence), (2) bladder overactivity (urge incontinence), and (3) urethral overactivity/bladder underactivity (overflow incontinence).

Diagnosis

Diagnosis is based primarily on patient complaints and a thorough history and physical.

Signs and Symptoms

Symptoms of stress incontinence include the loss of small amounts of urine during activities such as sneezing, coughing, laughing, or running. Symptoms of urge incontinence include urinary urgency and frequency that may be associated with the loss of large or small amounts of urine. Overflow incontinence is associated with the loss of a large amount of urine which may be accompanied by symptoms of frequency, nocturia, hesitancy, or weak urinary stream.

Guidelines

Because a nationally recognized guideline for the treatment of urinary incontinence does not currently exist, the following represents general recommendations for treatment of the various subtypes based on multiple primary and tertiary resources.

Summary of Treatment Recommendations

- General
  - Nonpharmacological therapy is important as either monotherapy or an adjunct to pharmacotherapy. Options such as Kegel exercises and scheduled voiding are common.
- Stress incontinence
  - Options for treatment include topical estrogen, alpha agonists, and tricyclic antidepressants. Alpha agonists carry the risk of elevating blood pressure and heart rate, and will be used only with caution in patients with pre-existing hypertension or heart conditions.
- Urge incontinence
  - Options for the treatment of urge incontinence include anticholinergic medications and imipramine.
- Overflow incontinence
  - Treatment options are varied based upon the determined etiology. Since many cases of overflow incontinence are secondary to benign prostatic hyperplasia (BPH), the treatment of choice includes either an alpha antagonist (terazosin, prazosin, doxazosin), a selective alpha 1A antagonist (tamsulosin, alfuzosin, silodosin), or a 5α reductase inhibitor (finasteride or dutasteride).
  - Alpha antagonists are the agents of choice in most cases of BPH. The use of a selective agent is most commonly indicated in patients who experience orthostatic hypotension with the nonselective agents. 5α Reductase inhibitors are reserved for patients with significantly enlarged prostates (50–60 g).

Drugs for Urinary Incontinence

Generic	Brand	Dose & Max	Contra-indications	Primary Side Effects	Key Monitoring Parameters	Pertinent Drug Interactions	Med Pearls	Top 200
Topical vaginal estrogen preparations: used in the treatment of stress incontinence (first-line) and urge incontinence (third-line); see HRT drug chart above for more detailed information								
Tricyclic antidepressants: imipramine and desipramine are the most commonly used in incontinence; used primarily in urge incontinence and stress incontinence; see drug charts in psychiatric disorders chapter for detailed information								
Anticholinergic agents								
• Oxybutynin • Syrup	Ditropan	2.5–5 mg PO TID–QID	• Urinary retention • Gastric retention • Narrow-angle glaucoma	• Dry mouth • Dry eyes • Constipation • Urinary retention • Somnolence • Blurred vision • Increased intra-ocular pressure	Presence of adverse effects	Additive effects with other anticholinergic medications	Side effects less common with extended-release version and transdermal	Yes
• Extended-release	Ditropan XL	5–30 mg PO daily						
• Transdermal	Oxytrol	3.9 mg/day apply 2x/wk						
Tolterodine Extended-release	Detrol	1–2 mg PO daily					Side effects less common with extended-release	Yes
	Detrol LA	2–4 mg PO 1x/day						
Darifenacin	Enablex	7.5–15 mg PO daily				• CYP450 3A4 inhibitors increase levels • Additive effects with other anticholinergic medications	Do not exceed 7.5 mg daily in combo with enzyme inhibitors	Yes
Solifenacin	Vesicare	5–10 mg PO daily						Yes
Fesoterodine	Toviaz	4–8 mg once daily				• CYP3A4 inhibitors increase levels • Doses above 4 mg not recommended concomitantly	• Dose adjusted for CrCl < 30 mL/min • Max dose of 4 mg daily with CYP3A4 inhibitors	No
Alpha agonists								
Pseudoephedrine	Sudafed, many	• 30–60 mg PO q4–6 hours PRN • Max: 240 mg/24 hrs	• MAOI therapy • Hypersensitivity • Uncontrolled hypertension (HTN)	• Increased blood pressure • Increased heart rate • Increased blood sugar • Irritability • Insomnia	• Blood pressure and heart rate periodically • Blood sugar if diabetic	MAO inhibitors	• Increases blood pressure and heart rate • Use with caution in HTN or pre-existing cardiac conditions	No
Phenylephrine	Many	10–20 mg q4 hrs PRN						No

Drugs for Urinary Incontinence *(cont'd)*

Generic	Brand	Dose & Max	Contra-indications	Primary Side Effects	Key Monitoring Parameters	Pertinent Drug Interactions	Med Pearls	Top 200
Alpha antagonists								
Doxazosin	Cardura	1–8 mg PO daily at bed time (HS)	Hypersensitivity	• Hypotension • Orthostasis • Syncope • Dizziness	• Blood pressure (BP) • Presence of orthostasis • Efficacy	• Phosphodiesterase inhibitors: combination may result in dangerous hypotension • Additive BP lowering with other antihypertensives	Dosed at HS to prevent dizziness/falls during the day	Yes
Terazosin	Hytrin	1–10 mg PO daily (HS)						Yes
Prazosin	Minipress	2–10 mg daily PO (BID–TID)					Not used often due to need for multiple daily dosing	No
Selective Alpha 1A antagonists								
Tamsulosin	Flomax	0.4 mg 1x daily	Hypersensitivity	Headache, dizziness, orthostasis	• Presence of side effects • Efficacy • Periodic BP	Cimetidine increases tamsulosin levels	Expensive relative to nonselective agents	Yes
Alfuzosin	Uroxatral	10 mg PO daily	• Hypersensitivity • Moderate to severe hepatic disease	• Dizziness • Fatigue • Headache • Potential for hypotension (rare)	• Presence of side effects • Efficacy • Periodic BP	Levels with CYP3A4 inhibitors: ketoconazole, itraconazole, and ritonavir	• Hepatically eliminated • Tablets are extended-release; do not crush or chew	Yes
Silodosin	Rapaflo	4–8 mg PO daily	• Severe renal impairment (CrCl < 30 mL/min) • Severe hepatic impairment (Child-Pugh ≥10) • Concomitant administration with CYP3A4 inhibitors	• Postural hypotension • Retrograde ejaculation • Dizziness • Diarrhea • Headache	• Response to treatment • BP	• CYP3A4 inhibitors (ketoconazole, itraconazole, clarithromycin, ritonavir) increase plasma silodosin levels • Concomitant use with PDE5 inhibitors can cause significant hypotension	• Renal dose adjustment required • Inform ophthalmologist prior to eye surgery due to risk of intraoperative floppy iris syndrome	No
5α Reductase Inhibitors								
Finasteride	Proscar	5 mg PO daily	• Female sex • Hypersensitivity	• Decreased libido • Erectile dysfunction • Gynecomastia	• Obtain PSA prior to therapy initiation • Agents can decrease PSA, thereby decreasing utility to detect cancer	None	• Should not be handled by pregnant women—teratogenic potential	Yes
Dutasteride	Avodart	0.5 mg PO daily	• Female sex • Hypersensitivity			• Metabolized by CYP450 3A4 • Unknown but suspected interactions with potent inhibitors and inducers	• Onset of effect can be up to 6 mos	Yes

Storage and Administration Pearls

- Store all medications at room temperature and out of the reach of children.
- Alpha-blockers should be taken at bedtime to avoid side effects of syncope and orthostasis while awake.

Patient Education Pearls

- If receiving an alpha-blocker, rise slowly from seated position to avoid potential dizziness associated with the medication.
- If receiving an alpha reductase inhibitor, know that reaching full benefit of this medication may take up to 6 months. An adequate trial should be allowed.
- Anticholinergic medications may make patient drowsy and experience dry mouth, dry eyes, blurred vision, or constipation.

LEARNING POINTS

- Oral contraceptives are highly effective when taken appropriately. Pharmacists should be able to educate patients on potential adverse effects, appropriate administration, and missed-dose instructions.
- Many varieties of contraception exist. It is important to identify adverse effects related to estrogen and progestin components in order to determine the most appropriate therapy change if a patient experiences adverse effects.
- Postmenopausal HRT is primarily indicated in patients with vasomotor symptoms. Because of results from large clinical trials, HRT is not indicated for the prevention of heart disease, for dementia, or as first-line therapy for osteoporosis.
- Progestin therapy should be used in patients who are on HRT and have an intact uterus.
- Although multiple therapies exist for the treatment of ED, phosphodiesterase inhibitors are the most commonly used agents. PDE5 inhibitors have significant drug interactions with nitrates and alpha-blockers.
- There are several subtypes of urinary incontinence, and therapy should be individualized on the basis of the identified etiology. Anticholinergic agents are among the most commonly used and may result in unpleasant side effects of dry mouth, dry eyes, constipation, and somnolence.

PRACTICE QUESTIONS

1. Which of the following is most accurate regarding the coadministration of sildenafil and nitroglycerin?

   (A) There is no drug interaction between the two medications.
   (B) There is a minor drug interaction between the two medications. The patient should be counseled to monitor for signs and symptoms of the interaction.
   (C) There is a major drug interaction between these two agents, but they can be safely coadministered as long as doses are separated by at least 1 hour
   (D) There is a major drug interaction between sildenafil and some forms of nitroglycerin. The specific formulation of nitroglycerin should be determined before the medications are taken.
   (E) There is a major, potentially life-threatening drug interaction between the two agents. Coadministration should be strictly avoided.

2. Which of the following is a progestin-only contraceptive?

   I. Ovcon-50
   II. NuvaRing
   III. Ovrette

   (A) I only
   (B) III only
   (C) I and II only
   (D) II and III only
   (E) I, II, III

3. In which of the following clinical scenarios would hormone replacement therapy be contraindicated?

   (A) Breast cancer
   (B) Obesity
   (C) Stage III chronic kidney disease
   (D) Diabetes mellitus
   (E) History of hysterectomy

4. Which of the following is the correct trade name for tadalafil?

   (A) Viagra
   (B) Levitra
   (C) Cialis
   (D) Caverject
   (E) Proscar

ANSWERS

1. **E**

There is a major, life-threatening drug interaction between these two medications. When coadministered, the two agents can result in a life-threatening drop in blood pressure. All forms of nitroglycerin carry this risk, and coadministration should be avoided for *at least* 24 hours.

2. **B**

Ovrette is a progestin-only oral contraceptive. Ovcon is a high-dose estrogen combination oral contraceptive. NuvaRing is a vaginal system with both estrogen and progestin components.

3. **A**

Hormone replacement therapy is contraindicated in patients with breast cancer due to the potential to exacerbate tumor growth. Obesity, kidney disease, and diabetes are not contraindications to hormone replacement therapy. Patients with a history of hysterectomy may take unopposed estrogen but do not need progestin.

4. **C**

Cialis is the trade name for tadalafil. Viagra is the trade name for sildenafil, Levitra is the trade name for vardenafil, Caverject is the trade name for alprostadil, and Proscar is the trade name for finasteride.

Clinical Lab Tests

16

 Suggested Study Time: **15 minutes**

Clinical lab tests are very important to pharmacists in that they are commonly used to measure the safety and efficacy of medications. It is imperative that a pharmacist have a working knowledge of the most commonly used clinical lab tests in order to be able to recommend testing when necessary, and to interpret the results obtained. Education of the patient regarding clinical lab tests may also be a role of the pharmacist in some instances.

ELECTROLYTES AND MINERALS

Among the most common laboratory tests, electrolyte concentrations are used to detect and assess many medical conditions and are measured most commonly as part of a basic metabolic panel, or chem 7.

Substance	Normal Reference Range	Most Common Uses/Comments
Sodium	136–145 mEq/L	• May detect hypo- or hypernatremia • Used to monitor serum osmolality to determine total body water balance
Potassium	3.5–5.0 mEq/L	• May detect hypo- or hyperkalemia • Used primarily to monitor safety of medications and renal function
Chloride	96–106 mEq/L	• May detect hypo- or hyperchloremia • Used in evaluation of acid-based balance and to monitor for safety of medications
Magnesium	1.5–2.2 mEq/L	• May detect hypo- or hypermagnesemia
Calcium	8.5–10.8 mg/dL	• May detect hypo- or hypercalcemia • Used to monitor renal osteodystrophy • Requires correction with serum albumin <4 g/dL
Phosphate	2.6–4.5 mg/dL	• May detect hypo- or hyperphosphatemia • Monitored along with calcium for renal osteodystrophy

RENAL

The kidneys are the body's major filter of toxins. Thus, the renal system plays a large role in the maintenance of physiological homeostasis. The kidneys also serve the role of producing and activating substances that have an impact on red blood cell production, blood pressure regulation, and mineral metabolism.

The following represent the most commonly used lab assays for evaluation of renal function. Urinary sodium, potassium, and chloride as well as hematologic assays and electrolytes may also be used in the assessment.

Substance	Normal Reference Range	Comments
Serum creatinine (SCr)	0.7–1.4 mg/dL	• Excretion of creatinine closely estimates the glomerular filtration rate (GFR) • Elevated serum creatinine is indicative of decreased GFR • Serum creatinine is used in the Cockroft-Gault equation to calculate CrCl • May be inaccurate in the very elderly due to decreased muscle mass
Creatinine clearance (CrCl)	90–140 mL/min	• Estimate of GFR • Can be measured over 24 hours or calculated using serum creatinine and ideal body weight
Blood urea nitrogen (BUN)	8–20 mg/dL	• Used along with other labs to monitor hydration, renal function, protein tolerance, catabolism • Most commonly used in BUN:SCr ratio to determine hydration status and renal function
BUN:SCr	1:1–20:1	• >20:1 indicates dehydration in most patients
Urine microalbumin	<30 mg:g creatinine	• Microscopic protein that escapes into the urine when significant glomerular injury is present • Most commonly used to identify nephropathy in patients with diabetes

HEPATIC

The functions of the liver are numerous and varied. Some of the primary functions include the synthesis of bilirubin, coagulation factors, and albumin; amino acid and carbohydrate metabolism; and cholesterol synthesis. Along with these activities, the liver is also the primary site of metabolism for the majority of drugs and hormones. Hepatic assays are important in assessing the overall liver function and also in monitoring the safety of many medications.

The following represent the most commonly used lab assays for the assessment of hepatic function. Viral antigens and antibodies are not reviewed in this chapter.

Substance	Normal Reference Range	Comments
Albumin	3.5–5 g/dL	• Reflects liver's synthetic ability, nutritional status, and hydration; if low, should be factored into serum drug concentrations of highly protein bound drugs such as phenytoin
Total protein	5.5–8.3 g/dL	• Represents estimated sum of albumin and globulin measurements
Prothrombin time (PT)	10–13 seconds	• Represents the time needed for a series of events in coagulation cascade to occur • Helps to determine synthetic ability of liver; if elevated, indicates potential decreased production of clotting factors
Alkaline phosphatase (ALP)	Varies with assay used	• Used to detect hepatocellular injury but is not specific, so should be combined with other tests
Aspartate aminotransferase (AST)	8–42 IU/L	• Aminotransferases are the most frequently used assays in monitoring hepatic disease and are sensitive indicators of hepatic injury • Elevations indicate injury • Used often to monitor potential hepatic damage of medications
Alanine aminotransferase (ALT)	3–30 IU/L	
Total bilirubin	0.3–1 mg/dL	• Elevations may indicate hepatocellular injury, but test is not sensitive
Ammonia	30–70 mcg/dL	• Elevations indicate an inability of the liver to remove ammonia from the blood • Used to identify hepatic encephalopathy
Amylase	44–128 IU/L	• Most commonly used to diagnose acute pancreatitis
Lipase	<1.5 U/mL	• Most commonly used in the late diagnosis of acute pancreatitis (3–4 days postonset)

ENDOCRINE

Disorders of the endocrine system most commonly result from the deficiency or excess of a hormone. These hormones act as regulators within the body by stimulating or inhibiting biological responses. The most common endocrine disorder is diabetes mellitus (DM), which is discussed in detail in a previous chapter. Thyroid disorders are also common.

The assays listed below represent the most commonly used measurements to monitor diabetes and thyroid disorders, and the medications used to treat these disease states.

Substance	Normal Reference Range	Comments
Fasting plasma glucose (FPG)	70–100 mg/dL	• Most commonly used assay for diagnosis of DM; must be repeated on another day to confirm diagnosis • Patients may also self-monitor this value • Used for disease-state monitoring and adjustment of medication
2-Hour postprandial glucose	100–140 mg/dL	• May be measured as part of an oral glucose tolerance test (OGTT) or by the patient at home • Used for disease-state monitoring and adjustment of medication
A1c	4–6%	• Represents blood sugar over an approximate 90-day time frame • Most common lab test to monitor glycemic control in DM • May be inaccurate in cases of severe anemia • Not used in diagnosis of DM • Although 4–6% is normal range, <6.5–7% is the goal for a patient with DM • A1c correlation to plasma glucose:
Free thyroxine (T4)	0.8–1.5 ng/dL	• Measures unbound T4 and is the most accurate representation of thyroid activity
Thyroid-stimulating hormone (TSH)	0.25–6.7 mcU/mL	• Low levels indicate hyperthyroid state; high levels indicate hypothyroid state • Used to monitor thyroid supplementation and need for dose adjustments

A1c%	Mean Plasma Glucose (mg/dL)
6	135
7	170
8	205
9	240
10	275
11	310
12	345

CARDIOLOGY

Laboratory tests are used both to detect and to monitor cardiac disorders. Because cardiovascular disease is the leading cause of death, it is imperative that pharmacists have a working knowledge of the markers used to evaluate these conditions.

The following measurements represent the most commonly used lab assays to detect acute cardiac conditions and to monitor chronic cardiac risk.

Substance	Normal Reference Range	Comments
Total cholesterol	<200 mg/dL	• Does not require that the patient fast but is most commonly measured as part of a complete fasting lipid panel • Not as useful as LDL and HDL in determining cardiovascular risk
Low-density lipoproteins (LDL)	Patient dependent-goals <160 mg/dL	• Highly atherogenic, known as "bad" cholesterol, used as the primary marker of cardiovascular risk • Higher values correlate with higher risk • Most often calculated rather than measured: LDL = Total cholesterol − HDL − Trigs/5 • Calculation inaccurate if triglycerides >400 mg/dL
High-density lipoproteins (HDL)	>40 mg/dL	• Antiatherogenic lipoprotein known as "good" cholesterol • Higher values associated with decreased cardiovascular risk
Triglycerides (Trigs)	<150 mg/dL	• High levels associated with cardiovascular risk • Very high levels associated with increased risk of pancreatitis
Troponin I	<1.5 ng/mL	• Elevated levels used to diagnose acute myocardial infarction (MI) • Elevation seen within 3–12 hrs and remain elevated for 5–10 days (I) or 5–14 days (T)
Troponin T	<0.1 ng/mL	
Creatine kinase–MB (CK–MB)	<12 IU/L	• Used to diagnose acute MI • Specific for cardiac tissue • Rises 3–12 hrs after onset and stays elevated for 2–3 days
B-type natriuretic peptide (BNP)	<100 pg/mL	• Secreted in response to cardiac stretching • Used to monitor heart failure
C-reactive protein (CRP)	≤1 mg/L	• Plasma protein synthesized by the liver • Biomarker of inflammation and cardiovascular risk
International normalized ratio (INR)	1.0	• Measure of coagulability • Goal is patient-dependent

HEMATOLOGY

The complete blood count (CBC) is among the most commonly ordered lab tests. The indices described below make up the CBC and are used to detect and monitor anemias and other hematologic disorders.

Indices	Normal Reference Range	Comments
Red blood cells (RBCs)	Males: 4.5–5.9 x 10^{12} cells/L Females: 4.1–5.1 x 10^{12} cells/L	• May be elevated in smokers
Hemoglobin (Hgb)	Males: 14–17.5 g/dL Females: 12.6–15.3 g/dL	• Indicates oxygen-carrying capacity of blood
Hematocrit (HCT)	Males: 42–50% Females: 36–45%	• Percentage of blood made up by erythrocytes; approximately 3 times Hgb
Mean cell volume (MCV)	80–96 fL/cell	• Hematocrit/RBC • Decreased in iron deficiency • Increased in vitamin B12 and folate deficiency
Mean cell hemoglobin concentration (MCHC)	33.4–35.5 g/dL	• Hgb/HCT • Decreased in iron deficiency
Reticulocyte count	0.5–2.5% of RBCs	• Reticulocytes are immature erythrocytes • Increased in blood loss (acute) • Decreased in iron deficiency and B12 and folate deficiency
RBC distribution width (RDW)	11.5–14.5%	• Variation in RBCs • Increased in iron deficiency
White blood cells (WBCs)	4.4–11 cells/mcL	• Made up of granulocytes and lymphocytes • Elevated in infection
Platelet count	150,000–450,000/mcL	• Important measure of coagulation

THERAPEUTIC DRUG LEVELS

Medications with narrow therapeutic indices and those with established therapeutic and/or toxic serum concentrations often require therapeutic drug monitoring. In general, serum concentrations are best obtained once the medication has reached steady state (in most cases a minimum of 5 elimination half-lives), just prior to an administered dose unless otherwise specified.

Drug	Therapeutic Concentration
Aminoglycosides: gentamicin, tobramycin, netilmicin	5–10 mcg/mL (peak) – efficacy <2–3 mcg/mL (trough) safety
Aminoglycosides: amikacin	15–30 mcg/mL (peak) – efficacy <10 mcg/mL (trough) – safety
Vancomycin	5–10 mcg/mL (trough) – efficacy 20–40 mcg/mL (peak) – safety
Digoxin	0.5–1.5 ng/mL (inotropic effects) 0.8–2.0 ng/mL (chronotropic effects)
Lidocaine	1.5–5 mcg/mL
Phenytoin	10–20 mcg/mL Must be corrected for hypoalbuminemia (Corrected phenytoin concentration = measured total concentration/[0.2*albumin] + 0.1)
Carbamazepine	4–12 mcg/mL
Valproic acid	50–100 mcg/mL
Phenobarbital/primidone	15–40 mcg/mL
Ethosuximide	40–100 mcg/mL
Cyclosporine	150–400 ng/mL
Lithium	0.6–1.4 mEq/L
Theophylline	10–20 mcg/mL

PRACTICE QUESTIONS

1. Which of the following lab tests is NOT used to monitor hepatic function?

    (A) Total protein
    (B) Ammonia
    (C) Prothrombin time
    (D) Alkaline phosphatase
    (E) Microalbumin

ANSWERS

1. **E**

There are many tests used for the assessment of hepatic function. Total protein (A) represents the estimated sum of albumin and globulin that are produced by the liver. Ammonia (B) is removed from the blood by the liver, and elevations indicate the liver is not able to remove it. The prothrombin time (C) helps determine the liver's ability to make clotting factors under normal circumstances (without anticoagulant therapy). Alkaline phosphatase (D) is used to detect hepatocellular injury and is often combined with AST/ALT. Microalbumin (E) is actually a test of the kidneys and is elevated when glomerular injury is present. Therefore, (E) is correct.

Over-the-Counter Medications

17

This chapter covers the following drug classes:

- **Top 10 herbals and supplements**
- **Decongestants**
- **Antihistamines and proton pump inhibitors**
- **Cough suppressants**
- **Antidiarrheals**
- **Constipation medications**
- **Athlete's foot medications**

The text also provides an overview of basic treatment for common ailments treatable by pharmacists. This chapter also makes recommendations as to when self-treatment is not appropriate.

 Suggested Study Time: **75 minutes**

TOP 10 HERBALS AND SUPPLEMENTS

Definitions

As they are being interviewed, asking patients about herbals and supplements is an important assessment measure. Data suggest that 1 in every 5 adults in the United States reports having used a natural product at least once in the previous 12 months.

The Dietary Supplement Health and Education Act of 1994 categorizes herbals, vitamins, protein bars, and shakes as dietary supplements. As a result, manufacturers are not required to demonstrate safety, purity, or efficacy of supplements. Labeling must include the FDA statement: "This statement has not been evaluated by the Food and

Drug Administration. This product is not intended to diagnose, treat, cure, or prevent any disease." Manufacturers cannot make specific claims on labels. The use of phrases such as "helps boost, support, enhance" are acceptable, though they essentially mislead the public and generate the need for healthcare assistance. It is important that you recommend only products that have undergone a standardization assurance.

Common Usage

- Saw palmetto
  - Used in men to improve symptoms of benign prostatic hyperplasia (BPH)
  - Effects of saw palmetto are comparable to symptomatic improvements
- Glucosamine and chondroitin
  - Used widely for treating osteoarthritis and joint structure support
  - Glucosamine: A precursor molecule important for maintaining elasticity, strength, and resiliency of the cartilage in articular (movable) joints
- Fish oils or omega-3 fatty acids
  - Used primarily for hypertriglyceridemia
  - Contain eicosapentaenoic acid (EPA) and docosahexaenoic acid (DHA), and are believed to be efficient in many people
- St. John's wort
  - Used for mild to moderate depression
  - Used in Europe for centuries for mild to moderate depression and its efficacy is comparable with tricyclic antidepressants; one study suggests it is no more effective than a placebo or sertraline in moderate to severe depression; it should not be used with other selective serotonin reuptake inhibitors (SSRIs).
- CoEnzyme Q10
  - Used for cardiovascular diseases, including angina, heart failure, and hypertension, and may help with myalgias due to statin therapy
- Melatonin
  - Used for insomnia, particularly when adjusting to shift-work cycles or jet lag
  - Naturally secreted from the pineal gland and appears to be the sleep-regulating hormone of the body; adults experience about a 37% decline in daily melatonin output between 20 and 70 years of age
- Echinacea
  - Used as an immune stimulant
  - Has been studied extensively in the area of flu and cold prevention/treatment
- Black cohosh
  - Used for women's health problems, especially postmenopausal symptom relief and painful menses

- Ginger
  - Used primarily for motion sickness, dyspepsia, and nausea
  - Lacks sedative affects of other antinausea treatments
  - Has been studied in pregnant women at less than 17 weeks' gestation
- Ginkgo biloba
  - Used for vascular dementia, Alzheimer's, and ischemic stroke
  - The ginkgolides are potent platelet-activating factor (PAF) antagonists
- Ginseng
  - Used to treat diabetes mellitus
  - Thought to also help with decreasing mental and physical stress

Over-the-Counter Medications

Generic	Brand	Dose & Max mg (frequency)	Contra-indications	Primary Side Effects	Key Monitoring Parameters	Pertinent Drug Interactions	Med Pearls
Mechanism of action – inhibits production of dihydrotestosterone (DHT), inhibits receptor binding, and accelerates the metabolism of DHT							
Serenoa repens	Saw palmetto	Prostate: 160 mg BID	Pregnancy or lactation	Transient nausea, vomiting, and gastrointestinal (GI) distress	Improvements in BPH symptoms	• Oral contraception • Estrogens • Finasteride and dutasteride • Warfarin	• Standardized to contain at least 80–90% fatty acid and sterol per dose • Decreases prostate size, but does not alter prostate-specific antigen (PSA) levels
Mechanism of action – glucosamine is an amino-sugar that is naturally produced and is a key substrate in the synthesis of macromolecules for connective tissues; chondroitin absorbs water, adding to cartilage thickness, and is found in natural physiologic connective tissue; inhibits synovial enzymes that may contribute to cartilage destruction							
Glucosamine/ chondroitin	Osteo Bi-Flex	• Gluc: 500 mg TID • Chon: 400 mg TID	• Gluc: allergy to shellfish • Chon: Hx of bleeding	• GI discomfort • Increased glucose • Increased bleeding time	• Arthritis pain • Glucose • Aspirin • Warfarin	Gluc: insulin and oral diabetes medications	Chon: discontinue 14 days before dental procedure
Omega-3 fatty acids	Fish Oils	Triglycerides 500–3,000 mg/day	• Active bleeding • Hx of anticoagulants	• GI upset • Loose stools • Nausea • Decrease glucose • Lower blood pressure	• Hypoglycemia • Blood pressure	• Warfarin • Aspirin • Antiplatelet agents	Mainly for treatment of triglycerides
Mechanism of action – increases concentrations of serotonin in the central nervous system (CNS) and may have some monoamine oxidase (MAO) inhibition affects							
Hypericum perforatum	St. John's wort	300 mg TID	• Pregnancy • Severe depression • MAOI contraindications	Nausea and vomiting	• Depression symptoms • International normalized ratio (INR) if on warfarin	• CYP450 3A4 inhibitor • Cyclosporine, azoles, statins • Digoxin, lithium, thyroid meds, anything that affects serotonin	• Standardized to contain 0.3–0.5% hypericin • Min of 4–6 wks of therapy is recommended before results seen
Mechanism of action – involved in adenosine triphosphate (ATP) generation and serves as a lipid-soluble antioxidant providing protection against free-radical damage within the mitochondria							
Ubiquinone	CoEnzyme Q10	20–300 mg/day	• Concurrent use with doxorubicin	Abdominal discomfort, headache, nausea, and vomiting	Bleeding time	Warfarin	

Over-the-Counter Medications *(cont'd)*

Generic	Brand	Dose & Max mg (frequency)	Contra-indications	Primary Side Effects	Key Monitoring Parameters	Primary Side Effects	Pertinent Drug Interactions	MedPearls
Mechanism of action—supplements the naturally deficient concentrations of melatonin								
N-acetyl-5-methoxy-tryptamine	Melatonin	1–5 mg at bedtime (HS)	Caution with warfarin	Morning sedation or drowsiness	INR with warfarin use		• CYP450 1A2 inhibitor • Theophylline • Caffeine • Clozapine 2⊝ • Warfarin	Drugs that deplete vitamin B6 may inhibit the ability of the body to synthesize melatonin
Mechanism of action — may stimulate white blood cell function, including cell-mediated immunity								
Echinacea purpurea/angustifolia/pallida	Echinacea	50–1,000 mg TID on day 1, then 250 mg QID	• Use for more than 10 days in acute infections • Immunosuppressed patients • Pregnancy		• Electrolytes • Improvements in symptoms		• CYP450 3A4 inhibitor • Cyclosporine • Tacrolimus, sirolimus • Methotrexate • Corticosteroids	• Standardized to contain 4% echinacosides or esters • Prophylaxis therapy should be 3 wks on, 1 wk off
Mechanism of action — contains phytoestrogens, which mimic estrogen								
Cimicifuga racemosa	Black cohosh	20–40 mg BID	• Hx of estrogen-dependent tumors • Endometrial cancer • Pregnancy		• Blood pressure • Serum hormones at baseline and 6 mos	• Nausea, vomiting • Hypotension • Headaches	• Oral contraceptives • Hormone replacement therapy (HRT) • Nonsteroidal anti-inflammatory drugs (NSAIDs) • anticoagulants	Standardized to 1 mg triterpene glycosides, calculated as 27-deoxyactein per dose
Mechanism of action — has local affects at the GI tract and in the CNS								
Zingiber officinale	Ginger	250 mg TID with food	Active bleeding		Increased bleeding time	Very few side effects	• Warfarin • Aspirin	Standardized to contain 4% volatile oils or 3% total pungent compounds

Over-the-Counter Medications *(cont'd)*

Generic	Brand	Dose & Max mg (frequency)	Contra-indications	Primary Side Effects	Key Monitoring Parameters	Pertinent Drug Interactions	Med Pearls
Mechanism of action – the flavonoid component of gingko protects neurons and retinal tissue from oxidative stress and injury							
Ginkgo biloba	Ginkgo biloba	120–240 mg/day divided into 2–3 doses	• Pregnancy • Bleeding disorders • Seizures • 2 weeks prior to surgery	• GI effects • Headache • Dizziness • Skin reactions • Bleeding	• INR • Blood glucose	• Anticoagulants • Trazodone • NSAIDs • Anticonvulsants	Products should contain 24% ginkgo flavone glycosides and 6% terpenoids and be free of ginkgolic acid
Mechanism of action – thought to reduce postprandial glucose levels and stimulate the release of insulin							
Panax quinquefolius	Ginseng	• Usual: 100–400 mg/day • Diabetics: up to 3 g/day, 2 hours before a meal	• Pregnancy • Patients taking warfarin	• Insomnia • Headache • Anorexia • CNS stimulation	• Blood pressure • Menstrual cycles	• Glucose-lowering drugs • Phenelzine • Anticoagulants • Antiplatelets • MAOIs	• Duration should be limited to 3 months • Can interfere with blood glucose lab tests

DECONGESTANTS

Definitions

Vasoconstrictive agents serve multiple roles in patient care including hemorrhoids, hypotension, ocular procedures and redness, and nasal congestion. Decongestants are the mainstay of therapy for colds and play an important role with allergic rhinitis. Nasal congestion can be treated with topical or oral adrenergic-agonist decongestants. Available agents include noradrenaline releasers (pseudoephedrine), alpha1-adrenergic agonists (phenylephrine), and alpha2-adrenergic agonists (naphazoline, oxymetazoline). This agonist effect causes vasoconstriction, which reduces the vascular blood supply to the sinuses, relieving intranasal pressure and reducing mucosal edema and mucus production. Decongestants are indicated for temporary relief of nasal congestion and cough associated with postnasal drip. They are no longer approved for sinusitis. Most recently, the FDA does not recommend over-the-counter (OTC) medications for children under the age of 2 years and includes decongestants because of the increased risk of death.

Signs and Symptoms

- Sinusitis
  - Tenderness over the sinuses; facial pain aggravated by postural changes; fever >101.5°F; tooth pain; halitosis; upper respiratory tract symptoms for >7 days with poor response to decongestants
- Common cold
  - Sore throat; nasal congestion; rhinorrhea; sneezing; common, low-grade fever; chills; headache; malaise; myalgia; cough
- Postnasal drip
  - Continued mucus accumulation in the back of the nose and throat leading to or giving the sensation of mucus dripping downward from the back of the nose

Guidelines

American Pharmaceutical Association. *Handbook of Nonprescription Drugs: An Interactive Approach to Self-Care*, 16th edition, 2009.

Adverse Effects

Appropriate FDA-approved doses should be used at all times since overdoses can cause excessive central nervous system stimulation and paradoxical depression. It is important to recognize any drug interactions that can occur with certain medications. The use of decongestants is contraindicated in patients taking MAO inhibitors. The main adverse effects of oral decongestants are cardiovascular stimulation and central nervous system stimulation.

Guidelines Summary

- Once the patient is excluded from the following bullet points, a pharmacist may appropriately recommend a decongestant.
  - Fever >101.5°F
  - Chest pain
  - Shortness of breath
  - Hypertension, arrhythmias, insomnia, and anxiety
  - Worsening of symptoms or development of additional symptoms during self-treatment
  - Concurrent underlying chronic cardiopulmonary disease
  - AIDS or chronic immunosuppressant therapy
  - Frail patients of advanced age
  - Children less than 2 years of age
  - Current medications such as MAOIs
- Topical decongestants should not be recommended for longer than 3–5 days due to the risk of rhinitis medicamentosa, a condition of rebound nasal congestion brought on by overuse of intranasal vasoconstrictive medications.

Decongestants

Generic	Brand	Dose & Max mg (frequency)	Contra-indications	Primary Side Effects	Key Monitoring Parameters	Pertinent Drug Interactions	Med Pearls
Oral decongestants							
Mechanism of action — alpha-adrenergic stimulator with weak beta-adrenergic activity							
Phenylephrine	• Neo-synephrine • Numerous others	• Topical: 1–2 sprays q4 hrs • Oral: 10–20 mg q4 hrs	• Hypertension • Ventricular tachycardia • Narrow-angle glaucoma • MAOI therapy within 14 days	• Reflex bradycardia • Restlessness • Hypertension • Tremor	• Blood pressure • Pulse • Anxiety	• MAOIs • Tricyclic antidepressants (TCAs) and methyldopa may enhance vasopressor effect	Avoid using with, or within 14 days of, MAOI therapy
Pseudoephedrine	• Sudafed • Numerous others	Oral: 240 mg/24 hrs					
Topical decongestants							
Oxymetazoline	• Afrin • Numerous others	• Intranasal: 2–3 sprays BID • Ophthalmic: 1–2 drops q6 hrs	• Hypersensitivity • Narrow-angle glaucoma	• Hypertension • Palpitation • Stinging	• Rebound congestion • Blood pressure	MAOIs	Not recommended for longer than 3–5 days
Naphazoline	Naphcon	• Nasal: 1–2 drops q6 hrs • Ophthalmic: 1–2 drops q6 hrs				• MAOIs • TCAs and methyldopa may enhance vasopressor effect	

ANTIHISTAMINES AND PROTON PUMP INHIBITORS

Definitions

Antihistamines can be used for multiple roles in patient care, including contact dermatitis, allergic rhinitis, common colds, insomnia, heartburn, and nausea and vomiting.

Three histamine receptors have been identified: Stimulation of histamine-1 receptors produces sneezing, pruritus, and mucus production. Histamine-2 receptors result in stomach acid production. Histamine-3 receptors are located in the brain and control the synthesis and release of histamine.

Antihistamines are classified into two categories: First-generation and second-generation. Second-generation antihistamines are nonsedating because they do not cross the blood-brain barrier.

Antihistamines against H_1 receptors are classified as either sedating (first-generation, nonselective) or nonsedating (second-generation, peripherally selective). These agents are commonly used to treat allergic rhinitis and common cold symptoms. H_2 receptor antagonists (H2RAs) are used to decrease gastric acid secretion by inhibiting histamine production of parietal cells. These agents are used to treat heartburn. Another class of drugs used to treat heartburn is proton pump inhibitors (PPIs). PPIs have more potent and prolonged effects than H2RAs, and therefore are indicated in more frequent, severe heartburn. They work by inhibiting H/K/ATPase, or the proton pump, which irreversibly blocks gastric acid secretion.

Signs and Symptoms

- Contact dermatitis: Papules, vesicles, erythema, crusting, and oozing
- Allergic rhinitis: Nasal stuffiness, rhinorrhea usually clear, pruritus of nose, sneezing, watering eyes, nasal drainage
- Common colds: Nasal stuffiness, sneezing, scratchy throat, cough, hoarseness, headache, fever
- Insomnia: Difficulty initiating sleep at usual time and/or wakefulness during usual sleep cycle, daytime tiredness
- Heartburn: Stomach and chest pain, choking with swallowing, relief with solids or liquids

Guidelines

American Pharmaceutical Association. *Handbook of Nonprescription Drugs: An Interactive Approach to Self-Care*, 16th edition, 2009.

Guidelines Summary

- Contact dermatitis
  - Identify the cause: chemical, acids, solvent, fragrances, metals, poison ivy, etc.
  - Clean the area with mild soap and water.
  - Refer patient to physician if the rash causes edema or invades the eyelids, external genitalia, anus, or massive areas of the body.
  - Treatment includes topical treatment with hydrocortisone, bicarbonate pastes, and antihistamines.
- Allergic rhinitis and common cold
  - Once the patient is excluded from the following, treatment recommendations can occur:
    » Symptoms of otitis media or sinusitis
    » Symptoms of lower respiratory tract infection
    » History of nonallergic rhinitis
- Insomnia
  - Transient or short-term insomnia but no underlying problems are okay to self-treat.
  - Discuss good sleep hygiene practices—no caffeine after 5 P.M., no exercise in the evening.
  - If diphenhydramine is recommended, it should be taken at bedtime only as needed.
  - Patients who complain of continuing insomnia after 14 days of treatment should be referred to a physician.
- Heartburn
  - Patient must be assessed for the following issues prior to self-treatment:
    » Frequent heartburn for more than 3 months
    » Heartburn while taking histamine-2 receptor agonist (H2RA) or proton pump inhibitor (PPI) or after initiating either one for 2 weeks
    » Nocturnal heartburn
    » Difficulty swallowing solid foods
    » Vomiting up blood or black material; or black, tarry stools
    » Chronic hoarseness, wheezing, coughing, choking
    » Unexplained weight loss
    » Pregnancy and nursing mothers
  - If the patient is a candidate, any of the following treatments are available—including antacids, which provide rapid relief versus the oral tablets, which have a slower onset of action.

Antihistamines

First-generation histamine H₁ antagonist

Mechanism of action – competes with histamine for H₁ receptor sites on effector cells in the GI tract, blood vessels, and respiratory tract

Generic	Brand	Dose & Max mg (frequency)	Contra-indications	Primary Side Effects	Key Monitoring Parameters	Pertinent Drug Interactions	Med Pearls
Clemastine	Tavist	• 1.34 mg TID • Max: 8.04 mg/day	Narrow-angle glaucoma	• Sedation • Anticholinergic • Dry mouth • Constipation • Blurred vision • Urinary retention	Mental alertness	May increase gastric degradation of levodopa	
Chlorpheniramine	Chlor-Trimeton	• 4 mg q4–6 hrs • Max: 24 mg/day					
Brompheniramine	• Dimetapp • Numerous others	1–2 tabs admin BID	• Hypersensitivity • MAOI within 14 days				
Diphenhydramine	• Benadryl • Sominex	• Allergic: 25–50 mg q6–8 hrs • Max: 400 mg/day • Insomnia: 50 mg HS	Acute asthma			• Acetylcholinesterase inhibitors • 2D6 substrates codeine, tramadol	
Doxylamine	Unisom	50 mg q HS	Hypersensitivity				
Fexofenadine	Allegra	60 mg BID or 180 mg once daily	Hypersensitivity			• Increased risk of QT prolongation when taken with other drugs that can prolong QT interval • Antacids • Azoles • Erythromycin	Avoid taking with fruit juices

Antihistamines *(cont'd)*

Second-generation histamine H$_1$ antagonist

Mechanism of action – long-acting tricyclic antihistamine with selectivity at H$_1$-receptor antagonistic properties; less blood-brain barrier penetration

Generic	Brand	Dose & Max mg (frequency)	Contra-indications	Primary Side Effects	Key Monitoring Parameters	Pertinent Drug Interactions	Med Pearls
Loratadine	Claritin	10 mg/day	Hypersensitivity	• Some sedation • Headache • Dizziness	• Relief of symptoms • Some sedation • Anticholinergic effects	Increases toxicity with CNS depressants and anticholinergics	
Cetirizine	Zyrtec	5–10 mg/day					
Azelastine	• Astelin • Astapro	Nasal spray: 1–2 sprays per nostril twice daily	Hypersensitivity	• Bitter taste • Nasal burning			Prime before initial use or after 3 days of storage

Histamine H$_2$ antagonist

Mechanism of action – competitive inhibition of histamine at H$_2$ receptors of the gastric parietal cells, resulting in reduced gastric acid secretion

Generic	Brand	Dose & Max mg (frequency)	Contra-indications	Primary Side Effects	Key Monitoring Parameters	Pertinent Drug Interactions	Med Pearls
Cimetidine	Tagamet	400 mg/day (OTC)	Hypersensitivity	• Gynecomastia • Increased liver function tests (LFTs) • Stevens-Johnson syndrome	• LFTs • Serum creatine (SCr) • Complete blood count (CBC)	• CYP450 • 2D6, 1A2, 2C19	• Shorter half-life • Renal adjustment required
Ranitidine	Zantac-OTC	Tabs: 75 mg or 150 mg BID		• Arrhythmias • Dizziness • Leukopenia • Aplastic anemia	• Gastric pH • GI bleeding • Bone density	• CYP450 • Inhibits 1A2, 2D6	Renal adjustment required
Famotidine	• Pepcid AC • Pepcid Complete	OTC: 10–20 mg BID		LFTs		May increase serum levels of -azoles	• Renal adjustment required • Pepcid Complete contains calcium carbonate, magnesium
Nizatidine	Axid AR	75 mg BID		Thrombocytopenia		• CYP450 • Inhibits 3A4	Renal adjustment required

Antihistamines *(cont'd)*

Mechanism of action – PPI; suppresses gastric basal and stimulated acid secretion by inhibiting the parietal cell H+/K ATP pump

Generic	Brand	Dose & Max mg (frequency)	Contra-indications	Primary Side Effects	Key Monitoring Parameters	Pertinent Drug Interactions	Med Pearls
Omeprazole	Prilosec OTC	20 mg/day	Hypersensitivity	Increased LFTs	Bone density	• CYP450 • Inhibits: 1A2, 2C9, 2C19, 2D6, 3A4 • Induces: 1A2	Treatment up to 14 days
Lansoprazole	Prevacid	15 mg/day		• Abdominal pain • Headache • Increased LFTS	• CBC • Liver function • Renal function • Serum gastric levels • Bone density	• CYPC19 • Indinavir • Iron salts • Azoles	Treatment up to 14 days
Omeprazole and sodium bicarbonate	Zegerid	20 mg & 1,100 mg		Same	Same	• Omeprazole same as above • Sodium bicarbonate: delavirine and nelfinavir	Sodium bicarbonate 1,100 mg = 300 mg = 13 mEq per capsule

COUGH SUPPRESSANTS

Definitions

A cough is caused by irritants or stimuli stimulating receptors located throughout the respiratory tract. The larynx is more sensitive than the trachea and bronchi. When activated, the receptors send signals through the brain-stem reflex pathway, the voluntary cerebral cortex pathway, or both. The signals eventually end up in the "cough center" of the medulla oblongata. The overall objective is to expel the irritant or stimuli.

Diagnosis

- A cough can be classified in the following ways:
  - Acute: duration less than 3 weeks
    - » Most commonly caused by a virus
  - Subacute: duration greater than 3 to 8 weeks
    - » Caused by infection, bacterial sinusitis, asthma
  - Chronic – duration longer than 8 weeks
    - » Smoking, post nasal drip, asthma, and gastroesophageal reflux disease (GERD)
- Angiotensin-converting enzymes (ACE) cause a dry cough in 20% or more of treated patients.
- Systemic and ophthalmic B-adrenergic blockers may cause cough in chronic obstructive pulmonary disease (COPD) patients.

Signs and Symptoms

- Productive
  - A wet or "chesty" cough, which expels secretions from the lower respiratory tract
  - Secretions may be clear, purulent, discolored, or malodorous
- Nonproductive
  - A dry or "hacking" cough that serves no useful physiologic purpose
  - Nonproductive coughs are caused by viral respiratory tract infections, atypical bacteria, GERD, cardiac disease, and some medications.

Guidelines

American Pharmaceutical Association. *Handbook of Nonprescription Drugs: An Interactive Approach to Self-Care*, 16th edition, 2009.

Guidelines Summary

- The primary goal of treating a cough is to reduce the number and severity of cough episodes.

- Codeine and dextromethorphan are the drugs of choice for nonproductive cough.

- Diphenhydramine is a better choice for coughs associated with allergies but is highly sedating.

  - Consider Claritin and/or Zyrtec, as there is less sedation.

- Guaifenesin is marketed only as an expectorant and should not be used to treat effectively productive coughs.

- Patients should be excluded from self-treatment if they have any of the following:

Cough with thick yellow sputum or green phlegm	Fever >101.5°F	Unintended weight loss
Drenching nighttime sweats	Hemoptysis	History of asthma, COPD, CHF
Foreign-object aspiration	Cough greater than 7 days	Cough worsens during self-treatment

Cough Suppresants

Generic	Brand	Dose & Max mg (frequency)	Contra-indications	Primary Side Effects	Key Monitoring Parameters	Pertinent Drug Interactions	Med Pearls
Mechanism of action – serves as antitussive agent by depressing the medullary cough center							
Dextromethorphan	• Robitussin • Delsym • Several others	• Cough: 10–20 mg q4 hrs or 30 mg q6–8 hrs • Extended-release: 60 mg BID • Max: 120 mg/day	Do not use within 2 wks of an MAOI	• Abdominal discomfort • Coma • Constipation • Dizziness • Respiratory depression		• CYP450 • Inhibits 2D6	• Withdrawn from OTC market for children under age 2 • Chemically related to morphine; lacks narcotic properties except in overdose
Mechanism of action – expectorant; irritates the gastric mucosa and stimulates respiratory tract secretions, thereby increasing fluid volumes and decreasing mucous viscosity							
Guaifenesin	• Mucinex • Several other combination products	• IR: 200–400 mg q4 hrs • ER: 600–1,200 mg BID • Max: 2.4 g/day	Hypersensitivity	• Dizziness • Kidney stone formation		None	More effective with water intake
Mechanism of action – causes cough suppression by direct central action in the medulla; produces CNS depression							
Codeine phosphate		• 10–20 mg q4–6 hrs • Max: 120 mg/day	Pregnancy	• Nausea and vomiting • Constipation • Sedation	• LFTs • CNS depression	• CYP450 • 2D6 inhibitor • Alcohol	10% of a codeine dose is demethylated in the liver to form morphine

ANTIDIARRHEALS

Definitions

Diarrhea is defined as an abnormal increase in stool frequency or liquidity. Each individual has a different frequency, which is affected by many variables. The typical range of stool frequency can be three times per day to once every 2 days. More than three bowel movements per day is considered to be abnormal.

Diagnosis

- Diarrhea is defined and characterized by more than three bowel movements in 1 day.
- Diarrhea may be acute, persistent, or chronic in nature.
- Acute diarrhea is defined as an episode of less than 14 days' duration.
- Persistent diarrhea is diarrhea of 14-day to 4-week duration.
- Chronic diarrhea lasts more than 4 weeks.

Signs & Symptoms

- Abdominal pain, cramping, and frequency are signs.
- Stool is approximately 75% water and 25% solid material.
- Stool contains unabsorbed food residue and minerals, bacteria, desquamated epithelial cells.

Guidelines

American Pharmaceutical Association. *Handbook of Nonprescription Drugs: An Interactive Approach to Self-Care*, 16th edition, 2009.

Guidelines Summary

- Acute diarrhea can be managed with fluids, electrolyte replacement, dietary interventions, and nonprescription drug treatment.
- Persistent and chronic diarrhea requires medical care, and patients are not candidates for self-treatment if this is present.
- Patients should be excluded from self-treatment if any of the following apply:
  - <6 months of age
  - Severe dehydration
  - >6 months of age with persistent high fevers greater than 102.2°F
  - Blood, mucus, or pus in the stool
  - Protracted vomiting, severe abdominal pain
  - Pregnancy
  - Chronic or persistent diarrhea

Antidiarrheals

Mechanism of action – decreases pain through inhibition of central cyclooxygenase, which in turn inhibits prostaglandin synthesis

Generic	Brand	Dose & Max mg (frequency)	Contra-indications	Primary Side Effects	Key Monitoring Parameters	Pertinent Drug Interactions	Med Pearls
Loperamide	Imodium	Initial: 4 mg, followed by 2 mg after each loose stool, up to 16 mg/day	• Abdominal pain without diarrhea • Children <2 yrs • Primary tx for acute dysentery, acute ulcerative colitis, and other colitis	• Constipation • Abdominal cramping • Abdominal distention	• CNS depression • Urinary retention • Paralytic ileus • Monitor for dehydration	• CYP450 • 2B6 substrate • May decrease levels of saquinavir	Toxicity can be treated with 100 g activated charcoal through nasogastric tube, and Naloxone

Mechanism of action – inhibits both antisecretory and antimicrobial and antiviral action; provides some anti-inflammatory action

Generic	Brand	Dose & Max mg (frequency)	Contra-indications	Primary Side Effects	Key Monitoring Parameters	Pertinent Drug Interactions	Med Pearls
Bismuth	• Kaopectate • Pepto-Bismol	524 mg q30 min to 1 hr PRN; up to 8 doses/24 hrs	• Influenza or chickenpox due to risk of Reye's syndrome • Hx of GI bleed • Pregnancy: third trimester	• Discoloration of tongue and feces (grayish) • Impaction of feces • Hearing loss, tinnitus		May decrease level and/or effects of tetracycline derivatives	

Mechanism of action – helps re-establish normal intestinal flora; suppresses the growth of potentially pathogenic microorganisms by producing lactic acid, which favors the establishment of an aciduric flora

Generic	Brand	Dose & Max mg (frequency)	Contra-indications	Primary Side Effects	Key Monitoring Parameters	Pertinent Drug Interactions	Med Pearls
Lactobacillus	• Culturelle • Lactinex	• Culturelle: 1 caplet QD or BID • Lactinex: 4 tabs 3–4x daily	Hypersensitivity	Flatulence	Improvement	None	Lactinex must be stored in refrigerator
Lactase enzyme	• Lactaid • Lactrase	1–2 capsules taken with milk or meal	None	No common side effects reported at this time	Improving diarrheal symptoms	No known drug interactions	• Used in the treatment of lactose intolerance • Prevents osmotic diarrhea

CONSTIPATION MEDICATIONS

Definitions

Constipation is a symptom-based disorder that is described as a decrease in the frequency of fecal elimination characterized by the passage of hard, dry stools. The Rome III Criteria requires a patient to have experienced at least two of the following symptoms over the past three months: (1) fewer than three bowel movements per week; (2) straining; (3) lumpy/hard stools; (4) the sensation of an obstruction; (5) sensation of incomplete defecation; or (6) manual maneuvering required to defecate. Its occurrence increases as the patient ages in both men and women. However, it tends to be more commonly reported in women. Over half of the elderly population is affected by constipation. It is also a main complaint during pregnancy and after childbirth.

Constipation can be caused by various medical conditions, psychological and physiological conditions (menopause, dehydration), and lifestyle characteristics. There are several medications that can induce constipation, including: analgesics, antacids, anticholinergics, antidepressants, antidiarrheals, benzodiazepines, calcium channel blockers, iron supplements, monoamine oxidase inhibitors, opiates, parkinsonism agents, and sucralfate.

Diagnosis

- There are three clinical subgroups of constipation:
  - Normal transit constipation
    - » Most common form—59%
  - Slow transit constipation
    - » Accounts for 13%—delayed colonic transit
  - Pelvic floor dysfunction
  - Combination syndrome
- Less frequency of stooling than the "normal" 3–5 times/week
- Harder stool than "normal"
- Smaller stools than "normal"
- Colonoscopy if age >50, alarm signs, or additional symptoms present

Signs and Symptoms

- Lack of passing a bowel movement
- Very hard stools, lumpy stools
- Need for performing manual maneuvers to pass stools
- Anorexia, dull headache, low back pain, abdominal distention

Guidelines

American Gastroenterological Association Medical Position Statement: Guidelines on Constipation. *Gastroenterology*, no. 119 (2000): 1761–78.

American Pharmaceutical Association. *Handbook of Nonprescription Drugs: An Interactive Approach to Self-Care*, 16th edition, 2009.

Cassagnol M, Saad M, Ahmed E, and Ezzo D. Review of Current Chronic Constipation Guidelines. *US Pharm*. 2010;35(12):74–85.

Guidelines Summary

- Educate patient about high fiber and increased hydration in diet.
- Lifestyle modifications:
  - Encourage patients to avoid postponing defecation.
  - Monitor bowel habits with a daily diary.
  - Encourage patients to maintain moderate exercise.
- Patients should be excluded from self-treatment if they have any of the following:
  - Marked abdominal pain or significant distention or cramping
  - Marked or unexplained flatulence
  - Fever
  - Nausea and/or vomiting
  - Paraplegia or quadriplegia
  - Daily laxative use
  - Unexplained changes in bowel habits and/or weight loss
  - Bowel symptoms that persist for 2 weeks
  - History of irritable bowel disease
- Pharmacology begins with bulk-forming agents, proceeds to osmotic laxatives.
- If these options are not helpful, stimulant laxatives should be considered.
- Enemas, suppositories, and lubricants are also available as options.

Drugs for Constipation

Generic	Brand	Dose & Max mg (frequency)	Contraindications	Primary Side Effects	Key Monitoring Parameters	Pertinent Drug Interactions	Med Pearls	Top 200
Mechanism of action – bulk-forming by absorbing water in the intestine to form a viscous liquid that promotes peristalsis								
Psyllium	Metamucil	1 tbsp TID 2–6 caps TID 1–2 wafers TID	• Fecal impaction • GI obstruction	• Abdominal cramps • Diarrhea	• Improvement • Diarrhea	• Warfarin • Digitalis • Diuretics	• Affects absorption of other meds • Take with full glass of water	No
Calcium polycarbophil	FiberCon	2–4 tabs QD						No
Methylcellulose	Citrucel	1–2 caps 6x/day 1 scoop TID						No
Mechanism of action – osmotic agent that causes water retention in the stool								
Polyethylene glycol 3350	MiraLax	17 g in 8 oz of water QD	• GI obstruction	• Abdominal cramps • Diarrhea • Bloating	• Improvement • Diarrhea	None	Can reconstitute with 8 oz of water, juice, cola, or tea	No
Mechanism of action – stimulates peristalsis by directly irritating the smooth muscle of the intestine								
Senna	Senokot	2 tabs QD to 4 tab BID	• Fecal impaction • GI obstruction	• Abdominal cramps • Diarrhea • Bloating	• Improvement • Diarrhea	None		No
Bisacodyl	Dulcolax	5–15 mg QD				Milk and antacids may decrease the effect of bisacodyl		No
Mechanism of action – reduces surface tension of the oil–water interface of the stool, resulting in enhanced incorporation of water and fat and allowing for stool softening								
Docusate sodium	Colace	100 mg BID	• Concomitant with mineral	• Intestinal obstruction • Diarrhea • Cramping	• Improvement • Diarrhea	None	Take with full glass of water	No
Docusate calcium	Surlak	240 mg QD	• Fecal impaction • GI obstruction					No
Mechanism of action – promotes bowel evacuation by causing osmotic retention of fluid which distends the colon with increased peristaltic activity								
Magnesium hydroxide	Phillips Milk of Magnesia	1–2 tbsp QD or BID	Hypersensitivity	Diarrhea	• Improvement • Diarrhea		Caution with impaired renal function	No
Mechanism of action – eases passage of stool by decreasing water absorption and lubricating the intestines								
Mineral oil	Fleet	1–2 tbsp HS	• Colostomy • Ileostomy • Appendicitis • Ulcerative colitis	• Abdominal cramps • Diarrhea • Bloating		May impair absorption of fat-soluble vitamins (A, D, K, E)	Aspiration is possible, especially in elderly population	No

ATHLETE'S FOOT MEDICATIONS

Definitions

Athlete's foot is a fungal infection called tinea pedis. The infection can range from mild itching to a severe inflammatory process characterized by fissuring, crusting, and discoloration of skin.

There are four types of tinea pedis.

- Chronic, intertriginous type
  - Most common form
  - Usually found in the lateral toe webs; however, infection is possible of spreading to the sole or instep of the foot
- Chronic, papulosquamous type
  - Found on both feet
  - Characterized by mild inflammation and diffuse, moccasin-like scaling
- Vesicular type
  - Occurs most often in the summertime
  - Characterized by small vesicles or vesicopustules near the instep and on the mid-anterior plantar surface
- Acute, ulcerative type
  - Caused from an overgrowth of gram-negative bacteria

Diagnosis

- Typically found in the lateral toe webs
- Can then spread to the sole or instep of the foot

Signs and Symptoms

- Fissuring and scaling
- Maceration in the interdigital spaces
- Malodor
- Stinging and burning sensation

Guidelines

American Pharmaceutical Association. *Handbook of Nonprescription Drugs: An Interactive Approach to Self-Care,* 16th edition, 2009.

Guidelines Summary

- Patients should be excluded from self-treatment if they have any of the following:
  - Causative factor unclear
  - Nails or scalp involved
  - Face, mucous membranes, or genitalia involved
  - Signs and symptoms of possible secondary bacterial infection
  - Excessive and continuous exudation, fever, malaise
- Apply a thin layer of medication to affected area for 2 weeks, even after the signs and symptoms disappear.

Athlete's Foot Medications

Mechanism of action – squalene epoxidase inhibitor results in deficiency of ergosterol within the fungal cell

Generic	Brand	Dose & Max mg (frequency)	Contraindications	Primary Side Effects	Key Monitoring Parameters	Pertinent Drug Interactions	Med Pearls
Butenafine	• Lotrimin Ultra • Mentax	Apply QD	Hypersensitivity	• Burning • Contact dermatitis • Erythema • Irritation • Stinging	Clinical signs of improvement	Minimal systemic absorption	• E. floccosum • T. mentagrophytes • T. rubrum
Terbinafine	Lamisil	Apply QD					

Mechanism of action – binds to phospholipids in the fungal cell membrane, altering cell wall permeability and resulting in loss of intracellular elements

Generic	Brand	Dose & Max mg (frequency)	Contraindications	Primary Side Effects	Key Monitoring Parameters	Pertinent Drug Interactions	Med Pearls
Clotrimazole	Lotrimin AF 1%	Cream; apply BID	Hypersensitivity	• Burning • Contact dermatitis • Erythema • Itching	Clinical signs of improvement	Minimal systemic absorption	• E. floccosum • T. mentagrophytes • T. rubrum • Candida albicans
Miconazole	Micatin	Apply BID x 4 wks					

Mechanism of action – distorts the hyphae and stunts mycelial growth in susceptible fungi

Generic	Brand	Dose & Max mg (frequency)	Contraindications	Primary Side Effects	Key Monitoring Parameters	Pertinent Drug Interactions	Med Pearls
Tolnaftate	Tinactin	Spray: BID	Hypersensitivity	• Burning • Contact dermatitis • Erythema • Itching	Clinical signs of improvement	Minimal systemic absorption	• E. floccosum • T. mentagrophytes • T. rubrum

Mechanism of action – inhibits conversion of yeast to the hyphal form (active form) and interferes with fatty-acid biosynthesis

Generic	Brand	Dose & Max mg (frequency)	Contraindications	Primary Side Effects	Key Monitoring Parameters	Pertinent Drug Interactions	Med Pearls
Undecylenic acid	• Cruex • Fungi-Nail • Blis-To-Sol	Applied BID	None	High alcohol concentrations may cause burning	Clinical signs of improvement	Minimal systemic absorption	• Fungistatic against C. albicans, Trichophyton spp, and E. inguinale • Contains 5% undecylenic acid and 20% zinc undecylenate

LEARNING POINTS

- The Dietary Supplement Health and Education Act of 1994 categorizes herbals, vitamins, protein bars, and shakes as dietary supplements. As a result, manufacturers are not required to demonstrate safety, purity, or efficacy of supplements.

- Decongestants are the mainstay of therapy for colds and play an important role with allergic rhinitis.

- ACE inhibitors cause a dry cough in 20% or more of treated patients.

- Having more than three bowel movements per day is considered to be abnormal.

- Constipation can be caused by medications (anticholinergics, analgesics, benzos, sucralfate, calcium channel blockers, and more), menopause, dehydration, psychologic condition, depression, and more.

- When treating athlete's foot, a 2-week treatment period is typically required.

PRACTICE QUESTIONS

1. Which of the following would NOT be the case with levothyroxine administration?

    (A) Insulin level should be increased due to hyperglycemic effect.
    (B) Ciprofloxacin causes decreased absorption.
    (C) Calcium and antacids cause decreased absorption.
    (D) Iron causes increased absorption.
    (E) Both (A) and (D) are correct.

ANSWERS

1. **D**

Iron causes a decrease, not an increase, in the absorption of levothyroxine, so (D) is correct. Levothyroxine causes a hyperglycemic effect, and insulin doses should be increased accordingly (A). Ciprofloxacin, calcium, and antacids all cause a decrease in the absorption of levothyroxine (B and C). Patients should be advised to take levothyroxine on an empty stomach, preferably before the first meal to avoid drug interactions.

Part Three

Pharmaceutical Sciences, Mathematics, and Biostatistics

Pharmaceutics

 Suggested Study Time: **1.5 hours**

Pharmaceutics encompasses a number of disciplines, including dosage form design, biopharmaceutics, and pharmacokinetics. This chapter focuses on dosage form design (drug dosage forms, and the physical and chemical properties that allow these products to be manufactured).

A key concept to keep in mind is that patients don't simply take drugs, they take dosage forms: The active ingredient is not the only substance involved.

PHYSICAL PHARMACY

Physical pharmacy is a branch of pharmaceutics that deals principally with the physical and chemical properties of drugs. It is a highly mathematical subject, but the Board exam is not concerned with these aspects except as they relate to chemical kinetics. As you study, focus mainly on how specific properties of drugs make particular types of formulations more or less suitable. A simple example would be antibiotic suspensions that arrive at the pharmacy in dry powder form. The reason for this is that many antibiotics are chemically unstable in liquid formulations; if the water is added only at the time of dispensing, the drug will remain effective long enough for the patient to finish the bottle. If the product were manufactured as a liquid, the drug would be degraded by the time the bottle was processed, shipped, and stored in the pharmacy prior to dispensing.

Preformulation

Preformulation is an important stage of drug development where the pharmaceutical company characterizes many of the physicochemical properties of the drug. Preformulation allows the company to make the best decisions about how to formulate the drug into a usable dosage form.

Solubility and Lipophilicity

Drugs must be in solution before they can be absorbed by the body. Drugs must possess at least some aqueous solubility in order to be effective; poorly soluble compounds show incomplete and unpredictable absorption. However, at least some lipophilicity must also be present, as drugs must be able to pass through biological membranes in order to reach their sites of action. Salts or esters of drugs may be formed to increase or decrease the solubility, depending on the characteristics needed in a particular case. For example, the benzathine salt of penicillin G has a very low solubility, which causes the drug to dissolve slowly after injection, which prolongs the duration of action.

Dissolution rate is improved by decreasing particle size, which increases the surface area of the drug that comes into contact with the body fluids. A more in-depth treatment of factors that influence dissolution rate and absorption is contained in the biopharmaceutics chapter.

Ionization Behavior

Ionization behavior is one of the most important factors in drug development. It applies only if a drug is an electrolyte; when such a drug goes into solution, a fraction of the molecules dissociate into ions (i.e., charged compounds). The proportion of ionized to un-ionized drug is very important because the two behave very differently in the body:

- Ionized drug: More soluble, but cannot cross body membranes
- Un-ionized drug: Less soluble, but can cross body membranes

Remember: Until the drug is absorbed across the body membranes it cannot get to the site of action, but it needs to go into solution before that can happen. The equilibrium between the more soluble ionized form and the more absorbable un-ionized form of the drug is crucial.

The Henderson-Hasselbalch equation (below) can be used to calculate exact ratios of ionized to un-ionized drug, but the following table will give you a rough estimate of the ionization behavior of weak acids and bases when comparing pH of absorption site to the pKa. In most cases, you will be able to obtain a sufficiently accurate answer by using the table instead of the actual equation, saving valuable exam time.

$$pH = pKa + \log \frac{[base]}{[acid]}$$

Ionization Behavior of Weak Acids and Bases

	Acid	Base
pH > pKa	More ionized	More un-ionized
pH = pKa	Equal	Equal
pH < pKa	More un-ionized	More ionized
Note that for pH more than 2 units away from pKa, expect complete ionization/un-ionization.		

Salts are often preferred over the weak acid or base because they dissolve more quickly, are more stable on storage, and are easier to crystallize and handle during processing. Different salt forms may have very different properties, and pharmaceutical companies may intentionally modify drugs into more useful salts for a given purpose. Calcium salts, for example, show wide variation in absorption and possible efficacy.

A final note on acid/base determinations: It is impossible to tell if a drug is an acid or a base by looking only at the pKa. Some acids have higher pKa (phenytoin = 8.3) than do some bases (morphine = 8.0). You can tell if a drug is an acid or base, however, by what type of salt it forms. Weak acids form sodium, calcium, potassium, or other cationic salts; weak bases form hydrochloride or other anionic salts.

Stability

Physical, chemical, and microbiological stability are all very important in preformulation studies. While physical instability does not generally result in decreased drug concentration, it can lead to problems with dose uniformity and pharmaceutical elegance (eg., the mottled appearance that can develop in tablets over time, or the formation of a nonsuspendable sediment in a liquid dosage form). Polymorphism and anhydrous-to-hydrate conversions can be considered types of physical instability and are discussed in greater detail in the following section.

Chemical instability does result in loss of drug or excipient molecules. This can lead to either undertreatment, when a patient does not receive the full dose intended, or toxicity from toxic degradation products. In some cases, chemical instability can lead to microbiological instability if a preservative degrades and can no longer protect the formulation from bacterial or fungal overgrowth. The main types of degradation that occur in drug products are:

- Hydrolysis: Occurs in presence of water; typically no change in formulation appearance
- Oxidation: Occurs in presence of atmospheric oxygen; often results in insoluble precipitates or colored compounds

- Photochemical decomposition: Occurs on exposure to light; often results in colored compounds

Temperature, humidity, and light often hasten the degradation process, and drug companies use this fact to perform accelerated stability testing and to assign product expiration dates. Finished products must retain 90% of the labeled dose during their shelf life, so studies are performed at extreme storage conditions, and mathematical equations are used to estimate the degradation rate constants at normal conditions. A good estimate, however, is that every 10°C rise in temperature doubles the rate constant.

Most drugs degrade by either zero- or first-order kinetics (see "Rate and Half-Life Equations" table, below). Drugs following zero-order degradation have a constant degradation rate that is independent of the drug concentration. First-order degradation, however, is concentration-dependent—the amount of drug degrading per unit of time is not constant. Suspensions degrade by pseudo–zero order kinetics, because only the drug molecules that are actually in solution can degrade. The concentration of drug in solution is in equilibrium with that in suspension, and the concentration of drug in solution is maintained at a constant level; suspended particles go into solution to replace the degraded drug. This continues as long as some solid is still present.

Rate and Half-Life Equations

Order	Rate Equation		Half-Life Equation
Zero	$C = C_0 - k_0 t$		$t_{1/2} = 0.5 \dfrac{C_0}{k_0}$
First	$\log C = \log C_0 - \dfrac{k_0 t}{2.303}$	$C = C_0 e^{-kt}$	$t_{1/2} = \dfrac{\ln 2}{k_1} = \dfrac{0.693}{k_1}$

Solid-State Properties

Because most drugs are given as solid-dosage forms, many properties specific to the solid state are important in pharmacy.

Crystallization

Solids are present in crystalline or amorphous forms, or as a combination of the two. Crystalline forms show fixed geometric patterns, whereas the atoms in amorphous solids are randomly placed (as they would be in a liquid). The most important things to remember about crystalline versus amorphous solids for the purposes of this test are as follows:

- Crystalline solids have definite melting points, whereas amorphous solids melt over a range of temperature.

- Amorphous solids are more soluble than the corresponding crystalline forms.
- Solids tend to revert to the more stable crystalline form on storage.

Solvates are crystalline structures that contain trapped solvent; when the solvent is water, they are called hydrates. Typically, hydrates are less soluble than their anhydrous counterparts, whereas solvates are more soluble.

Polymorphism

Polymorphs are one of several crystalline structures that have the same chemical formula. The properties they exhibit can vary substantially, however, and this leads to pharmaceutical companies patenting different polymorphic forms based on variations in solubility, bioavailability, solid-state stability, or processing behavior (such as improved powder flow or tablet compaction).

Metastable polymorphs will revert to the most stable form over time; in some instances, however, the metastable form might have more favorable properties than the stable form (e.g., better solubility). In those cases, even though it is not the most stable form, it may be the best one to market, provided the stability is at least acceptable.

The classic example of excipient polymorphism is cocoa butter, which is often used in suppository and troche formulations. Four polymorphs exist; only the β form is stable. When cocoa butter is heated above 34°C, some of the β form converts to unstable polymorphs. The unstable polymorphs are liquid at room temperature. The cocoa butter is never able to remain solid outside of the refrigerator in those cases. This explains why chocolate or cocoa butter that has been overheated does not fully solidify when cooled.

Another pharmacy-related example is ritonavir (Norvir), a protease inhibitor used to treat HIV. Initially, it was thought to exist in only one polymorphic form, with relatively poor aqueous solubility. It was marketed in a soft gelatin capsule, which contained an ethanol/water cosolvent system. After drug approval, several batches failed quality control tests. It was discovered that a second polymorphic form with even lower solubility had formed, causing the drug to precipitate out of the cosolvent system. The product had to be reformulated to include Cremophor (polyethoxylated castor oil) as a solubilizing agent.

Rheology

Rheology is the science of flow properties, especially important when discussing liquid and semisolid dosage forms. During manufacturing, rheology is important when mixing and packaging materials. Once the products reach the consumer, the rheology affects the removal of the product from its container, whether by pouring, extruding from a tube, or passing through a syringe needle.

Viscosity and fluidity are two common terms associated with rheology. Viscosity refers to the resistance offered when part of the liquid flows past another part; fluidity is essentially the opposite. Viscous liquids are thick and slow-moving; fluid liquids are thin and flow more readily.

Rheological behavior is divided into two main types: Newtonian flow and non-Newtonian flow. Newtonian materials do not change viscosity with changes in stirring speed; they do, however, become less viscous when heated. True solutions and pure liquid compounds such as water and oil are examples of Newtonian materials. Non-Newtonian materials do change viscosity when stirring speed changes. Three types of non-Newtonian behavior exist: Dilatant, plastic, and pseudoplastic. Dilatant materials become more viscous when stirred more rapidly, which can cause manufacturing equipment to malfunction. Plastic and pseudoplastic materials become more fluid when stirred. Plastic flow is best illustrated by a nonpharmacy example: Tomato catsup. It doesn't pour until shaken enough for contacts between adjacent particles to be broken but then acts much like a Newtonian material. Concentrated suspensions show similar behavior. Pseudoplastic flow differs in that flow can start immediately on stirring or shaking; the harder the bottle is shaken, the more fluid the material becomes. Polymer solutions often exhibit pseudoplastic flow.

Thixotropic products are a special case and are actually the ideal situation for pharmaceutical suspensions. They are viscous at rest but become fluid when shaken. Because of this, the suspension settles only slowly, but the liquid pours easily when shaken. After shaking stops, thixotropic products gradually become viscous again. Both plastic and pseudoplastic materials can show thixotropic behavior.

Testing

Numerous quality assurance tests exist for dosage forms, though only four will be discussed here. These four are used to test tablets and sometimes capsules.

Disintegration testing is performed by placing tablets into mesh-bottomed cylinders that are immersed in a solution and agitated at a specified rate. The tablets are considered to have disintegrated when the particles are small enough to fall through the mesh screen. It is not a good measure of in vivo behavior, but is a frequently used quality-control measure for tablets.

A better measure of in vivo behavior is dissolution testing. Here, the tablets or capsules are immersed in appropriate dissolution liquids (typically, simulated gastric fluid) and samples are taken at specific time points to determine how much of the drug has gone into solution. While this test is still not a true predictor of in vivo behavior—because it does not demonstrate absorption—it is an improvement over disintegration testing, as the drug must go into solution with body fluids before being absorbed.

Friability and hardness testing evaluate the ability of tablets to withstand manufacturing, packaging, and shipping. Hardness testing measures the force required to cause a tablet to break, and friability testing measures what percentage weight of a tablet is lost after it is tumbled for a specified amount of time in a friabilator. Tablets that are too soft or fragile will suffer too much damage during manufacturing and shipping to be useful, even if they have excellent dissolution and absorption behavior.

PHARMACEUTICAL DOSAGE FORMS

What things need to be considered when a drug company designs a dosage form for a particular drug? Some of the primary considerations are:

- Nature of the illness
- Manner in which the illness is treated
- Age of the patient
- Condition of the patient
- Stability of the drug

Suppose a patient suffers from motion sickness and is getting ready to go on a cruise. Would a tablet be the best dosage form in which their antinausea medication should be formulated? Probably not, as there is a risk that they could vomit and lose the medication before it had a chance to be absorbed by the body. For this reason, scopolamine is formulated into transdermal patches for motion sickness.

Some drugs can be used to treat different conditions based on their formulation and route of administration. An example is the antifungal product terbinafine (Lamisil). It is given as cream for surface conditions such as athlete's foot, and as tablets for more deep-seated fungal infections of the toenails and fingernails.

Age of the patient plays a large role in development of dosage forms. Young children and the elderly are much more likely than adults and teenagers are to have difficulty swallowing. Therefore, most medications for small children are marketed as easy-to-swallow dosage forms such as liquids and chewable or rapid-dissolve tablets. Other groups of patients may also lack the ability and willingness to swallow. Patients with psychiatric conditions will often refuse to swallow medication, and rapid-dissolve formulations or injections may be required to ensure that they receive treatment. Severely debilitated or comatose patients cannot swallow and may receive medicine through nasogastric tubes or by injection.

Oral Delivery: Solids

Solid dosage forms are the most commonly prescribed—over 80% of dosage forms are tablets or capsules. These products are convenient for the patient and are the preferred route for giving nonemergency medications. Some benefits of solid dosage forms are that they are already divided into accurate doses and are easy to handle. Taste is generally less of an issue than with liquid dosage forms and can be masked by coating the product, as long as the dosage is not designed to be chewed or dissolved in the mouth.

Solid products, however, are not perfect. If a very rapid response is needed, traditional tablets and capsules are not the best option because they take time to dissolve and become absorbed by the body. If formulated improperly, the absorption of the active ingredient(s) may be irregular or incomplete.

Traditional Release

The simplest type of solid dosage form is the powder. Powders taken orally have a few advantages: They are absorbed more rapidly than tablets and capsules because they do not have to undergo a disintegration step, they are easier to swallow than large tablets and capsules, and they are more chemically stable than liquids. It is easier to give large doses of drug in a powder than in a tablet. One gram of drug plus excipients is much easier to stir into water and swallow than it would be if formulated into a tablet.

On the other hand, it is very difficult to mask the taste or smell of unpleasant drugs when they are given in powder form. They are also highly inconvenient to handle and, if provided in bulk containers (such as Metamucil), may be subject to dose inaccuracy. Therefore, potent drugs should not be given as powders. If a drug is hygroscopic, it also should not be formulated into a powder dosage form as it will pick up too much moisture from the air. Finally, contrary to expectations, powders can be more expensive to produce than other solid dosage forms; there is a fairly substantial risk of explosion when working with large quantities of powder, and special handling equipment may be necessary to offset this risk.

Granules have many of the same advantages and disadvantages as powders. The primary difference between the two substances is that granules are prepared agglomerations of smaller particles. They behave as single particles but are irregularly shaped and have a larger particle size than the associated powders. Granules therefore flow better than powders and are more easily wetted by fluids, whether in manufacturing, in administration of the drug, or in the body. A simple example of the differences in properties of granulated versus powdered solids is sugar. Granulated (common table) sugar flows much more readily and dissolves easily in coffee or other liquids. Powdered sugar tends to clump, not flow freely, and dissolve slowly.

Granules are used more as a component of tablets and capsules than they are as dosage forms in their own right. They can be made by wet or dry methods. Wet granulation involves forming a dough of powder and liquid, pressing that dough through a mesh screen to form appropriately sized particles, and drying. In dry granulation, dry powders are compacted together, without the presence of liquid, into ribbons or oversized tablets that are then ground to size.

Capsules are a much more frequently dispensed type of solid dosage form and contain drug and excipients enclosed inside a gelatin, starch, or cellulose shell. They, like tablets, have many advantages over powders and granules. Since capsules are essentially unit-of-use products, they have excellent dose accuracy and the ability to mask the taste and smell of unpleasant drugs. They are also easy to administer, as the active ingredient does not need to be measured out. It is also easy to formulate products with multiple active ingredients. One advantage that capsules have over tablets is that they can be extemporaneously prepared in the pharmacy in instances where the prescriber requests a nonstandard dose of drug.

Capsules do have some disadvantages. They are permeable to moisture and may not be a suitable dosage form for moisture-sensitive drugs. They are also not suitable for water- or alcohol-based preparations, as those bases would dissolve the capsule shell. Some liquids, however, can be dispensed in capsules. Oil or nonaqueous water-miscible liquids such as polyethylene glycol (PEG) 400 can be used to dissolve or suspend drugs and vitamins that are then placed into soft gelatin capsules. Finally, gelatin may be inappropriate for certain patient populations who wish to avoid animal (particularly pork-based) products. In those cases, vegetarian capsule shells made of starch or cellulose may be substituted. Many dietary supplements and herbal products are manufactured in such capsules for this reason.

Tablets are the most frequently prescribed dosage form and are preferred for many reasons. In addition to the advantages they share with capsules, they are easy to make in a variety of shapes and colors, aiding in product identification. They are also inexpensive and quick to produce, especially when compared to most other dosage forms.

In order to make a drug into a tablet, however, the drug needs to be compressible. In other words, when force is placed on the powders in tableting equipment, they must be able to stick together sufficiently to make a durable tablet. Not all powders possess this property. If only small amounts of noncompressible active ingredient are needed, a compressible diluent can be used. Failing that, some materials can be granulated to improve compressibility. This does not work in all cases; if the material remains noncompressible, it may be best to formulate the product as a capsule instead of a tablet.

Types of Immediate-Release Tablets

Type of Tablet	Key Features	Example
Compressed	All ingredients contained in a single layer; designed to be swallowed whole; may or may not be coated	Various
Multi-compressed	Contain separate layers of drug, for various reasons (incompatibility of drugs, immediate- plus extended-release in the same tablet, etc.)	Mucinex (guaifenesin)
Chewable	Disintegrate rapidly when chewed; usually mannitol-based (pleasant mouth feel, sweet taste)	Children's vitamins Dilantin Infatabs (phenytoin)
Buccal	Dissolved in cheek cavity; may be designed to erode slowly or quickly	Fentora (fentanyl)
Sublingual	Dissolve under the tongue; erode quickly and are absorbed rapidly	Nitroglycerin tablets
Effervescent	Contain drug that dissolves rapidly after adding to water; results in carbonated liquid that masks taste	Alka Seltzer

Many immediate-release tablets are coated. This process can help mask unpleasant tastes and odors, as well as improve the appearance of the tablet, protect the drug from the atmosphere, and allow it to be swallowed more easily. The two types of coating used for immediate-release products are sugar and film coatings. Sugar coating produces a very attractive tablet that is typically much larger than the uncoated product, due to the several layers of sugar, color, flavor, and waterproofing shellac added. The process is very time-consuming, and batch variations are common in the coated tablets. The coatings are applied manually in coating pans, not mechanically, by highly skilled personnel. Film coatings are much thinner, and leave a coat of opaque, colored polymer on the surface of the tablet. Although they are customarily machine-applied, requiring less skill in application, many coating defects are possible:

- Picking and peeling: Film fragments flake from the tablet surface
- Orange-peel effect: Coating leaves rough surface on the tablet
- Mottling: Coating has uneven color distribution
- Bridging: Score lines or logos present on tablet are filled in by coating
- Erosion: Coating solution is in contact with tablet for too long and disfigures the core

Extended Release

Extended-release oral products maintain more constant blood levels than do immediate-release products. Because of this, patients can take the drugs less often (once or twice a day instead of up to four times), which improves adherence. Adverse effects are usually fewer and less severe, as the concentration of the drug in the blood does not vary as widely from peak and trough as much as with immediate-release products. There is a risk of dose-dumping, however, especially if the patient chews the medicine instead of swallowing it whole.

Drugs that are best suited for extended release are usually given in fairly small doses, as the practical limit for the amount of drug to be contained in an individual tablet or capsule is 500 mg. The drug should also not have either a particularly fast or slow rate of absorption: Drugs that absorb too quickly require too large a dose, and drugs that absorb slowly are inherently long-acting and an extended-release formulation is not needed. Because of the risk of dose-dumping, the drug should have a good margin of safety and be uniformly absorbed from the GI tract. Different methods of achieving extended release are given in the table below.

Types of Extended-Release Tablets and Coatings

Type of Tablet		Key Features	Example
Enteric coat		Coating remains intact until drug reaches small intestine; can protect drug from stomach acid and enzymes, or stomach from irritating drugs	Enteric-coated aspirin
Diffusion-controlled reservoir system		Beads or pellets are coated with polymer that releases drug at varying speeds; may involve several release rates	Theo-Dur (theophylline)
Diffusion-controlled matrix system		Drug is mixed into an inert plastic matrix; drug dissolves and leaves matrix	
	Wax	Remains intact in GI tract and is eliminated in feces; inform patient that this is normal	Desoxyn Gradumet (methamphetamine)
	Hydrophilic	Water causes matrix to swell; drug diffuses through gel layer, and may also be released as matrix erodes	Slo-Niacin (niacin)
Dissolution-controlled system		Rate of release affected by dissolution and tablet or bead erosion (some hydrophilic matrices fall into this category as well as diffusion-controlled)	Cardizem CD (diltiazem)
Ion-exchange resin		pH conditions of GI tract cause drug to be released from resin	Ionamin (phentermine resin)
Osmotically controlled system		Tablet pulls water into system, then releases drug at controlled rate by osmotic pressure; tablet shell eliminated in feces	Glucotrol XL (glipizide)
Complex formation		Drug is combined with other agents, forming a slowly soluble chemical complex	Rynatan allergy products

Rapid Release

Rapid-release products are becoming more important, particularly in the over-the-counter (OTC) industry. Because they can be taken without water, they are convenient for the patient, and they have a rapid onset of action. Some of the products are very soft, however, and they may require expensive protective packaging.

Types of Rapid-Release Solid Dosage Forms

Type of Product	Key Features	Example
Tablets	Product can contain large doses of drug	Claritin RediTabs
Strips	Dissolves before sick children can spit it out; cannot put large doses of drug into product	Triaminic Thin Strips
Lollipops	Absorbed through buccal mucosa	Fentanyl Actiq

Oral Delivery: Liquids

Oral liquid dosage forms have the same advantages as other oral products, with the additional advantage of being easy to swallow for small children and others who cannot easily swallow solid dosage forms. Several disadvantages exist as well. Liquids are less portable and convenient than solids. Incorrect doses are much more likely, as patients or caregivers could measure using an inappropriate measuring device (i.e., not all spoons are standard size), and product may be spilled before being consumed. Also, taste can be a large issue, as more of the drug will reach a patient's taste buds than with the same drug in a tablet or capsule.

Solvents

Water is the most common solvent for pharmaceutical products; purified water prepared by distillation, reverse osmosis, or ion-exchange treatment is acceptable for oral use. Other commonly used solvents include ethyl alcohol, glycerin, sorbitol, propylene glycol, and some edible oils. Typically, solvents other than water are included to improve solubility and, in some cases, add sweetness to the final product (glycerin, sorbitol, and propylene glycol). Only small amounts of sorbitol and glycerin should be present in a given dose of liquid, however, as they may act as osmotic laxatives in higher quantities.

Types of Liquids

Single-phase liquid dosage forms are all variants of the solution. One or more soluble substances are dissolved in one or more solvents, including water. Therefore, the drug(s) must be water-soluble and stable in aqueous solution. The presence of other excipients in varying amounts results in the following designations:

Types of Single-Phase Liquid Dosage Forms

Type of Product	Key Features	Examples
Syrups	• Contain sugar or sugar substitutes • Little or no alcohol • Thickeners improve mouth feel and physically conceal the drug from taste buds • Taste pleasant; often used with children	• Various cough/cold preparations
Elixirs	• By definition alcoholic, but some nonalcoholic commercial products are mislabeled as elixirs • Slightly sweet; artificial sweetener usually used since sucrose is not very soluble in alcohol • Less viscous than syrups	• Diphenhydramine • Phenobarbital • Digoxin
Tinctures	• 15–80% alcohol • Usually consist of drug extracted from plant material • Unpleasant taste; not commonly used today	• Laudanum (opium tincture; 1,000 mg morphine/100 mL) • Paregoric (camphorated opium tincture; 40 mg morphine/100 mL)
Spirits	• Alcoholic solutions of aromatic or volatile substances • High concentration of alcohol • Active ingredient may precipitate out when added to aqueous preparations	• Flavoring agents
Aromatic waters	• Aqueous solutions of volatile oils • Very dilute	• Flavoring and perfuming agents
Fluid extracts	• Similar to, but more potent than, tinctures • Used as drug source, not as dosage form	

Multiphase liquids are more complicated than single-phase liquids. They still possess most of the advantages and disadvantages of other liquid dosage forms but have the additional disadvantage of being nonhomogenous. Because of this, suspensions and emulsions should always have "Shake Well" labels attached.

Suspensions are multiphase products that contain finely divided solid particles distributed through the liquid phase. They can be used on the skin, used in the ear or eye, or given by intramuscular (IM) or subcutaneous (SC) injection, but are most commonly given by mouth. Some advantages exist over single-phase liquids: Drugs that have an unpleasant flavor are preferred as suspensions, since the drug does not interact with the taste buds as much when it is not dissolved. Also, drugs that have poor stability in water do not degrade as readily in suspension as they do in solution.

The primary concern with making suspensions is to have a particle size that is small enough to remain suspended in the dispersion medium of choice while not being so small that the particles start to attract each other and form clumps that will not resuspend. This can be achieved by two techniques, used separately or in combination: Use of structured vehicles and controlled flocculation.

- Structured vehicles: Increase viscosity and slow the sedimentation of suspended particles. Natural and synthetic polymer solutions are often used (cellulose gels, acacia, bentonite).
- Controlled flocculation: Add materials that promote loose aggregation of suspended particles, but that keep their surfaces apart, by charge or interaction of polymer chains. Settle, but loosely, and resuspend easily.

Emulsions are dispersions that consist of nonmiscible liquids. The dispersed phase is also called the internal phase, and the dispersion medium is called the external phase. These products are very thermodynamically unstable and require an emulsifying agent to keep them combined properly. A good nonpharmacy example is mayonnaise. Lemon juice or vinegar serves as the external phase, and the lecithin from the egg yolk emulsifies the product so that the oil that is added does not separate out.

Only oil-in-water (O/W) emulsions are used for oral dosage forms, as water needs to be in the external phase to be palatable to the patient; otherwise, all the patient would taste would be the oil in the outer portion of the product. Topical products can be either O/W or W/O. When prepared in the pharmacy, emulsions are made by rapid stirring in a mortar and pestle, shaking in a bottle (though only with reasonably thin oils), or using a hand blender, or by heating the phases separately and then mixing them. Three types of emulsifiers are used, depending on the product being made:

- Surfactants: Contain hydrophilic and hydrophobic portions, which remain at the interface of the oil and water phases to stabilize the product. Often used in combination.
- Hydrophilic colloids: Water-soluble polymers that form a film around oil droplets in O/W emulsions. Tend to increase viscosity of the product.
- Finely divided solids: Form a film of particles around the droplets of the dispersed phase, but allow interaction with the dispersion medium as well.

The exact quantity of surfactant needed can be determined by the hydrophilic-lipophilic balance (HLB) system. Surfactants and the ingredients to be emulsified have been assigned experimentally determined HLB numbers, and the exact amount of emulsifier needed can be determined algebraically if a formula has not already been determined.

Topical Delivery

Topical products are used for three primary reasons: To protect injured areas of the skin from the environment, to hydrate the skin, and to apply medication to the skin for local effect. In some cases, drug may reach the blood supply and be systemically absorbed; this is not desired with topical delivery. Systemic absorption of a drug applied to the skin is known as transdermal drug delivery and is discussed later in this chapter.

Powders and liquids are used as topical delivery systems, though not as frequently as semisolid preparations. Of the types of liquids mentioned in the oral delivery section, solutions, suspensions, and emulsions may all be used topically. Two external-use–only liquid products are:

- Liniments: Alcoholic solutions used to irritate the skin and relieve more deep-seated pain or discomfort (Heet, Absorbine Jr), or oleaginous emulsions used as emollients or protective agents. Liniments are applied by rubbing and are not suitable for application to bruised or broken skin.

- Collodions: Contain pyroxylin in an alcohol/ether base that evaporates, leaving an occlusive film on the skin; used to hold edges of incised wounds together.

Ointment Bases

Five types of ointment bases exist:

- Hydrocarbon/oleaginous: Greasy, petroleum-based products used for emollient effect (Vaseline, petrolatum)
- Anhydrous absorption: Greasy products that form W/O emulsions when aqueous solutions are added; can be used to incorporate solutions into an otherwise lipophilic base (hydrophilic petrolatum, anhydrous lanolin)
- W/O emulsion: Similar to anhydrous absorption bases, but already contain some water (hydrous lanolin, cold cream)
- O/W emulsion (water-removable): Creamy emulsions that are easily washed from the skin; may be diluted with water to form lotions (hydrophilic ointment, Lubriderm)
- Water-soluble: Greaseless, water-washable bases containing no oleaginous compounds; cannot add large amounts of water or will soften too much (polyethylene glycol ointment)

Particular bases are chosen on the basis of the desired rate of drug release, stability of the drug in the base, the need for an occlusive barrier, and ability to wash the ointment easily from the skin. When preparing ointments in a pharmacy, if a levigating agent is needed, it should be compatible with the type of ointment base used. For instance, mineral oil will mix well with any ointment base containing hydrocarbons (all except water-soluble bases). Water-miscible liquids such as glycerin and PEG will be more appropriate when using bases that contain water, such as water-soluble or emulsion bases. If solutions need to be incorporated into an ointment base, acceptable options are anhydrous absorption base or either type of emulsion base.

Other topical product definitions are:

- **Creams:** Terminology often used to describe emulsion bases; soft, cosmetically acceptable topical products

- **Pastes:** Very thick semisolids containing at least 20% solids by weight
- **Gels:** Jelly-like dispersions that are water-soluble, water-washable, and greaseless

Rectal, Vaginal, and Urethral Delivery

Rectal, vaginal, and urethral dosage forms such as suppositories and enemas are less frequently prescribed than many other types of dosage form, but they do have an important place in certain types of therapy. They can be useful for local therapy in rectal or vaginal conditions, or when protecting susceptible drugs from GI tract degradation or first-pass metabolism.

Rectal conditions amenable to local therapy with suppositories, enemas, or other rectally administered dosage forms include hemorrhoids, rectal itching, ulcerative colitis, and constipation.

Rectal suppositories can also be used to administer drug for systemic absorption. Usually, this is done when the patient cannot or will not take medication by mouth. Infants, small children, and severely debilitated patients cannot easily swallow. Patients with severe nausea (as a symptom of a condition such as gastroenteritis or migraine, or as a side effect of chemotherapy or anesthesia) cannot hold down oral antiemetics long enough for the medication to take effect; several medications (chlorpromazine, prochlorperazine, and trimethobenzamide) are given rectally to avoid this problem.

Vaginal dosing, including suppositories, creams, and other dosage forms, is usually used for local effect, either for treatment of local infections (clindamycin and -azole antifungals) or for contraception (nonoxynol-9). Hormone replacement may also be administered via vaginal cream or suppository, and will have local effects on the vaginal mucosa. Systemic absorption may be seen with higher estrogen doses.

Urethral suppositories are seldom seen. Alprostadil was approved in 1997 for use in impotence (as Muse urethral suppository) but is not commonly used now that oral medications are available and more readily acceptable to patients.

The most common bases used in suppositories are fatty bases similar to cocoa butter that melt at body temperature, and water-soluble bases such as polyethylene glycol and glycerinated gelatin bases that dissolve slowly in body fluids. Fatty bases are more soothing but do not mix well with body fluids and have a tendency to leak from body orifices. For this reason, they are not suitable for vaginal or urethral delivery. Water-soluble bases can be irritating to the mucosa because they take up water from the area. They are frequently used for vaginal or urethral delivery, but seldom for rectal. Different bases release drugs differently based on the water/oil partition coefficient of the base and of the drug. Lipophilic drugs are released slowly from oleaginous bases but more quickly from water-soluble bases. Hydrophilic drugs, on the other hand, are released extremely quickly from fatty bases but more slowly from water-soluble bases.

Pulmonary Delivery

The lung is an increasingly popular delivery site and is no longer reserved only for pulmonary conditions. The lungs possess a large surface area for drug absorption and a good blood supply that bypasses first-pass metabolism. Even though the first inhaled insulin (Exubera) was a market failure, it proved that large-molecule drugs could be delivered effectively via the lung for systemic use. Continued improvement in delivery devices should cause the field of pulmonary delivery to grow rapidly.

Metered-Dose Inhalers

Metered-dose inhalers (MDIs) are primarily used to deliver medications for the treatment of asthma and chronic obstructive pulmonary disease (COPD): Bronchodilators, steroids, and mast cell stabilizers. While MDIs are portable and able to deliver precise quantities of potent drugs, many patients have difficulty using them properly. MDIs have undergone rapid changes in the last few years, due in part to federal legislation restricting the use of chlorofluorocarbon (CFC) propellants due to their link to ozone depletion. Beginning in 2009, medical device exemptions will no longer be allowed for these propellants, so companies have redesigned their products as either hydrofluoroalkane (HFA) propellant devices or dry-powder inhalers. Significant engineering challenges were involved in converting products to use these new delivery devices.

Dry-Powder Inhalers

Dry-powder inhalers (DPIs) avoid some of the difficulties with MDIs: They are generally easier for patients to use correctly, since the device can be primed before use and the patient does not have to coordinate breath with device actuation. Ease of use, however, depends significantly on the particular type of device. One study indicated that 92% of patients learned to use the Diskus device correctly, whereas only 74% were able to learn proper use of the Turbohaler.

The Diskus is a classic example of the discrete-dose style of DPI. Individual doses are contained in foil packets, protecting them from humidity and allowing for dose consistency if the device is dropped. Some discrete-dose devices are single-dose units, and the drug is added when the device is ready to be actuated (Rotahaler, Aerosilizer, Handihaler); this is often a necessity if a drug is heat-sensitive and must be kept refrigerated until use, such as Spiriva (tiotropium bromide). The Twisthaler, on the other hand, is an example of a reservoir device. All of the doses are contained in a central compartment; and if the device is dropped or exposed to humidity, all doses are affected. Of currently marketed products, only the Twisthaler and Flexhaler are reservoir devices.

Nebulizers

Nebulizers allow the drug to be delivered directly to the lung in high concentration and without the use of propellant. They are particularly useful for uncoordinated or unabled patients, including those who are intubated. Two types exist: Jet and ultrasonic. Jet nebulizers can be used with either solutions or suspensions, and operate by the Bernoulli principle: Compressed air from the machine flows at high speed over the medicated liquid, atomizing it and carrying it to the patient. Ultrasonic nebulizers can only be used with solutions. Ultrasonic nebulizers use the vibrations of high-frequency sound waves to move liquid from the machine through the face mask. Vibrations are timed to coincide with inhalation, so less medication is lost than with the jet nebulizers.

Nasal Delivery

Nasal delivery shares many of the advantages of pulmonary delivery: Drugs that are inactivated by the GI tract or that undergo first-pass metabolism are protected, and large-molecule drugs can be absorbed across the nasal mucosa. The nose has a dense vasculature, which aids in absorption. Viscosity enhancers and mucoadhesives are often included in the formulations to increase residence time, as nasal drainage can be a problem. In addition to the many drugs available via nasal delivery (e.g., oxytocin, desmopressin, calcitonin, and butorphanol tartrate), the route shows promise for vaccine delivery, with FluMist being the first approved example.

The most commonly used nasal products are saline solutions for dry nasal mucosa, nasal decongestants, and intranasal steroids. Nasal decongestants are adrenergic agents that constrict the nasal vasculature, shrinking the nasal mucosa and making breathing easier. Overuse can lead to a phenomenon called rhinitis medicamentosa (rebound congestion), so patients should be cautioned to use the products only as directed and for no longer than 3 to 5 days. Intranasal steroids are commonly prescribed for allergic rhinitis; they may be administered in pump spray containers or as metered-dose aerosols.

Parenteral Delivery

Injectable products have many advantages over other dosage forms but also have more potential complications. No drug is lost to first-pass metabolism or acid- or enzyme-mediated degradation in the GI tract, which makes injection a particularly useful route for protein drug delivery. The rate of delivery can be accurately controlled; and drug, nutrients, and fluids can be given when other routes cannot be used. However, injectable drugs must be prepared and administered by highly trained personnel and cannot be retrieved once given. Additionally, the products must be sterile, free from undesired particulate matter, and pyrogen-free.

Sterilization Methods Used in Industry

Method	How Does It Work?	Advantages	Disadvantages	Products Sterilized by This Method
Steam sterilization	Heat coagulates and kills microorganisms	• Method of choice when applicable • Lower heat than dry heat sterilization	• Cannot use with heat- or moisture-sensitive drugs • Autoclave can have cools spots	• Aqueous solutions in closed containers • Surgical Instruments • Glassware
Dry heat sterilization	Heat coagulates and kills microorganisms	• Useful for moisture-sensitive material	• Cannot use with heat-sensitive drugs • Autoclave can have cool spots	• Glassware • Surgical equipment • Oleaginous materials • Powders • Moisture-sensitive material
Filtration	Bacteria and particulate matter are physically removed by membrane filters	• Inexpensive	• Technique failure • Membrane defects • Drug can absorb to membrane	• Small volumes of thin liquid • Heat-sensitive liquid formulations
Ionizing radiation	Gamma radiation mutates and kills bacteria		• Expensive setup	• Sterilizing plastic medical devices
Gas sterilization	Ethylene and propylene oxide gases alkylate microbial protein	• Good for heat- and moisture-sensitive materials	• Possibility of toxic residue • Explosion hazard • Expensive setup • Cannot penetrate glass to sterilize material in sealed containers	• Heat-sensitive material • Moisture-sensitive material • Medical and surgical equipment wrapped in plastic

Multiple-dose injectable products must contain preservative in order to ensure that the product remains sterile after the initial use. Large-volume, single-use products, however, cannot contain preservative, as the amount required to reach an effective concentration would lead to preservative-related toxicity. In addition to sterilization and preservation intended to decrease the likelihood of microbial growth in the product, steps must be taken to ensure that pyrogens (lipopolysaccharides from gram-negative bacterial cell walls that cause high fever, hypertension, and chills) are not present.

The main routes of injectable delivery are intravenous (IV), subcutaneous (SC), and intramuscular (IM). Intravenous products must be solutions or O/W emulsions (e.g., Intralipid, a component of total parenteral nutrition), as particulate matter could lead to phlebitis and other complications. SC and IM injections may be solutions or emulsions; however, they may also be suspensions, which exhibit slower absorption since the drug must go into solution in the tissue before being absorbed into the bloodstream. In the case of some injectable suspensions, such as the contraceptive Depo-Provera (medroxy-progesterone acetate), release of medication can continue for several months, improving patient convenience. Some products are given by other injectable routes: Allergy tuberculosis testing is handled by intradermal injection; hydrocortisone is frequently injected directly into the joint (intra-articular) in arthritic patients; anesthesia is often injected into the epidural space (around the nerve roots of the spine); and anesthetics, some drugs used to treat meningitis, and some chemotherapy agents are injected into the intrathecal (subarachnoid) space (into the cerebrospinal fluid) to bypass the blood-brain barrier.

Ocular and Otic Delivery

Drug delivery to the eye is complicated by two factors: Drug loss due to blinking and lacrimal drainage, and poor drug penetration through the corneal membrane. Polymers are typically used as viscosity enhancers to prolong retention time and reduce lacrimal drainage; some, such as hyaluronic acid, have mild adhesive properties that prolong retention time even further. Drop size reduction can also serve to improve ocular availability; only about 10 mcL of fluid remains in the conjunctival cul-de-sac after blinking, so dose volumes larger than this lead to waste.

Drug penetration into the eye can be improved by creating a prodrug that is more lipophilic than the original compound. It is then converted to the active substance by enzymes in the body.

Most ocular products are solutions, but suspensions, ointments, and gels may also be used. These dosage forms prolong drug contact with the eye and may be preferable in some situations. Drug contact may also be prolonged by the use of an ophthalmic insert (Pilocarpine Ocusert system); these small inserts are placed in the cul-de-sac of the eye and release the drug over a 7-day period, improving patient adherence with glaucoma therapy.

Ocular products must be sterile when dispensed, and all multidose products must contain preservative. This helps prevent serious ocular infections, which can lead to corneal ulcers and blindness.

Otic products are generally solutions or suspensions, which frequently contain glycerin or propylene glycol to increase viscosity and maximize contact between the product and the ear canal. The hygroscopic nature of these solvents also helps them draw moisture out of the tissues, which can reduce inflammation and decrease the amount of moisture available for any microorganisms to grow. Most otic products fall into one of the following categories:

- Anti-infective and anti-inflammatory products: May contain analgesics and local anesthetics to reduce pain associated with otitis externa or otitis media

- Ear-wax removal agents: Contain surfactants (which emulsify ear wax) or peroxides (which release oxygen and disrupt the integrity of the ear wax), allowing easy removal

Transdermal Delivery

Transdermal delivery differs from topical delivery in that the drug is intended for systemic use. The drug molecules must therefore be small enough to penetrate the stratum corneum and reach the general circulation. Some transdermal ointments (nitroglycerin ointment) exist, but most products are available as transdermal delivery systems (patches).

Patches

Transdermal patches attach to the skin with adhesive and contain the drug either in a polymer matrix or in a drug reservoir covered by a rate-controlling membrane. An excess of drug is typically present to ensure that a concentration gradient exists, causing drug to exit the patch and enter the skin passively. Patches provide more uniform blood levels than conventional release products and can improve patient compliance since, depending on the drug, they can be worn for 1 to 7 days. GI absorption problems and first-pass metabolism are avoided. A wide range of drugs are now available in patches, including nitroglycerin, nicotine, and hormones (for birth control or hormone replacement therapy).

Ultrasound

Drug can be transported across skin by mixing it with a coupling agent and using ultrasonic energy to disrupt the stratum corneum and increase penetrability. This method of delivery is not common, but high-dose hydrocortisone can be delivered in this fashion.

Iontophoresis

This method of transdermal delivery is not widely used but is gaining popularity. It involves delivery of charged compounds across the skin by applying an electrical current. Since the skin is disrupted, larger molecules may pass than is possible with transdermal patches. Local anesthesia (Numby Stuff) and fentanyl (IONSYS) are available in small iontophoretic patches, and the method is being investigated to deliver protein drugs.

LEARNING POINTS

- A drug cannot work until it is absorbed. It cannot be absorbed until it is dissolved.

- Ionized, hydrophilic drugs dissolve more readily; un-ionized, lipophilic drugs are absorbed more easily.

- Focus on why a particular dosage form might work better for a particular condition or with a particular drug.

- Consider nonoral routes for drugs that undergo extensive first-pass metabolism.

- At this time, protein drugs can be given only by injectable or pulmonary routes. There is future potential with nasal delivery.

PRACTICE QUESTIONS

1. Which of the following dosage forms must be sterile?

    (A) Ophthalmic suspension
    (B) Oral suspension
    (C) Topical suspension
    (D) Suspension for rectal administration
    (E) Otic suspension

2. A 15-year old patient with ADHD who had been stable on a dose of 10 mg BID of Focalin is transitioning to Focalin XR 20 mg QD. After 2 weeks, he returns to the doctor complaining of distractedness during school and a jittery feeling in the morning an hour or two after taking his medication. When asked how he is taking his medication, he states that due to difficulty swallowing he has been opening the capsules of Focalin XR and mixing them with chunky applesauce, which he chews before swallowing. How do you explain the patient's current symptoms?

    (A) The new dose of Focalin XR is too high and should be reduced.
    (B) The patient is experiencing dose-dumping because he is opening the capsules.
    (C) The patient is experiencing dose-dumping because he is chewing the capsule contents with the applesauce.
    (D) The severity of the patient's ADHD has increased and he is suffering from a new-onset anxiety disorder.
    (E) The patient is experiencing dose-dumping because the capsule contents are interacting with the applesauce.

3. What environmental advantage do HFA inhalers have over CFC inhalers?

    (A) They contain less packaging.
    (B) They are less likely to lead to ozone depletion.
    (C) They do not contain mercury.
    (D) They are a pump spray instead of an aerosol spray.
    (E) They do not use petroleum-based mineral oil as an emulsifier.

ANSWERS

1. **A**

All ophthalmic dosage forms must be sterile, and either packaged in single-dose containers or formulated to contain a preservative. Sterility is not required for any of the other routes, as the drug is being applied either to an epithelial surface (topical, otic) or to the GI mucosa (oral, rectal). These surfaces are not sterile in their natural state, and dosage forms applied to them need not be sterile.

2. **C**

Focalin XR derives its extended-release properties from a coating on the beads contained within the capsule. It is therefore appropriate to open the capsule and consume the contents with food or in liquid; applesauce is specifically mentioned in the manufacturer instructions as appropriate. However, crushing or chewing the beads destroys the coating, causing dose-dumping. The patient's jitteriness in the morning and inattention later in the day are symptomatic of too high a dose being absorbed in the morning, and too little medication remaining in his system later in the day.

3. **B**

HFA inhalers were designed to replace CFC inhalers, which are being phased out due to the Montreal Protocol and the effect of CFCs on ozone depletion. HFA inhalers are similar in size to CFC inhalers. Neither type of product contains the other excipients mentioned in the question.

Biopharmaceutics

 Suggested Study Time: **2–3 hours**

Biopharmaceutics deal with the relationship between the physicochemical properties of a drug; the dosage form in which the drug is available; and its route of administration, with the rate and extent of its absorption and elimination from the body. It is the science that links together traditional pharmaceutics (physical pharmacy and dosage form design) with pharmacokinetics. The acronym LADME (liberation, absorption, distribution, metabolism, and excretion) is often used to describe the main processes addressed by biopharmaceutics.

DRUG LIBERATION AND ABSORPTION

A key concept to remember is that drugs are administered as dosage forms, not individual chemicals. Once taken, they must first be liberated from the dosage form in question and absorbed into the bloodstream before they become available in the systemic circulation. The exception is intravenously administered drugs, as they are delivered directly into the systemic circulation.

Liberation from a dosage form can be as simple as powder from a capsule being released from the capsule shell after ingestion, or as complicated as the slow release of drug from a tablet or transdermal patch matrix. Oral compressed tablets are the most commonly dispensed dosage form; in this case, liberation of the drug requires disintegration of the tablet into smaller drug particles that then undergo dissolution.

If the drug is not already in solution within the dosage form (as in an oral syrup or elixir), it must first undergo dissolution. Undissolved drug particles cannot cross biological membranes and are therefore trapped at their location of administration. For oral dosage forms, this means the gastrointestinal (GI) tract; any drug not absorbed is lost in the feces. In the case of an eyedrop given in suspension form, the drug particles remain on the corneal surface until the drug either dissolves and passes through the corneal membrane or is lost via lacrimal drainage. Similarly, topical products remain on the skin surface, and intramuscular and subcutaneous injections remain in the tissues until the drug is dissolved in the body fluids.

The rate and extent to which the drug contained in the dosage forms described above is absorbed into the systemic circulation is the bioavailability. This property plays a very important role in the biopharmaceutics and pharmacokinetics of drugs. The liberation and dissolution of a drug can be affected by processing factors and excipients, which can in turn affect bioavailability. Other factors affecting bioavailability are addressed later in this chapter.

One physicochemical property that can affect bioavailability is particle size. Decreasing the particle size of a drug formulation increases the surface area, which leads to more rapid dissolution. This is an important factor for drugs with low water solubility; finely milling or micronizing drugs such as griseofulvin and nitrofurantoin can dramatically improve their oral bioavailability.

Many excipients can affect product bioavailability. Some examples are listed in the table below.

Excipients That Affect Product Bioavailability

Excipient Category	Examples	Effect on Drug Particles	Effect on Bioavailability
Disintegrants	Starch, microcrystalline cellulose	Breaks tablet into smaller particles, increases dissolution	Possible increase
Surfactants	Tweens, Spans	Low concentration: Decrease surface tension and increase dissolution rate	Possible increase
		High concentration: Form micelles with drug inside, decrease dissolution	Possible decrease
Lubricants	Magnesium stearate	Has tendency to waterproof particles in large concentration, making them less soluble	Possible decrease

Drug Transport Across Membranes

There are several ways for drugs to cross body membranes that you should be aware of: Passive diffusion, carrier-mediated transport, endocytosis, and drug efflux. In passive diffusion, the drug crosses cell membranes based on a concentration gradient, moving from regions of higher concentration to areas of (relatively) lower concentration. For this mechanism to be practical, the drug must be small enough to be absorbed across cells and lipid-soluble enough to interact with the cell membranes. The rate of transport is described by Fick's first law of diffusion:

$$\frac{dC}{dt} = \frac{DA(C_s - C)}{h}$$

While it is unlikely that the exam will require you to perform calculations based on this equation, you should be familiar with the items that affect it: The concentration gradient ($C_S - C$), the thickness of the membrane being crossed (h), the surface area of the membrane (A), and the diffusion coefficient of the drug (D).

As would be expected, drugs diffuse more slowly through thicker membranes. Body locations with larger surface area tend to promote faster diffusion, as there is more available membrane through which the drug molecule can diffuse. The small intestine is thus a prime location for drug absorption, as the surface area is very large due to the presence of villi and microvilli.

Another key factor to remember is that the GI membranes are more permeable to drug in the un-ionized form. Solubility of weakly acidic drugs therefore increases as the drug moves from the stomach to the intestines; solubility of weakly basic drugs decreases. Because of this, poorly soluble, weakly basic drugs may be poorly absorbed if taken with drugs that reduce gastric acid secretion. Ketoconazole and dipyridamole both exhibit reduced rate and extent of absorption when taken with H_2 blockers such as cimetidine or with proton pump inhibitors such as omeprazole.

Not all drugs are absorbed by passive diffusion; many undergo carrier-mediated transport processes. Active transport, which requires input of energy and occurs against a concentration gradient, is the most common type. Unlike passive diffusion, the process can be saturated or competitively inhibited by chemically similar substrates. Many drugs are transported via transport systems designed to move amino acids and vitamins across cell walls (see table on next page). Some drugs undergo simultaneous passive diffusion and active transport.

Active Transport Mechanisms for Drugs in the Body

Transporter	Drugs Transported
Peptide	• Penicillins • Cephalosporins • ACE inhibitors
Nucleoside	• Anticancer/antiviral nucleosides
Amino acid	• L-dopa • Methyldopa

Facilitated diffusion is another carrier-mediated transport process; it differs from active transport in that it occurs only from high to low concentrations. As with active transport, the transporter may bind to structurally similar inhibitors, which will decrease the transport rate of the drug. If the inhibitor is present in high concentration, the transporter may become saturated. Furosemide, morphine, and dopamine are examples of drugs that undergo facilitated diffusion.

Macromolecules are most likely to cross cell membranes by endocytosis, a process in which substances are transported across cell membranes by formation of vesicles. Most endocytosis is receptor-mediated; nonreceptor-mediated endocytosis is called either phagocytosis (engulfment of solid particles) or pinocytosis (engulfment of liquid), and is often seen in the GI tract and lungs. Protein and peptide drugs such as insulin, erythropoietin, and growth hormone are transported in this fashion. Polio and other oral vaccines are absorbed from the GI tract by phagocytosis, a specific type of endocytosis that is not receptor mediated.

The final method of drug transport with which you should be concerned is drug efflux. In this case, transporters pump drugs and other substances out of cells rather than into them. P-glycoprotein is the key efflux protein, and is linked to multidrug resistance in tumor cells. In this case, resistance occurs because the transporter pumps drug back out of the tumor before it can accumulate to an effective concentration. In addition, p-glycoprotein can reduce net absorption (and hence bioavailability) of other drugs by routing them out of the plasma and back into the lumen of the GI tract. Digoxin, steroids, and immunosuppressive agents are just a few of the drugs that can be affected in this way.

Barriers to Drug Absorption

Several factors can affect drug absorption. Not only must the drug dissolve initially, it must stay in solution during the absorption process itself. The pH of the GI tract varies significantly, and a drug that is in solution at the low pH of the stomach may be less soluble in the higher pH of the small intestine. Food intake can affect absorption and bioavailability in a variety of ways, including increasing the pH in the stomach, which can in turn affect drug dissolution and absorption (increasing dissolution and absorption for weak acids, and decreasing both for weak bases). Chemical stability may be affected as well, which can in turn lower the amount of drug available for absorption.

Food-Related Absorption and Bioavailability Variations

Process	Explanation	Examples
Food-drug complexation	Can bind and make drug insoluble; prevent absorption	Tetracycline complexes with calcium and iron in food and supplements
Alteration of pH	Food acts as buffer in stomach; increases pH	• Increases dissolution (and subsequent absorption) of weak acids • Decreases dissolution of weak bases
Gastric emptying	Foods (especially fatty ones) and some drugs slow gastric emptying and delay drug onset	
Gastric acid secretions	• Pepsin may increase drug metabolism • Bile salts increase dissolution of poorly soluble drugs, but can form complexes with other drugs	Bile acid-drug complexes: Neomycin, kanamycin, nystatin
Competition for specialized absorption mechanisms	Competitive inhibition of drugs by nutrients with similar chemical structures	
Increased volume and viscosity of GI contents	Presence of food can lead to: • Slower drug dissolution • Slower diffusion of dissolved drug from GI tract	
Food-induced changes in first-pass metabolism	Increased bioavailability due to inhibited cytochrome P450 (primarily CYP3A)	Grapefruit juice ingestions lead to increased bioavailability of: • Cyclosporin • Saquinavir • Verapamil
Food-induced changes in blood flow	• Giving some drugs with food increases bioavailability due to increased blood flow to the GI tract and liver following a meal • A larger fraction of drug escapes first-pass metabolism because the enzyme system becomes overwhelmed	Drugs with metabolism sensitive to rate of presentation to liver: • Propranolol • Hydralazine

DRUG DISTRIBUTION

Once in the bloodstream, some drug may be bound to the plasma proteins while the remainder remains unbound. A key point to remember is that only drug that is unbound can pass out of the plasma to reach the site of action. The amount of drug that is bound to plasma protein is in dynamic equilibrium with the amount that is not.

Volume of Distribution

In the average 70-kg (~155-lb) patient, blood volume is approximately 5 L and total body water is about 40 L. After absorption, a drug will distribute into the body fluids; since the total amount of drug placed into the body is known and the concentration of drug in the body can be measured, the volume of fluid through which the drug seems to have distributed can be determined. This volume is referred to as the *apparent* volume of distribution, because it is not a physical volume. Rather, it is a calculated number, dependent on physicochemical properties of the drug, which helps compare the behavior of different drugs.

$$V_d = \frac{dose}{C_p}$$ when dose = IV bolus and C_p is measured immediately after injection

Different types of drugs show very different apparent volumes of distribution:

- Macromolecules: Too large to distribute into the capillaries; V_d will equal plasma volume of individual (about 3 L)
- Small polar drugs: Not lipophilic enough to enter intracellular fluid; V_d will equal plasma + interstitial fluid volume (about 12 L)
- Small lipophilic drugs: Can diffuse into cells; V_d will equal total body water (about 40 L)

Plasma Protein Binding

The above examples all assume that the drug does not bind to plasma proteins. Most drugs do, however, exhibit protein binding, and this greatly affects their volume of distribution. Proteins are large molecules that cannot leave the capillaries; therefore, the drug-protein complex remains in the plasma. However, since the concentration of protein-bound drug is not usually measured, protein binding will cause a decrease in the free plasma concentration of the drug, increasing the apparent volume of distribution. As protein binding is reversible, equilibrium exists between bound and free drug. As free drug distributes out of the bloodstream, bound drug is released from plasma proteins to maintain the equilibrium.

Although plasma proteins are relatively nonspecific in their binding behavior, the different proteins do tend to bind to different types of drug:

- Albumin: Weak acids
- α_1-acid glycoprotein: Weak bases
- Lipoproteins: Basic and neutral drugs
- Globulins: Steroids, vitamins, metal ions

Dosing a highly protein-bound drug based only on physiological volumes (plasma volume, interstitial volume, or total body water) may not produce a high enough concentration at the site of drug action to yield adequate pharmacological response. Therefore, a higher dose may need to be given. The protein-drug complex may also act as a drug reservoir, prolonging action in the body. These factors must be considered when determining dose and dosing frequency. Certain disease states can alter the levels of plasma proteins significantly enough to require drug dose adjustments. Additionally, if a patient is receiving several drugs that all bind to the same plasma protein, one drug may displace another, leading to higher-than-expected drug concentrations and possible toxicity. This is most important in drugs that are more than 95% bound, particularly if they have a narrow therapeutic index. Warfarin (99% bound) is an excellent example of this.

Some Disease States and Physiological Conditions That Affect Plasma Protein Concentration

Decrease plasma protein concentration	• Liver disease • Trauma (albumin) • Surgery (albumin) • Burns • Renal failure (albumin) • Hyperthyroidism • Age (neonate, geriatric) • Pregnancy
Increase plasma protein concentration	• Hypothyroidism • Schizophrenia • Rheumatoid arthritis • Renal failure (α_1-acid glycoprotein) • Trauma (α_1-acid glycoprotein) • Surgery (α_1-acid glycoprotein)

DRUG METABOLISM

Drugs are eliminated from the body by two processes: Metabolism and excretion. Metabolism, also referred to as biotransformation, leads to the chemical conversion of drug to active or inactive compounds called metabolites. These metabolites are generally more polar (and hence more water-soluble) than the parent drugs. This allows the metabolites to be more efficiently cleared in the urine. Not all drugs undergo metabolism.

Metabolism is most likely to occur in organs that contain high levels of enzymes. Many microsomal enzymes, including the cytochrome P450 (CYP450) mixed-function oxidases, are found in the liver, which is the primary site of biotransformation. Metabolizing enzymes are found in many other locations of the body, and significant biotransformation of some drugs can occur in the intestinal tract, kidney, and brain. Drugs administered via nasal, pulmonary, or dermal routes often also show significant biotransformation in the nasal tissue, lung, or skin.

One concern with oral delivery of certain drugs is presystemic, or first-pass, metabolism. Because the venous outflow of the GI tract travels directly to the liver via the portal vein, drugs administered via the GI tract are susceptible to hepatic metabolism before they reach the systemic circulation. Bioavailability is decreased, so the drug must be given either in a higher dose or by a delivery route that bypasses the GI tract. Nitroglycerin, for example, is almost completely degraded by first-pass metabolism and is therefore usually formulated as sublingual tablets or spray, or transdermal ointment or patches. Oral extended-release capsules are also available and are believed to work by saturating the hepatic enzymes responsible for metabolism and by producing metabolites that possess some activity.

Phase I Reactions

Metabolism is classified into Phase I and Phase II reactions. In many cases, a drug may undergo metabolism by competing pathways, leading to multiple metabolites. The metabolites may in turn undergo metabolism. Some of these metabolites may possess therapeutic activity. Some medications are deliberately administered as inactive prodrugs, and the therapeutic component results from the metabolism of the prodrug. Formulating a medication as a prodrug can improve its pharmaceutical, pharmacodynamic, or pharmacokinetic properties.

Phase I reactions are so named because they generally occur before Phase II reactions. They are nonsynthetic and introduce or expose a functional group. The primary types of Phase I reactions are oxidation, reduction, and hydrolysis. Oxidation is the most common type of metabolism, and many of these reactions are catalyzed by enzymes in the CYP superfamily.

Phase II Reactions

Phase II reactions are synthetic reactions. They are often called conjugation reactions, as a reactive group on the drug is attached to a polar molecule or group originating inside the body. This generally leads to a polar, water-soluble metabolite. While most drugs undergo Phase I metabolism prior to Phase II, this is not required provided the drug already possesses one or more reactive groups.

Examples of Phase II reactions are listed in the table on the next page, with glucuronidation being the most common example. Since these reactions involve enzymes, the reactions may be capacity limited. If the concentration of drug approaches or exceeds the metabolic capacity of the enzyme, nonlinear drug metabolism may be observed.

Two types of conjugation reactions (methylation and acetylation) lead to metabolites that are less polar, and therefore less soluble, than the original compound. Less soluble metabolites will have extended elimination half-lives. This can extend the duration of action in cases where an active metabolite is formed, such as *N*-acetylprocainamide. Toxicity may also occur from increased blood or tissue levels of toxic metabolites. For example, at high concentrations the acetylated metabolites of sulfonamides can precipitate in the kidney tubules and lead to kidney damage and crystalluria.

Phase II Reactions

Type of Phase II Reaction	Drugs Metabolized by This Route
Glucuronidation	• Chloramphenicol • Meprobamate • Morphine
Sulfation	• Acetaminophen • Estradiol • Methyldopa • Minoxidil
Amino acid conjugation	• Salicylic acid
Acetylation	• Isoniazid • Procainamide • Sulfonamides • Hydralazine
Methylation	• Catecholamines • Niacinamide • Thiouracil
Glutathione conjugation	• Chlorambucil

Factors Affecting Biotransformation

Several factors can affect metabolizing enzyme activity in the body. Disease state, age, gender, or chemical and nutritional exposure to a variety of substances can lead to enzyme inhibition or enzyme induction. Genetic variability also plays a role. Drug–drug interactions are a common result of the metabolic process, as most marketed drugs are metabolized by multiple pathways, and drugs that inhibit or induce enzyme activity can affect the metabolism of many other drugs.

Enzyme Inhibition

Enzyme inhibition describes the situation when an enzyme is prevented from binding with its substrate. The substrate is therefore unable to be properly metabolized, and plasma levels rise, possibly to toxic levels. In cases where a prodrug must be activated by metabolism, enzyme inhibition may limit, delay, or prevent drug activity. Enzyme inhibitors can act by competitive or noncompetitive means.

Drugs that are metabolized by the same metabolic pathways frequently act as competitive inhibitors to each other. Drug metabolites, herbal products, and foods can also act as enzyme inhibitors. Compounds containing imidazole, pyridine, or quinolone groups in particular are often found to be enzyme inhibitors. The table below contains an incomplete list of common enzyme inhibitors.

One of the most widely known drug–food interactions results from enzyme inhibition. Grapefruit juice is an inhibitor of CYP3A, the isozyme responsible for metabolism of a host of drugs, including macrolide antibiotics, benzodiazepines, calcium channel blockers, and HIV protease inhibitors. While a single portion is unlikely to lead to problems, patients receiving drugs metabolized by this isozyme should be cautioned to avoid grapefruit juice.

Drugs Involved in Inhibition of Metabolic Enzymes

Calcium channel blockers	• Diltiazem • Verapamil
Macrolide antibiotics	• Erythromycin
Quinolone antibiotics	• Ciprofloxacin • Ofloxacin
Imidazole antifungals	• Ketoconazole • Fluconazole • Lansoprazole • Miconazole
Metronidazole	
Omeprazole	
Cimetidine	

Enzyme Induction

Enzyme induction is essentially the opposite of enzyme inhibition. Enzyme inducers stimulate enzyme activity, which leads to decreased plasma levels of the enzyme's targets. In most cases, this means a decrease in both activity and adverse effects. If active or toxic metabolites are produced, however, drug activity and toxic effects may be increased. A number of commonly prescribed drugs induce metabolic enzymes, as do ethanol, tobacco, marijuana, and certain herbal products, most notably St. John's wort. This can lead to clinically significant drug interactions. For example, triazolam is extensively metabolized by CYP3A4. St. John's wort, rifampin, and several seizure medications (carbamazepine, phenytoin, and phenobarbital) induce this isozyme. Using any of these agents with triazolam or other drugs metabolized by 3A4 will lead to significantly reduced plasma concentrations and therapeutic effect.

Some drugs undergo a phenomenon called auto-induction, wherein they stimulate their own metabolism. Carbamazepine is a key example of a drug of this type. Due to auto-induction, long-term administration of carbamazepine can lead to decreased blood levels and therapeutic activity.

Drugs Involved in Induction of Metabolic Enzymes

Seizure medications	• Carbamazepine • Phenytoin • Phenobarbital • Secobarbital
Tuberculosis medications	• Rifampin • Isoniazid
Prednisone	
Omeprazole	
Modafinil	

Genetic Variability

Genetic polymorphisms lead to a number of metabolism-related issues. "Fast" and "slow" metabolizers exist for particular drugs. Dosage adjustments must be made in order to avoid subtherapeutic consequences or toxic effects, depending on the population into which a patient falls.

CYP enzymes in particular possess a high level of polymorphism. The table on the next page lists select drugs metabolized by the most common CYP enzymes. CYP2D6 in particular can be problematic, as individuals can be classed as poor, intermediate, extensive, and ultrarapid metabolizers. The percentage of poor metabolizers varies somewhat by ancestry, comprising approximately 5–10% of Caucasians, 4% of Blacks, and 1% of Asians. One of the drugs metabolized by CYP2D6 is codeine; in this case, poor metabolizers receive less benefit from the drug, as codeine must be metabolized into morphine to take effect. Pharmacists should be aware of this variability, since poor metabolizers may be falsely labeled as drug-seekers when in fact codeine is an ineffective analgesic for them. These patients should instead be placed on analgesics not activated by CYP2D6, such as morphine itself.

Common Drugs Metabolized by This Pathway

CYP Class	Common CYP Enzymes
1A2	• Caffeine • Theophylline
3A4	• Macrolide antibiotics • Calcium channel blockers • Benzodiazepines – Alprazolam – Midazolam – Triazolam • HIV protease inhibitors
2C9	• Glipizide • Warfarin • Phenytoin
2C19	• Omeprazole • Diazepam
2D6	• Select opioids – Codeine – Dextromethorphan – Hydrocodone – Oxycodone • Fluoxetine • Haloperidol • Tricyclic antidepressants

Glucose-6-phosphate dehydrogenase is an enzyme with over 300 reported polymorphic variants, leading to individuals possessing low, normal, or increased levels of the enzyme. As this enzyme protects red blood cells from oxidative stress, deficiency in combination with certain environmental or pharmacological stresses—such as eating fava beans or taking certain drugs—can lead to life-threatening hemolytic anemia. Prevalence of this deficiency is highest among those of African, Asian, and Mediterranean ancestry, with more severe variants occurring in Mediterranean populations. The high gene frequency in certain populations is believed to be related to its protective effect against malaria.

Substances to Be Avoided in Glucose-6-Phosphate Dehydrogenase Deficiency

> - Oxidant drugs
>   - Primaquine
>   - Chloroquine
> - Sulfonamides
> - Quinolones
> - Aspirin
> - Probenecid
> - Vitamin K
> - Nitrofurantoin
> - Fava beans
> - Mothballs

Acetylation is another important instance of genetic variability in drug metabolism. Rapid-metabolizing and slow-metabolizing polymorphic variants of *N*-acetyl-transferase-2 can have therapeutic implications for several drugs, most notably the tuberculosis drug isoniazid. Slow acetylators do not metabolize the drug quickly, and must be given lower doses in order to prevent toxic effects. Rapid acetylators require substantially higher doses, and therapeutic failure rates are more common than with normal or slow acetylators.

DRUG EXCRETION

The other process by which the body eliminates substances is excretion. Unlike metabolism, excretion eliminates substances without further chemical change. The kidney is the primary organ involved, and most substances are excreted in the urine. Polar, water-soluble drugs are usually excreted unchanged; lipophilic drugs are generally excreted as metabolites. There are three components to renal excretion:

1. Glomerular filtration:
   - Blood passes through the capillary network (glomerulus) inside Bowman's capsule.
   - Fenestrated endothelium allows paracellular transport of most solutes (other than macromolecules) into Bowman's capsule.
   - Filtrate (including drug) moves from Bowman's capsule into renal tubules.
   - All nonprotein-bound, small-molecule drugs undergo glomerular filtration; the concentration of drug or metabolite in the filtrate will be equal to the concentration of unbound drug in the plasma.

2. Tubular reabsorption:

- Many nutrients and ions are actively reabsorbed into the bloodstream.

- Water is reabsorbed, and filtrate becomes more concentrated as it moves along the tubule.

- No transporters exist for reabsorption of drug; passive diffusion process is dependent on filtrate pH. Acidic (citrus fruits, cranberry juice, aspirin) and basic (milk products, sodium bicarbonate) foods and drugs can alter urine pH enough to affect reabsorption.

  » In alkaline urine: Acidic drugs are ionized → less reabsorbed → more readily excreted

  » In acidic urine: Basic drugs are ionized → less reabsorbed → more readily excreted

  » Pentobarbital (weak acid) overdose: Treated by alkalinizing urine with sodium bicarbonate injection

3. Tubular secretion:

- This occurs simultaneously with tubular reabsorption.

- This removes certain substances from the blood and secretes them back into the filtrate.

- This occurs against concentration gradients and is an energy-requiring process that uses protein transporters.

- Only ionized drugs are bound to and secreted by the transporter proteins; drugs that are highly ionized at pH 7.4 will be secreted to a greater extent.

- Plasma protein binding has little effect on this process; transporters can strip drug off of protein.

  » Competitive process; can lead to drug interactions

    - Desirable: Probenecid and penicillin

    - Undesirable: Cimetidine and procainamide

    - Saturable process; at high dose, process plateaus → less drug excreted → higher plasma concentration than expected

The rate of renal excretion of drugs is the net result of the above processes. It depends on blood flow in addition to the physicochemical properties of the drugs in question. More rapid blood flow through the nephron generally leads to an increase in all three processes, with an overall higher drug excretion rate. Glomerular filtration rate (GFR) is normally about 120 mL/min, but may vary widely with the patient's age, size, and disease state. GFR for an individual is determined by calculating the clearance of creatinine, an endogenous substance that is not reabsorbed or secreted. This value gives an indication of kidney function.

Renal clearance is a measure of the efficiency of renal excretion in removing unchanged drug in the urine. It is an indirect measurement expressed by the following equation, where C_U and V_U are concentration of drug in the urine and volume of urine formation per unit time:

$$CL_r = \frac{excretion\ rate\ in\ urine}{plasma\ concentration} = \frac{C_U V_U}{C_p}$$

Nonrenal Excretion

Drugs may also be excreted by the liver into the bile; at this point, one of two things can happen:

- Biliary excretion: Bile (including drug) is emptied into the small intestine, where it is eventually excreted from the body in the feces.
- Enterohepatic recycling: The drug is partially reabsorbed from the intestines (based on pKa and partition coefficient) and re-enters the bloodstream. Drugs undergoing this process may show a secondary peak in plasma concentration; with multiple dosing regimens, the blood-level curve can be altered significantly.

Some drugs are excreted into other fluids, though this is usually not a significant route:

- Saliva: Swallowed, leading to salivary recycling; routine and noninvasive way of monitoring for levels of certain drugs
- Breast milk: Mostly occurs by passive diffusion (primarily of weak bases); can lead to drug transfer to breastfeeding infants
- Sweat: Small volume, so not a significant mode of drug excretion; could become a convenient method for detecting use of illegal or restricted drugs (cocaine, amphetamines, morphine, and ethanol)
- Expired air: Significant route of excretion for volatile drugs (anesthetics, ethanol); drug volatility is more important than polarity for this method of excretion

LEARNING POINTS

- The prime body location for drug absorption is the small intestine, due to the high surface area; the drug must be dissolved in order to be absorbed, however, and factors affecting dissolution in the small intestine (i.e., pH) may prevent this from being the prime absorption location for a particular drug.

- Only drugs that are unbound to plasma protein can pass from the plasma to reach the site of action.

- Enzyme inhibition can often lead to toxicity; enzyme induction can lead to inadequate blood levels of drug.

- Genetic variations in CYP metabolism lead to fast and slow metabolizers of a variety of drugs; dosage adjustments or alternate therapies must be made in some cases.

- Tubular reabsorption decreases drug and metabolite concentration in the urine, while tubular secretion increases the amount. Water-soluble, ionized drugs are more likely to be excreted.

PRACTICE QUESTIONS

1. A single IV dose of a drug is given and the AUC is calculated. After an adequate washout period, a single oral dose of the same drug is given. If the doses are the same size, which of the following results is possible?

   (A) $AUC_{PO} = AUC_{IV}$
   (B) $AUC_{PO} > AUC_{IV}$
   (C) $AUC_{PO} < AUC_{IV}$
   (D) A and B
   (E) A and C

2. The quality control test required for tablets, intended to reflect the absorption of the drug, is the

   (A) weight variation test.
   (B) content uniformity test.
   (C) dissolution test.
   (D) disintegration test.
   (E) friability test.

3. A 15-year-old patient taking Focalin XR for his ADHD is experiencing inattention later in the day. He admits that after having a cold 2 weeks ago, he started taking 2 g of vitamin C per day to "boost his immune system." What do you think is causing his symptoms?

   (A) He is experiencing vitamin C toxicity.
   (B) The vitamin C is acidifying his urine, causing decreased excretion of Focalin XR.
   (C) The vitamin C is acidifying his urine, causing increased excretion of Focalin XR.
   (D) The vitamin C is inducing CYP2D6, causing increased metabolism of Focalin XR.
   (E) The vitamin C is inhibiting CYP2D6, causing increased metabolism of Focalin XR.

ANSWERS

1. E

Because the bioavailability of a drug administered intravenously is 1, by definition, the oral bioavailability of a dosage form containing the same drug may be as high as the IV bioavailability (assuming complete absorption and no first-pass metabolism). It will usually be lower than the IV dose. However, because bioavailability can never be greater than 1, the oral bioavailability may never exceed the IV bioavailability. The AUC_{PO} may, therefore, be less than or equal to the AUC_{IV}, but never greater.

2. C

The quality control test intended to reflect the absorption of the drug is the dissolution test. It is only an approximation; going into solution is the last step before absorption. Weight variation and content uniformity tests assess the distribution of the active ingredients across the tablets and ensure that each dose is approximately the same weight. The disintegration test evaluates how quickly or slowly a tablet disintegrates; disintegration is a necessary step prior to dissolution. The friability test determines how well tablets will hold up to handling.

3. C

Focalin (dexmethylphenidate) is a weakly basic drug primarily excreted via the renal route. Acidification of the urine will cause trapping of the ionized form of the drug in the urine, increasing urinary excretion. Although some quantity of Focalin is metabolized by CYP2D6, vitamin C does not induce this enzyme. Symptoms of vitamin C toxicity do not include inattention.

Pharmacokinetics and Graph Interpretation

20

 Suggested Study Time: **2 hours**

Pharmacokinetics is the mathematical study of drug concentration in the body. It is dependent on the absorption, distribution, metabolism, and excretion (ADME) discussed in this book's biopharmaceutics chapter and is the quantitative description of what happens to the drug in the body. Clinical pharmacokinetics applies the concepts directly to individual patients, making individualized drug therapy and therapeutic drug monitoring possible.

Many equations are employed in pharmacokinetics. The more complicated of these are unlikely to be used in calculations on the NAPLEX due to time constraints, but you should be familiar with their concepts because they could form the basis for theoretical questions. Study for this section of the exam should focus primarily on being able to perform calculations related to the basic pharmacokinetic parameters discussed below and being able to properly interpret graphs of blood level data. Calculations involving drugs most likely to be monitored clinically (phenytoin, aminoglycosides) are the most important to focus on.

PLASMA DRUG CONCENTRATION PROFILES

Plasma level-versus-time curve charts are used extensively in pharmacokinetics. A known dose of drug is given to a patient, and blood samples are taken at various time intervals following drug administration. The concentration of drug in plasma is measured and plotted in the figure below. The shape of the curve depends on the relative rates of absorption, distribution, and elimination of the drug.

Figure 20-1: Blood Level-versus-Time Curves for Intravenous and Oral Drug Administration

PK MODELING (Compartmental)

From a pharmacokinetic perspective, the body is considered to consist of compartments, inside each of which the drug can be considered evenly distributed. These compartments are interconnected, and the drug moves between them at defined rates. Although compartments are completely theoretical (consisting of groups of tissues with similar blood flow and drug affinity, not actual body regions), they serve a useful purpose in simplifying calculations. Several models exist, but only two are likely to be considered on the NAPLEX:

- One-compartment model:
  - » Body consists of homogenous central compartment.
  - » Drug distributes rapidly and uniformly to this compartment.
  - » This is generally the preferred model.
- Two-compartment model:
  - » Central compartment is still present, and includes highly perfused organs (liver, kidneys).
  - » There is a slow distribution of drug into a peripheral compartment of poorly perfused tissue (muscles, connective tissue).

Multicompartmental models exist (hydromorphone [Dilaudid] is best described by a three-compartment model), but the calculations become very complex, and it is generally possible to group a few compartments together and still obtain an adequate description of the data.

Figure 20-2: **One-Compartment Versus Multicompartment Models**

One-Compartment Model | Multi-Compartment Model

BASIC PHARMACOKINETIC PARAMETERS

Most calculations you are likely to see on the NAPLEX involve the parameters listed below.

Bioavailable Fraction

Bioavailable fraction (F) is the portion of dose administered that reaches the systemic circulation. For IV administration, $F = 1$. Drug given by any other route can have a bioavailable fraction ranging from 0 to 1; the bioavailable fraction will never be greater than 1. Two factors can decrease the bioavailable fraction of a drug:

- Incomplete absorption
- First-pass metabolism

The equation governing bioavailable fraction is given below. *fa* represents the fraction of administered dose absorbed into the bloodstream, and *ffp* represents the fraction of absorbed drug escaping first-pass metabolism.

$$F = ffp \cdot fa$$

Hepatic Extraction Ratio

The hepatic extraction ratio (E) is the fraction of drug in the blood that is metabolized during each pass of blood through the liver.

$$(1 - E) = ffp$$

High-*E* drugs are extensively metabolized by liver enzymes. Low-*E* drugs are metabolized by sluggish enzymes with relatively low affinity for the drug. Knowing a drug's *E* value is useful in predicting the effects of first-pass metabolism, disease states, and drug–drug interactions on the metabolism of the drug.

Plasma Level

The plasma level of the drug (*C*) can be determined by a number of equations. The most basic version, for a drug following a one-compartment model, is given below in three formats. You should remember and be able to use at least one of these equations:

$$\log C = \log C_0 - \frac{kt}{2.3}$$
$$\ln C = \ln C_0 - kt$$
$$C = C_0 e^{-kt}$$

When calculating plasma levels following an intravenous (IV) bolus dose, these are the equations you should use.

Elimination Rate Constant

The first-order elimination rate constant, *k*, represents the fraction of drug eliminated per unit time, and thus has units of reciprocal time (i.e., hr^{-1}). It can be obtained graphically (see figure below) or from the drug half-life:

$$k = \frac{\ln 2}{t_{1/2}} = \frac{0.693}{t_{1/2}}$$

Figure 20-3: **Graphical Calculation of Elimination Rate Constant**

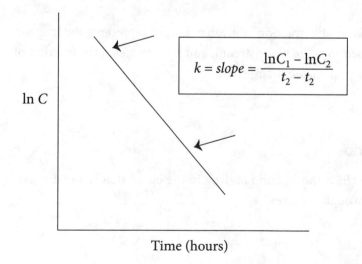

$$k = slope = \frac{\ln C_1 - \ln C_2}{t_2 - t_2}$$

ln C

Time (hours)

Half-Life

The elimination half-life of a drug is the time required for its serum concentration to decrease by half. It can be obtained mathematically or graphically:

$$t_{1/2} = \frac{\ln 2}{k} = \frac{0.693}{k}$$

Half-life can also be calculated from clearance and volume of distribution (see sections below). While these parameters do not influence or depend on one another, half-life depends on both of them:

$$t_{1/2} = 0.693 \cdot \left(\frac{Vd}{CL}\right)$$

Clearance

Clearance refers to the efficiency of the body in removing drug from the blood. The liver and kidney are the primary organs involved, and body clearance refers to the sum of the hepatic and renal clearances, plus any clearance from other organs, usually negligible:

$$CL = CL_h + CL_r$$

Some drugs are cleared primarily by one organ (propranolol has a hepatic clearance of 840 mL/min and a total clearance of only 848 mL/min), while others show more mixed clearance (procainamide has a hepatic clearance of 268 mL/min and a renal clearance of 303 mL/min). Knowledge of drug clearance can help determine when dosage adjustments are needed in patients with liver or kidney disease. Using the above examples, patients with kidney disease would need dose adjustments for procainamide but not propranolol. Patients with liver disease would need dose adjustments for both drugs.

If clearance increases, the drug is more efficiently removed from the body and the drug half-life decreases.

Population clearance values are typically based on body weight; clearance corresponds to ideal, not actual, body weight (IBW):

- Tall, lean individuals have larger eliminating organs à higher clearance than a shorter lean person.
- Adipose tissue does not affect the size of eliminating organs à actual body weight should not be used to determine clearance in obese patients (use IBW).

$$IBW(males) = 50kg + [2.3 \cdot (\text{\# of inches of height} > 60")]$$
$$IBW(females) = 45kg + [2.3 \cdot (\text{\# of inches of height} > 60")]$$

Volume of Distribution

Apparent volume of distribution (V_d) describes the volume of body fluids required to account for all drugs in the body. As mentioned in the biopharmaceutics chapter, it is not a real volume but a calculated number that helps compare the behavior of different drugs. Several equations can be used to calculate V_d, depending on the information you have available:

$$V_d = \frac{dose}{C_{peak}} - \frac{F \cdot D_0}{AUC \cdot k} = \frac{CL \cdot t_{1/2}}{0.693}$$

Volume of distribution has the following effect on half-life:

- Small V_d:
    - » Drug mostly located in blood
    - » Liver and kidneys can only clear drug in blood
    - » Fewer passes needed to rid body of drug
    - » Shorter half-life
- Large V_d:
    - » Drug extensively distributed into extravascular tissues
    - » More passes required to clear drug from blood
    - » Longer half-life

Area under the Curve

Area under the curve (AUC) is a measure of the extent of drug bioavailability. It is defined as the area under the drug plasma level – time curve from $t = 0$ to infinity. It can be calculated by the trapezoidal rule (unlikely to appear on the NAPLEX, due to time constraints), or by the other listed equations, and has units of concentration/time. S is the salt factor for a given drug formulation and refers to the percentage of administered product that is the active moiety (the acid or base, not the salt). A commonly used example of a drug with a salt factor is aminophylline ($S = 0.8$), as compared to theophylline ($S = 1$).

Trapezoidal rule:

$$AUC = \frac{C_{n-1} + C_n}{2} (tn - t_{n-1})$$

Other equations:

$$AUC = \frac{F \cdot S \cdot D_0}{CL} = \frac{F \cdot D_0}{k \cdot V_D}$$

AUC is often directly proportional to dose, such that increasing the dose of a drug from 500 mg to 1,000 mg will lead to a two-fold increase in *AUC*. This is not always the case, however. If a pathway for drug elimination becomes saturated, as can happen with the enzyme-dependent metabolism of certain drugs (such as phenytoin and salicylates), increasing the dose can lead to a disproportionately large increase in *AUC*.

ORAL DOSING

Most immediate-release oral dosage forms follow a first-order absorption model, as do some nonoral dosage forms such as suppositories and intramuscular (IM) injections. When plotting log *C* versus time (see figure below), the following equation of the "y = mx + b" format applies:

$$\log C = \log \frac{F \cdot K_a \cdot D}{V_D(k_a - k)} = \frac{kt}{2.3}$$

Figure 20-4: First-Order Blood Level-versus-Time Curve

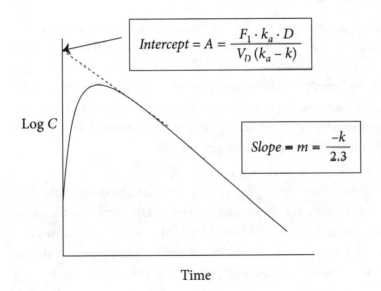

$$Intercept = A = \frac{F_1 \cdot k_a \cdot D}{V_D(k_a - k)}$$

$$Slope = m = \frac{-k}{2.3}$$

The above equation may also be expressed as:

$$C = \frac{F \cdot K_a \cdot D}{V_D(k_a - k)} = (e^{-kt} - e^{-k_at}) \quad or \quad C = Ae^{-kt} - Be^{-k_at}$$

The absorption rate constant, k_a, cannot be measured directly. It can be calculated by several methods, which are fairly lengthy mathematical processes and are unlikely to be tested on the NAPLEX. General questions about the methods could be asked, however.

- Method of residuals (feathering, peeling)
  - » The difference between the extrapolated line in the above graph and the point directly below it on the absorption portion of the curve (the residual) is plotted versus time.
  - » The slope of this line is equal to $-k_a / 2.3$.
- Wagner-Nelson method
  - » Plots fraction of drug unabsorbed versus time
  - » Can use blood level and/or urinary excretion data
- Loo Riegelman method
  - » Plots percent of drug unabsorbed versus time
  - » Used for two-compartment model drugs
  - » Must give drug intravenously and orally in order to obtain all necessary information

MULTIPLE DRUG DOSING

Most drugs are not given as single doses but are administered in multiple doses over prolonged periods of time. Since plasma levels must be maintained within certain levels in order to achieve maximum effectiveness and to limit toxicity (minimum effective concentration [MEC] and minimum toxic concentration [MTC]), drug accumulation must be considered. Knowing basic pharmacokinetic parameters for a given drug (k, V_d, and/or CL), as well as the dose (D) and dosing interval (τ), it is possible to predict the plasma level at any time after beginning the dosage regime.

The most common model used in calculating drug levels in the setting of multiple-dosage regimens is that of superposition. It assumes that early doses do not affect the pharmacokinetics of subsequent doses, and that the blood levels after subsequent doses will overlay the previous doses. In other words, the blood level after each dose can simply be added to the level remaining in the system from prior doses. First-order elimination kinetics are assumed.

If the same dose of drug is given at a fixed-dose frequency, eventually the plasma level curve reaches a plateau and a steady-state plasma level is reached (C_{SS}). At this point, the rate of the drug entering the body equals the rate of drug leaving the body. Blood levels are constant from interval to interval provided the patient's pharmacokinetic parameters do not change and the dose and dosing interval stay the same. Ninety percent of the steady-state concentration has been attained after three half-lives; after five half-lives, 97% has been attained. These numbers are very important to remember as they will allow you to estimate some answers on the NAPLEX. Calculation of C_{SS} is discussed below, but two other terms must be accounted for first.

MULTIPLE DOSING FACTOR AND ACCUMULATION FACTOR

The extent of accumulation can be predicted by using the multiple dosing factor (MDF), where N = the number of doses:

$$MDF = \frac{1 \cdot e^{-N \cdot k \cdot t}}{1 - e^{-k \cdot t}}$$

Single-dose equations can be converted to multiple-dose equations simply by multiplying each exponential term that contains time as a variable by the MDF.

At steady state, the MDF simplifies to the following accumulation factor:

$$MDF = \frac{1}{1 - e^{-k \cdot t}}$$

As the equation for AF shows, two things affect how much drug accumulates between the first dose and a dose at steady state:

- Elimination constant or half-life
- Dosing interval

We cannot control the half-life; it is dependent on the drug in question. However, the dosing interval can be adjusted in order to increase or decrease the drug accumulation factor. A simple estimation of this can be described by:

- Dosing interval < drug half-life → C_{SS} will be much higher than the concentration after the first dose.
- Dosing interval = drug half-life → C_{SS} will be twice as high as the concentration after the first dose.
- Dosing interval > drug half-life → C_{SS} will be similar to the concentration after the first dose (because the drug is almost completely washing out before the next dose is given).

Steady-State Equation and Peak-to-Trough Ratio

The steady-state equation is given below. It may be easily rearranged to solve for CL or dose rate (dose/dosing interval):

$$C_{SS,avg} = \frac{F \cdot S \cdot (S/t)}{CL}$$

Another useful equation is the peak-to-trough ratio:

$$P : T = e^{+k(t - T_{max})}$$

Shorter dosing intervals for a particular dose will lead to a decreased $P:T$ ratio, meaning that less fluctuation in peak-to-trough is occurring.

The peak-to-trough ratio can be especially useful when predicting the effect of switching a patient from a regular to a sustained-release formulation. T_{max} represents time to peak concentration within the dosing interval; it is smaller for immediate-release formulations than for sustained-release, as the drug is liberated and absorbed more quickly, and so the peak concentration occurs sooner.

Loading Doses

Loading doses are often used to achieve target plasma drug concentrations as quickly as possible. These large initial doses (which may be given as either a single dose or divided doses over a specified period of time) are especially important in life-threatening conditions such as myocardial infarction, status asthmaticus, and status epilepticus. Loading doses should not be used when there is not an urgent need to achieve target blood levels immediately or the patient cannot be supervised for possible toxicity. Loading doses for narrow-therapeutic-index drugs should ideally occur within a clinical setting.

Loading doses that are given slowly can be calculated by the equation given below. If given rapidly (by bolus injection, for example), the volume of the central compartment (V_c) should be used instead of V_d. Lidocaine is an example of a drug that would require a fast loading dose, due to its use in the treatment of life-threatening arrhythmias.

$$LD_{slow} = \frac{(C_{target} - C_{onboard}) \cdot V_d}{F \cdot S}$$

$C_{onboard}$ is included in case the patient is already taking the drug. If this is not the case, that term drops out and the equation simplifies. It is primarily included as a safety factor to avoid overshooting the upper limit of the therapeutic range.

When patients are within 20% of their IBW, total body weight (TBW) should be used when calculating loading dose. For obese patients, the decision to use IBW versus TBW depends on the drug and its ability to partition into adipose tissue.

- Drug fully partitions into fat: V_d will increase with weight gain à use TBW
  - » Example: Lidocaine
- Drug does not partition into fat: V_d does not change with weight gain à use IBW
  - » Example: Digoxin
- Drug that partially partitions into fat: an intermediate value should be used
  - » Example: Theophylline

Constant IV Infusion

Constant-rate infusions do not generate fluctuations in plasma concentration. Determining the rate for such infusions is relatively simple:

1. Determine the target steady-state plasma concentration.
2. Find the appropriate population CL.
3. Look up S (if drug is a salt).
4. Calculate infusion rate (R).

$$R = \frac{CS \cdot CL}{S}$$

Clearance adjustment factors may be available for some drugs. Some conditions that may have corresponding clearance adjustments include patient age, smoking status, and concurrent use of certain drugs. If available, these factors should be used in order to better predict blood levels in the individual patient.

If a drug is infused at a faster rate, a higher steady-state concentration will result. However, the time to steady-state is based on half-life and will remain the same. In order to achieve and maintain immediate steady-state concentrations:

- Give IV loading dose of R/k.
- Begin IV infusion.

Intermittent IV Infusion

Short IV infusions separated by time for drug elimination are often given to prevent high drug concentration and associated adverse effects. The drug may not reach steady-state in such cases.

$$C = \frac{R}{V_d \cdot k} (1 - e^{-kt})$$

The rate of infusion is equal to the dose/infusion period. After the infusion has stopped, drug concentration at a particular time can be determined by the following equation, given the concentration at the time the infusion was stopped.

$$C = C_{stop} (1 - e^{-kt})$$

Intermittent Oral Dosing

Dose rate in intermittent oral dosing is calculated in a similar fashion to IV infusions. Remember to take F into account with oral dosing, however, since bioavailability may not be equal to IV products. After the dosing rate is determined, dose can be calculated based on the preferred dosing interval.

$$\frac{D}{t} = \frac{C_{SS} \cdot CL}{F \cdot S}$$

NONLINEAR PHARMACOKINETICS

So far, this chapter has referred to general pharmacokinetic principles. These principles are applicable to most drugs without significant modification, and they result in linear mathematical models. Several assumptions are made when different or multiple doses are given:

- Drug clearance remains constant.
- Doubling the dose à doubled C and AUC.

These assumptions are not always accurate. With some drugs, giving a single low dose of the drug leads to the expected linear pharmacokinetics. However, when higher doses are given, or when the medication is taken chronically, the drug no longer fits the linear pharmacokinetic profile.

Figure 20-5: **Pharmacokinetic Relationships: Linear versus Nonlinear**

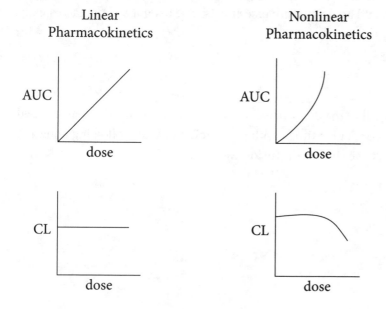

Nonlinear pharmacokinetics generally occur when one or more enzyme- or carrier-mediated systems are saturated. These systems are often referred to as capacity-limited.

- Active drug absorption: Absorption of riboflavin involves saturable gut wall transport
- Drug distribution: Saturable protein binding of salicylates
- Drug metabolism: Saturable metabolism of phenytoin
- Drug excretion: Active secretion of penicillin G

Most elimination processes can be saturated if enough drug is given. Certain drugs (phenytoin in particular) show nonlinear behavior even at normal drug doses.

For drugs exhibiting nonlinear behavior, dose increases lead to half-life increases, and AUC is not proportional to the amount of bioavailable drug. The behavior is described by the Michaelis-Menten equation:

$$\frac{dC}{dt} = \frac{V_{max} - C_{SS}}{K_M + C_{SS}}$$

V_{max} (the maximum elimination rate) and K_M (the Michaelis constant, equal to one-half the concentration at V_{max}) are dependent on both the drug and the enzyme system. Two general situations can apply:

- $C \gg K_m$; rate of change simplifies to V_{max}, a constant → zero-order kinetics
- $C \ll K_m$; rate of change is concentration dependent → first-order kinetics

In order to determine K_m and V_{max}, steady-state concentrations are measured as the result of two different doses given at different times. Recall that at steady-state, the rate of drug metabolism is assumed to be the same as the rate of drug input. In other words, the change in concentration over time is equal to the dosing rate (DR). As most nonlinear calculations that you will encounter involve phenytoin, remember that the salt factor (S) for phenytoin sodium is 0.92, and the dose must be multiplied by this number when the salt form (capsules and injection) is used.

$$DR = \frac{V_{max} - C_{SS}}{K_M \cdot C_{SS}}$$

K_m may be obtained in two ways:

1. Graph the data and obtain K_m from the slope.
2. Solve simultaneous equations using two dosing rates and respective C_{SS} (algebraic determination; see below).

$$DR_1 = V_{max} - Km \cdot \frac{DR_1}{C_{ss1}}$$

$$-(DR_2 = V_{max} - Km \cdot \frac{DR_2}{C_{ss2}})$$

Subtracting the second equation from the first, V_{max} will drop out and the equation can be solved for K_m.

V_{max} may be obtained in two ways as well:

1. Graph the data, and determine the y-intercept from the graph.
2. Use the dosing rate, C_{ss}, and the newly calculated K_m to solve mathematically.

Graphical data, if available, is the faster way to obtain K_m and V_{max}.

Figure 20-6: Graphical Determination of K_m and V_{max}

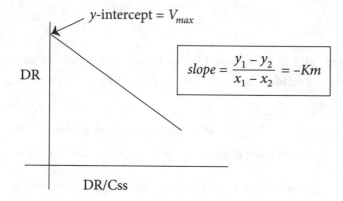

LEARNING POINTS

- Ninety percent of steady-state blood levels have been achieved after three half-lives; 97% after five half-lives.
- Increasing the infusion rate will lead to higher steady-state concentrations, but the drug will not reach steady state more quickly.
- The main parameters you should be able to calculate are half-life, k, CL, V_d, plasma concentration (simple cases), and R.
- When calculating loading doses, the tendency of drug to partition into fat must be considered when determining whether to use TBW or IBW for obese patients (use TBW for drugs that partition heavily into fat).

- Increasing the dose for nonlinear drugs such as phenytoin increases the half-life and can increase AUC above what would be expected for drugs exhibiting linear behavior. Pharmacokinetic monitoring is especially important in such cases.

PRACTICE QUESTIONS

1. A patient is being started on digoxin. What plasma level would you expect after a loading dose of 0.75 mg? Patient weight = 65 kg. V_d = 6 L/kg

   (A) 167 mcg/L
   (B) 2.6 mcg/L
   (C) 125 mcg/L
   (D) 1.95 mcg/L
   (E) 11.5 mcg/L

ANSWERS

1. **D**

Use $C = \dfrac{dose}{V_d} = \dfrac{0.75\ mg}{\dfrac{6L}{kg} \cdot 65\ kg} = \dfrac{1000\ mcg}{1\ mg} = \dfrac{1.95\ mcg}{L}$

Calculations

 Suggested Study Time: **2 hours**

This section contains a quick review of the types of calculation questions likely to be covered on the NAPLEX. Practice is the key to this section. Keep in mind that you will be restricted to using a basic calculator (provided by testing centers).

If you would like additional review, older editions of pharmacy calculation text books will be helpful—the techniques involved have not changed. Two suggestions are *Pharmaceutical Calculations* by Ansel and Stoklosa, and *Pharmaceutical Calculations* by Zatz and Teixeira.

PROBLEM-SOLVING TECHNIQUES

Ratio-Proportion and Dimensional Analysis

There are two techniques that can be used to solve most pharmaceutical calculations: Ratio-proportion and dimensional analysis. Either of these techniques is acceptable, and you should use whichever one you find most comfortable.

Ratio-proportion is a one-step calculation technique that is probably the easiest to use for simple (one- or two-step) calculations. In this process, you set up a likeness between a fraction involving known quantities and one that includes your unknown, and solve the equation by cross-multiplying. An example is given below, illustrating how to convert 3 fluid ounces to milliliters:

$$\frac{29.6\ mL}{1\ fl\ oz} = \frac{x\ mL}{3\ fl\ oz} \quad (29.6\ mL)(3\ fl\ oz) = (x\ mL)(1\ fl\ oz) \quad \frac{(29.6\ mL)(3\ fl\ oz)}{(1\ fl\ oz)} = x\ mL$$

While ratio-proportion is often the most intuitive method, and is something with which you have been familiar since early grades of school, it has no inherent error-checking and it is not ideal for multistep calculations. When using ratio-proportion for multi-step problems, you will have to write down intermediate steps; rounding intermediate answers reduces your accuracy, and writing them down takes time. Both of these can be problems when taking exams, so dimensional analysis might be preferred for these reasons.

Dimensional analysis is a technique, often used in chemistry and other sciences, which allows you to set up long calculations in a single step. Using the short example given above, the problem would be solved:

$$3\ fl\ oz \cdot \frac{(29.6\ mL)}{(1\ fl\ oz)} = 88.8\ mL$$

As you can see, the fluid ounces cancel out and leave you with the correct units of milliliters. This serves as an internal error-check and is especially helpful in longer, more complex problems. Also, it saves you from having to write down intermediate steps, and helps prevent "kitchen-sink" syndrome (using every bit of information given, whether it will help solve the problem or not). Finally, it avoids the problem of rounding too early; you round once, when the problem is finished.

When you have completed a calculation, regardless of the method you choose, always ask yourself if the answer makes sense. You won't always be able to determine this, but in many cases you can tell if something has gone wrong in your calculation just by looking at the final answer. For example, it would be impractical to have an IV drip rate of 1,000 mL/min, or a dose rate of 52 tablets per day. If your answer doesn't make sense, check your calculation to find out where you went wrong.

Estimation

Estimation is not always appropriate; when working in pharmacy, you want the most accurate answer possible, especially when working with drugs with narrow therapeutic indices, or for dosing of infants and children. However, for exam purposes you will often be able to eliminate several, if not all, incorrect options by using estimates, particularly of some of the conversion factors listed in the upcoming section. This could allow you more time to focus on other portions of the exam. Use estimation with caution, however, especially if several foils are very similar to each other.

FUNDAMENTALS OF UNITS AND MEASUREMENT

The metric system is the standard system used for science worldwide. It is not, however, the only system used in pharmacy. The avoirdupois, or "common," system is the customary measure in the United States, and most patients will communicate with you in this system. Because of this, you will have to convert between systems of measurement. Unfortunately, cross-system conversions are inherently inexact. Convert from one system of measurement to another only once in a problem, not multiple times, and use the most direct conversion possible. Otherwise, the measurement error will be compounded.

A few key facts about systems of measurement are given below:

- Avoirdupois refers to solid measures only (pounds and ounces).
  - » 1 pound = 16 ounces
- Common or household liquid measurements start with the teaspoon:
  - » 3 teaspoons (tsp) = 1 tablespoon (T)
  - » 2 T = 1 fluid ounce (fl oz) = 1/8 cup
  - » 1 cup = 8 fl oz
  - » 1 pint = 16 fl oz (or 2 cups)
  - » 1 quart = 32 fl oz (or 4 cups)
  - » 1 gallon = 128 fl oz (or 16 cups)
- Apothecary measures, the measures pharmacists originally used (drams, grains, and scruples), are no longer used.
  - » Some medications (aspirin is one) were traditionally measured in grains, and you may still see strength listed this way; Roman numerals are used instead of Arabic (65 mg = 1 grain [gr]; a gr V aspirin tablet = 325 mg).
  - » The apothecary system adopted the common or household liquid measurements of pint, quart, and gallon.
  - » Note that the apothecary system has pounds and ounces. These are not the same size as avoirdupois pounds and ounces, and are seldom—if ever—used. The grain, however, is the same size in the avoirdupois and apothecary systems.

Some of the more common conversion factors are given below:

Avoirdupois System	Metric System
1 lb	454 g
2.2 lb	1 kg
1 oz	28.4 g
1 grain	64.8 mg

Apothecary System	Metric System
1 tsp	5 mL
1 'T'	15 mL
1 fl oz	29.6 mL (30 mL is an acceptable estimate)
1 cup	240 mL
1 pint	473 mL (30 mL/fl oz estimate is no longer exact enough)
1 quart	946 mL
1 gallon	3,785 mL (readjust for accuracy again)

DENSITY, SPECIFIC GRAVITY, AND SPECIFIC VOLUME

Density describes the relationship between the mass of a substance and the volume it occupies. This is a helpful concept in pharmacy, as it allows you to convert between measures of mass and measures of volume. This is most useful with liquid ingredients used in compounded formulations. In compounded recipes, you may see liquid amounts expressed as either weight or volume and, depending on the recipe and the equipment you have available, it might be easier to measure in one form over the other. For instance, viscous liquids might be hard to get out of a graduated cylinder and, if you don't have a dosing syringe in which to measure the liquid, it might be better to weigh the product in a weigh boat.

Density should be treated like a conversion factor, since you are converting between mass and volume. The following example will illustrate:

450 mL of phenol weighs 482.56 g. What is its density? Express your answer in g/mL.

$$\frac{482.56\,g\,phenol}{450\,mL} = 1.07\,g/mL$$

Specific gravity (SG) is a related concept, one that many pharmacy students find confusing. SG is simply the density of a substance relative to a reference substance (usually water). It is a unitless number, because it is equal to density divided by density—the units cancel out. Since water has a density of 1 g/mL, the SG will be numerically identical to the density expressed in g/mL. However, the SG of a substance is the same regardless of what units it was calculated from, so it allows you to compare the relative masses of equal volumes of substances. Also, some sources will list SG instead of density, so you need to be familiar with it to understand these sources. An example is given below:

150 mL of formaldehyde weighs 121.82 g. What is its specific gravity?

$$\frac{\dfrac{121.82\ g\ formaldehyde}{450\ mL}}{\dfrac{1\ g\ water}{1\ mL}} = 0.81$$

REDUCING AND ENLARGING FORMULAS

Most compounding formulas are for stock quantities, and how much the formula makes is rarely the amount you are actually wishing to prepare. However, it is simple to reduce or enlarge the formula to make the amount you need, provided you keep the ingredients in the same proportion with one another. In many ways, this is similar to doubling a recipe when you are cooking for a crowd. Compounding recipes come in two formats:

1. The amount of product produced is specified (formula makes 1,000 mL, for instance).
2. The quantity of each ingredient is specified, either in measured units or in parts. You figure out how much product will be made.

Say you wish to make 50 capsules from the following recipe:

> Rx   Ketoprofen 2.5 g
>   Phenyltoloxamine citrate 6 g
>   Caffeine 6 g
>   Lactose 70.5 g
>
>   M et div caps 200

First of all, how many doses is this recipe for? "M et div" means "mix and divide," so the recipe is for the entire amount of capsules (200), not for a single capsule. What do you do now? You can either reduce each ingredient by the same proportion (which is easy to figure out but involves lots of writing) or create a single conversion factor and apply it to each ingredient. Since you want 50 capsules and your recipes makes 200, your conversion factor would be 50 capsules/200 capsules = 0.25. Multiplying each ingredient by 0.25 yields:

2.5 g ketoprofen × 0.25	= 0.625 g
6 g phenyltoloxamine citrate × 0.25	= 1.5 g
6 g caffeine × 0.25	= 1.5 g
70.5 g lactose × 0.25	= 17.625 g

This method also works well if you do not have enough of a particular ingredient in stock. Say you have only 4 g of caffeine and want to use the above recipe, which calls for 6 g. You can reduce the recipe to fit the amount of your limiting ingredient. Simply multiply each ingredient by the conversion factor of 4 g/6 g = 0.667.

If you have a recipe that does not have a total amount calculated, you will need to add up the amounts represented by each ingredient to find your total. Remember that you must add like to like, using density if needed in order to make sure that all amounts are specified in the same units (usually either g or mL).

Finally, some recipes are given in parts rather than measurements. If total parts are given (total is listed on the recipe, or one or more ingredients is listed as "qs" or "ad"):

- Set total parts to the amount you want to make
- Solve for the value of one part
- Multiply the size of one part by the number of parts for each ingredient

If total parts are not given:

- Add the number of parts for each ingredient to obtain the total number of parts in the recipe
- Proceed as above

Try this example:

Rx	Bacitracin	105 parts
	Neomycin	35 parts
	Polymyxin B	5 parts
	Petrolatum	qs 10,000 parts

Calculate the quantities of all ingredients to make 30 grams

In this case, 30 g/10,000 parts = 0.003

Multiplying this factor times the other ingredients gives:

105 parts bacitracin × 0.003 = 0.315 g = 315 mg
35 parts neomycin × 0.003 = 0.105 g = 105 mg
5 parts polymyxin B × 0.003 = 0.015 g = 15 mg

The petrolatum needed may be found by subtracting the masses of the other ingredients from the 30 total grams desired:

30 g total – 0.315 g bacitracin – 0.105 g neomycin – 0.015 g polymyxin B = 29.565 g petrolatum

PERCENTAGE AND RATIO STRENGTHS

Since drugs are administered as dosage forms that contain more than just the active ingredient, the amount of the active ingredient needs to be expressed. There are several ways to do this:

- Amount per individual dosage form (capsule, tablet, suppository)
- Concentration per dosing volume (oral liquids, certain topical products)
- Percent
- Ratio strength
- Parts per million or billion

Percent describes the number of parts of active relative to 100 parts of the total. In pharmacy, simply stating % is incomplete; you must attach the appropriate descriptor from the following list:

- % w/w: g of active per 100 g of product
- % w/v: g of active per 100 mL of product
- % v/v: mL of active per 100 mL of product

You may also see concentrations expressed in milligram percent. In this case, the amount in the numerator, usually assumed to be in grams, is expressed in milligrams instead: 0.001% w/w = 1 mg% w/w. This value is the same as mg/dL, a commonly used unit in some blood tests (such as serum glucose).

Ratio strength is another way of expressing concentration, in terms of parts of active related to any number of parts of the whole. Ratio strength is usually expressed in terms of 1 part of active relative to the total number of parts of the product, as opposed to percent, which is any number of parts of active relative to 100 parts of product. For example, 5% means 5 parts per 100, or 5:100, or 1:20. Ratio strength is used for low-concentration solutions, and triturations of high-potency powders (e.g., 1:75 trituration of estradiol).

Express 1 g of epinephrine in 1 L of solution as a percent strength and as a ratio strength:

$$\frac{1\,g\,epinephrine}{1,000\,mL} \times \frac{100\,mL\,product}{g\,active} = 0.1\%\ w/v\ or\ 1{:}1,000$$

Using another example:

How much sodium benzoate do you need to preserve 10 L of a solution at a concentration of 1:10,000?

$$\frac{1\,g\,sodium\,benzoate}{10,000\,mL} \times \frac{1,000\,mL}{1L} \times 10L = 1g$$

Parts per million (ppm) is a special case of ratio strength. Instead of fixing the numerator as 1, in this case you fix the denominator constant as 1,000,000. Parts per billion (ppb) and trillion (ppt) are handled in the analogous fashion. These are used to express very small concentrations; for example, the EPA action level for lead in drinking water is 15 ppb (or 0.015 mg/L).

DOSAGE CALCULATIONS

Pharmacists frequently need to calculate the size of a dose or total amount of medication to dispense, even for noncompounded prescriptions. The following general equation applies:

Number of doses × size of dose = total amount

Example:

How many milliliters of a liquid medicine would provide a patient with 2 teaspoons three times a day for 7 days?

$$2\ tsp \times \frac{3\ doses}{day} \times 7\ days \times \frac{5\ mL}{tsp} = 210\ mL$$

DILUTION, CONCENTRATION, AND ALLIGATION

In some cases, you may receive a prescription in which you need to either dilute a product you have on hand or make a product more concentrated. These problems can generally be solved by:

1. Using the equation: (quantity) × (concentration) = (quantity) × (concentration)
2. Determining the quantity of active ingredient needed and then calculating the quantity of the available solution (usually a concentrated stock solution), which will provide the needed amount of active ingredient

When some ingredients are given as ratio strength, you should convert them to percentage strength before setting up the proportion. Whenever proportional parts enter the calculation, you should reduce them to their lowest terms before beginning (i.e., reduce 75 parts:25 parts to 3 parts:1 part). In both cases, this will simplify your calculations. Example:

If 250 mL of a 15% v/v solution of methyl salicylate in alcohol are diluted to 1,500 mL, what will be the percentage strength?

250 mL × 15% = 1,500 mL × X%   X = 2.5% v/v

Stock Solutions

Stock solutions are strong solutions of known concentration that allow the pharmacist to conveniently prepare weaker solutions. They are generally prepared on a w/v basis and their concentration is expressed as a ratio strength. Example:

How many milliliters of a 1% stock solution of certified red dye should be used in preparing 2,000 mL of an antiseptic that is to contain 1:5,000 of the certified red dye as a coloring agent?

First, how many grams of red dye are needed in the 2,000 mL of antiseptic solution?

$$\frac{1\ g\ red\ dye}{5,000\ mL} \times 2,000\ mL\ antiseptic\ solution = 0.4\ g$$

Next, how much of the 1% stock solution of red dye contains this amount of dye?

$$0.4\ g \times \frac{100\ mL}{1\ g\ red\ dye} = 40\ mL$$

Alligation

Alligation is a method of solving problems that involves mixing multiple products that have different percentage strengths. Two types of alligation exist: Alligation medial and alligation alternate.

Alligation Medial

This method allows the calculation of the weighted average percentage strength of a mixture of two or more substances of known quantity and strength. The technique is best shown via illustration:

What is the percentage strength (v/v) of alcohol in a mixture of 3,000 mL of 40% (v/v) alcohol, 1,000 mL of 60% (v/v) alcohol, and 1,000 mL of 70% (v/v) alcohol?

$$
\begin{aligned}
40 \times 3,000 &= 120,000 \\
60 \times 1,000 &= 60,000 \\
70 \times 1,000 &= 70,000 \\
\hline
\text{Totals: } 5,000 &= 250,000
\end{aligned}
$$

250,000 / 5,000 = 50% (v/v)

Alligation Alternate

This method allows calculation of the number of parts of two or more components of a given strength when they are mixed to prepare a mixture of a desired strength. Crosswise subtraction is used to determine the amounts needed of each component. This method can be used regardless of how concentration is expressed (mg/mL, ratio, parts, %). Example:

In what proportion should 20% benzocaine ointment be mixed with an ointment base to produce a 2.5% w/w benzocaine ointment?

Since there is no active drug in the ointment base, its strength can be expressed as 0%.

Strengths to Be Mixed	Desired	Difference in Strength Mixed (crosswise subtraction of absolute values)
20%		2.5 parts (2.5−0) of 20% ointment
	2.5%	
0%		17.5 parts (20 − 2.5) of ointment base

So 2.5 parts of the 20% w/w ointment should be added to 17.5 parts of the ointment base. Remember that the values are subtracted crosswise, but the identities of the substances are read across.

ELECTROLYTE SOLUTIONS

Electrolyte solutions are frequently prescribed for patients who have lost an essential ion through disease, as they play a critical role in maintaining normal body function. Sometimes the necessary amount of the appropriate salt will be stated on the prescription, but often the prescription will ask for a quantity of the needed ion in chemical units, and the pharmacist will need to calculate how much of the salt will contain the desired amount. Milliequivalents are the most common unit used.

Millimoles and Milliequivalents

A review of several chemistry concepts will be useful before beginning milliequivalent calculations.

- Moles (mol): Measurement of the amount of a substance; Avogadro's number of particles (6.023×10^{23})
- Atomic weight: Found on the periodic table; 1 mol of that atom weighs that many grams (also, 1 mmol of that atom weighs that many mg)
- Molecular weight (MW): The sum of all the atomic weights for all of the atoms in the molecule. 1 mol of the molecule weighs MW g; 1 mmol weight MW mg.
- Molar solution: 1 mol of solute in 1 L of solution
  - » Stock solutions often expressed this way
  - » 0.1 M = 0.1 mol of solute/1 L solution

What is the molar concentration of a 5% w/v $MgCl_2$ solution? MW $MgCl_2$ = 95.

$$\frac{1\ mol\ MgCl_2}{95\ g\ MgCl_2} \times \frac{5\ g\ MgCl_2}{100\ mL} \times \frac{1{,}000\ mL}{1\ L} = 0.53\ mol/L = 0.53\ M$$

What if you are interested in moles of atoms instead of moles of molecules? In this case, you need to look at the molecular formula. If there is more than one of an atom in a molecule (such as the chloride in the example above), you need to adjust your formula. In that example, you have 1 mol of $MgCl_2$, which contains 1 mol of Mg^{+2} and 2 mol of Cl^-. If you don't have a molecular formula, you can figure one out by balancing charges, provided you know the valencies of the ions involved. In the magnesium chloride example, Mg^{+2} is divalent; it takes two Cl^- to make as much negative charge as one Mg^{+2}. Therefore, the correct formula is $MgCl_2$, not $MgCl$. $NaCl$, however, is made up of two monovalent ions, so the charges are equal.

Electrolytes are commonly prescribed in terms of equivalents rather than mass. What does this mean? One mol of hydrogen has 1 mol of positive charge. One equivalent of an ion is the amount required to replace (in positively charged ions) or react with (in negatively charged ions) 1 mol of hydrogen. Monovalent ions (Cl^-, Na^+, K^+, NH_4^+, OH^-) therefore have 1 Eq/mol. Divalent ions like Ca^{+2} are 2 Eq/mol, as it takes 2 mol of hydrogen to replace the charge carried by 1 mol of calcium. Example:

How much potassium citrate powder would we weigh to compound 1 dose of the following prescription?

> Rx   Potassium citrate, 20 mEq of K^+, tid

Recall that potassium has a valence of +1 and citrate has a −3, so the formula must be $K_3(C_6H_5O_7)$ MW = 324.41 mg/mmol.

$$20\ mEq\ K^+ \times \frac{1\ mmol\ K^+}{1\ mEq\ K^+} \times \frac{1\ mmol\ K_3(C_6H_5O_7)}{3\ mmol\ K^+} \times \frac{324.41\ mg\ K^+}{mmol\ K^+} =$$

$$\frac{g}{1{,}000\ mg} = 2/16\ g\ K_3(C_6H_5O_7)$$

Be very careful with labeling when performing milliequivalent calculations! Millimoles of ions do not necessarily equal millimoles of molecules.

Osmolarity and Isotonicity

Osmotic pressure is the pressure that exists across a semipermeable membrane due to the free movement of solvent but not solute. Because cell membranes are semipermeable, this concept is important in patients. When administering parenteral drugs, you must balance the osmolarity of your medication with the osmolarity of the body. If not, tissue damage, pain, and possibly death can result due to cells swelling or shrinking with the movement of solvent.

Solutions are considered isotonic when each one has the same osmotic pressure; in pharmacy and medicine, the reference solution is the plasma (280–300 mOsm/L). Hypertonic solutions have higher osmotic pressure than this; hypotonic solutions have lower osmotic pressure. Some other facts you should remember about osmotic pressure are:

- It is a colligative property, based on the number of particles in solution.
- It can be calculated directly, using dissociation constants.
    - » NaCl dissociates 80% in aqueous solution.
    - » For every 100 particles, 80 will have dissociated (making 160 particles) and 20 will not → 180 particles.

    $$\frac{180 \; particles \; after \; dissociation}{100 \; particles \; before \; dissociation} = 1.8 = i$$

- It can be calculated by its effect on other colligative properties, including freezing point, boiling point, and vapor pressure.
    - » All colligative properties vary together.
    - » A solution with the same freezing point as a reference solution will have the same osmolarity as that reference solution.

Try this example:

A solute dissociates 50% in aqueous solution. Assuming each molecule of the solute dissociates into two parts, give the dissociation constant (i).

$$\frac{100 \; dissociated \; dissociation + 50 \; undissociated \; particles}{100 \; undissociated \; particles} = 1.5$$

You can use the ratio form of the dissociation constant as a conversion factor. If $i = 1.5$, 1 mol = 1.5 Osm, and 1 mmol = 1.5 mOsm.

Try another example: Calculate the osmolarity of NS in mOsm/L.

NS = normal saline = 0.9% w/v NaCl in water
MW NS = 58.5
$i = 1.8$

$$\frac{0.9 \; g \; NaCl}{100 \; mL} \times \frac{1 \; mol}{58.5 \; g \; NaCl} \times \frac{1000 \; mmol}{mol} \times \frac{1.8 \; mOsm}{mmol} \times \frac{1000 \; mL}{L} = 276.9 \; mOsm/L$$

Because NS is nearly isotonic with plasma, it is useful for comparison. If we know that a product is isotonic to NS, it will be isotonic to body fluids as well. Sodium chloride equivalents are therefore useful, and are for expression of the amount of NaCl it would take to exert the tonic effect of a particular active ingredient. Some baseline assumptions are:

- The tonic effects of solutes are additive and independent.
- The total tonic effect in the solution is the sum of the effect of each solute.

The following steps can be followed when adjusting tonicity:

1. Determine how much NaCl it would take to exert the tonic effect already seen in the solution.
2. Calculate how much NaCl is required to make the solution isotonic if NaCl is the sole tonicity agent. Compare this to the amount already present (step 1). Proceed only if the total amount of NaCl equivalent already present is less than the amount needed (i.e., solution is currently hypotonic).
3. Amount needed = Goal amount – Amount you already have
   a. If adjusting tonicity with NaCl, use amount in step 3.
   b. If adjusting tonicity with another substance, figure out how much of your substance is needed to deliver the required tonic effect, using the E value (1 g of substance has the same tonic effect as E g of NaCl).

If one of your ingredients is already isotonic, you can disregard that volume as you calculate your values.

For example, how much boric acid (E = 0.52) should be added to make 15 mL of a 3% w/v pilocarpine HCl (E = 0.24) eye drop solution isotonic?

Following the steps given above:

1. $$\frac{3\,g\,pilocarpine}{100\,mL} \times 15\,mL = 0.45\,g\,pilocarpine$$

$$0.45\,g\,pilocarpine \times \frac{0.24\,g\,NaCl(eq)}{1\,g\,pilocarpine} = 0.108\,g\,NaCl(eq)$$

2. $$\frac{0.9\,g\,NaCl}{100\,mL} \times 15\,mL = 0.135\,g\,NaCl$$

3. $$0.135\,g - 0.108\,g = 0.027\,g\,NaCl$$

$$0.027\,g\,NaCl \times \frac{1\,g\,boric\,acid}{0.52\,g\,NaCl(eq)} = 0.05192\,g = 0.52\,g\,boric\,acid$$

Another way to describe and calculate osmolarity and isotonicity is freezing-point depression. As mentioned above, this is a colligative property that varies along with other colligative properties of a solution. Some things to remember:

- Plasma freezes at −0.52°C.

- Solutions isotonic to plasma (such as NS) will also freeze at −0.52°C.

- Pure water freezes at 0°C. Therefore, an amount of solute that will make the solution isotonic depresses the freezing point by 0.52°C.

Given the following prescription, how much NaCl must be added to make the solution isotonic? The freezing point of a 1% w/v solution of procaine HCl is −0.122°C.

Rx	Procaine HCl	2% w/v
	NaCl	qs
	Sterile water	qs 30 mL

First, what would be the effect of a 2% w/v solution?

$$\frac{1.22°C}{1\%} \times 2\% = 0.244°C$$

Since the desired freezing point − The depression from the ingredients already in the formulation = The additional depression needed:

$$-0.52°C - (-0.244°C) = -0.276°C$$

So, the required concentration of sodium chloride is:

$$-0.276°C \, \frac{0.9\% \, NaCl}{-0.52°C} = 0.48\% \, NaCl \quad \text{or}$$

$$-30 \, mL \, \frac{0.48 \, g \, NaCl}{100 \, g \, NaCl} = 0.144 \, g \, NaCl$$

COMPOUNDING CALCULATIONS

Use of Prefabricated Dosage Forms in Compounding

When compounding, the source of active ingredient will often be prefabricated dosage forms (tablets, capsules, ointments). When performing such calculations, it is important to remember that if your calculation determines that you need 1.3 tablets as your source drug, you must actually crush 2 tablets and then weigh out a proportional amount of the resultant powder. Remember, a tablet contains far more ingredients than just the drug, so take that into account in your calculations.

> Rx   Aspirin   300 mg
>   Lactose   qs
>
> M.ft. cap DTD #60

Using 325-mg aspirin tablets (weighing 430 mg each) as the source drug, how many tablets are needed to compound this prescription? How much of the crushed powder should be weighed out?

$$300 \, mg \, ASA \times 60 \, capsules \times \frac{ASA \, tablet}{325 \, mg \, ASA} = 55.38 \, tablets \rightarrow 56 \, tablets$$

$$55.38 \, tablets \times 430 \, mg \, total \, tablet \, weight = 23.813 \, g \, required \, (of \, 24.08 \, g \, produced)$$

Suppository Calculations

The density factor method is often used when preparing suppositories. The density factor expresses the relationship between the mass of an ingredient and the volume of suppository base it displaces. Therefore, a drug will have a different density factor in each suppository base.

$$density \, factor = \frac{weight \, of \, drug}{weight \, of \, base \, displaced}$$

If a pharmacist needs to prepare six 30-mg phenobarbital suppositories in cocoa butter, how many grams each of cocoa butter and phenobarbital should be weighed? Density factor of phenobarbital in cocoa butter is 1.2. Blank suppositories (base only) weigh 2 g.

If one suppository contains 30 mg drug (0.03 g), it will replace:

$$\frac{0.03 \, g \, drug}{1.2 \, g} = 0.025 \, g \, cocoa \, butter$$

2 g – 0.025 g = 1.975 g cocoa butter / suppository × 6 suppositories = 11.85 g cocoa butter

0.025 g × 6 suppositories = 0.15 g phenobarbital

Reconstitution Calculations

Some medications, particularly antibiotics for oral suspension or parenteral use, come as powders for reconstitution. While the container or package will include instructions for reconstitution, including what and how much diluent to use, occasionally the prescriber will need to manipulate the final concentration of the drug. Some simple calculations can help you make these adjustments to provide a more dilute or concentrated product. First, a simple example:

Cefadroxil powder for oral suspension comes in a strength of 250 mg/5 mL. The reconstitution instructions are to add 70 mL of purified water to yield a final solution volume of 100 mL. How many grams of cefadroxil powder are in the bottle?

$$\frac{250\,mg\;cefadroxil}{5\,mL\;suspension} \times 100\,mL = 5{,}000\,mg = 5\,g$$

There are a few interesting things to pay attention to here. First, this is an easy example of a question that gives more information than you need to solve the problem (while the 70 mL is necessary for reconstitution, it is not needed to answer this particular question). Be sure to pay attention and use the correct numbers when extra information is given. Second, if you add only 70 mL of water, how do you get 100 mL of total suspension? The powder takes up space in the final product. This volume is called the powder volume: It is a calculated quantity, not corresponding to the physical volume. The powder volume may be greater than, equal to, or less than zero, depending on the drug and the way it was prepared.

When preparing a final concentration that is different from the package directions, you must first calculate the powder volume. The powder volume is equal to the difference between the diluent volume and the final solution volume. Take the following case:

Rx   Biaxin 100 mg/5 mL suspension
       Sig: 1 tsp PO q 12 hr × 10 days

Biaxin comes as a powder for reconstitution with instructions to prepare a final concentration of 125 mg/5 mL by adding 55 mL diluent to make a final volume of 100 mL. The amount of active ingredient in the bottle is 2,500 mg, and the powder volume = total volume – diluent, so 100 mL – 55 mL = 45 mL.

$$2500\,mg\;Biaxin\;\frac{5\,mL}{100\,mg\;Biaxin} = 125\,mL\;total$$

$$125\,mL\;total - PV = 125\,mL - 45\,mL = 80\,mL$$

Adding 80 mL of diluent will produce 125 mL of solution with a concentration of 100 mg/5 mL.

Drip Rate Calculations

IV medications are regulated by one of the following methods:

- Drip chambers
    - » Deliver drops of defined volume.
    - » Flow is adjusted by the nurse to a set number of *whole* drops per minute (gH).
    - » Standard sets are 10 gtt/mL or 15 gtt/mL.
    - » Pediatric and critical care drugs may use microdrop infusion sets: 60 gtt/mL.
- Infusion pumps
    - » Deliver a rate of mL/hr.
    - » Round to the nearest 0.1 mL.

17 mL of concentrated vancomycin solution is added to a 100-mL piggyback bag of NS. This solution is to be infused over 1 hour. What is the infusion rate?

$$\frac{17\,mL\ vancomycin + 100\,mL\ NS}{60\ min} = 117\,mL/60\ min = 117\,mL/hr$$

What is the infusion rate in drops/min if the drug is administered using an infusion set that delivers 10 gtt/mL?

$$\frac{117\,mL}{60\ min} \times \frac{10\,gtt}{mL} = 19.5\,gtt/min = 20\,gtt/min$$

Nutrition Calculations

Total parenteral nutrition (TPN) calculations involve many of the calculation techniques described throughout this chapter. Since electrolytes are commonly given via TPN, milliequivalent calculations may be useful. They also supply fluid, calories, essential fatty acids, and vitamins. One example is given below:

Glycerin is sometimes used as an alternative energy source in TPN formulations and produces 4.32 kcal of energy per gram. Given a commercial stock solution of electrolytes, amino acids, and 3% w/v glycerin, how many calories are present in 200 mL of this stock solution?

$$200\,mL \times \frac{3\,g\ glycerin}{100\,mL} \times 4.32\,kcal/g = 26\,kcal$$

LEARNING POINTS

- Always perform a "sanity" check on your answer. Does it make practical sense? If not, recheck your numbers.

- Remember crucial conversion factors (or at least approximations of these): 1 fluid oz = 30 mL, 2.2 lb/kg (*not* the reverse; remember, your weight is always a smaller number when measured in kilograms; if you get an answer to the contrary, you flipped your conversion).

- Valence of a molecule is equal to the total number of negative charges *or* the total number of positive charges, not the two numbers added together.

- When using prefabricated dosage forms as a drug source, fractions of a dosage form must always be rounded up to the next nearest whole.

- Drops must be rounded to the nearest whole drop. You cannot measure partials.

PRACTICE QUESTIONS

1. How many milliliters of water should be mixed with 240 mL of syrup containing 85% w/v sucrose to make a syrup containing 60% w/v sucrose?

    (A) 80 mL
    (B) 100 mL
    (C) 160 mL
    (D) 240 mL
    (E) 340 mL

2. If 10 mL of a solution are to contain 3 mEq of sodium ion, how many 1-g sodium chloride (MW 58.5) tablets would be required to compound 250 mL of solution?

    (A) 2
    (B) 3
    (C) 4
    (D) 5
    (E) 6

3. You have been asked to prepare 500 mL of a benzalkonium chloride solution. The concentration of the solution you prepare must be such that if 20 mL of your solution are diluted to a liter, a 1:1,470 solution is formed. How many milliliters of a 17% benzalkonium chloride solution will you need to compound the solution?

    (A) 17 mL
    (B) 20 mL
    (C) 100 mL
    (D) 147 mL
    (E) 500 mL

4. A pharmacist has 75 grams of 3% w/w zinc oxide paste in stock, to which she adds 5 g of pure zinc oxide. What is the percent concentration of zinc oxide in the final product?

    (A) 2.4% w/w
    (B) 3% w/w
    (C) 7.25% w/w
    (D) 9.06% w/w
    (E) 9.67% w/w

5. How many milligrams of boric acid are needed to compound the following prescription? (The E values are as follows: zinc chloride 0.62, phenacaine HCl 0.17, and boric acid 0.52.)

Rx	Zinc chloride	0.2%
	Phenacaine HCl	1%
	Boric acid	qs
	Purified water qs	60 mL

(A) 92 mg
(B) 189 mg
(C) 339 mg
(D) 364 mg
(E) 698 mg

6. How many milligrams of sodium chloride are needed to compound the following prescription? (The E value of phenylephrine HCl is 0.32.)

Rx	Phenylephrine HCl	0.5%
	Sodium chloride	qs
	Purified water qs	30 mL

(A) 48 mg
(B) 86 mg
(C) 150 mg
(D) 222 mg
(E) 270 mg

7. How many mL of a 1% stock solution of epinephrine HCl are needed for the following prescription?

Rx	Epinephrine HCl sol. 1:500	60 mL

(A) 0.012 mL
(B) 0.12 mL
(C) 1.2 mL
(D) 12 mL
(E) 120 mL

8. Calculate the percentage (v/v) of witch hazel in the following prescription. Round to one decimal place.

   Rx   Sulfur ppt   15 g
         Witch hazel   45 mL
         Alcohol
         Calamine lotion qs   120 mL

   (A) 12.5%
   (B) 25%
   (C) 27.3%
   (D) 37.5%
   (E) 45%

9. A prescription calls for penicillin suspension to be administered: 1.5 teaspoonfuls PO TID for 12 days. How many mL of the suspension should be dispensed?

   (A) 23 mL
   (B) 54 mL
   (C) 90 mL
   (D) 270 mL
   (E) 810 mL

10. A 40-pound child is to receive Dilantin 2.5 mg/kg PO BID. How many mL of Dilantin suspension (125 mg/5 mL) should be dispensed for a 30-day supply?

    (A) 55 mL
    (B) 109 mL
    (C) 240 mL
    (D) 265 mL
    (E) 528 mL

11. A patient who weighs 167 pounds is receiving phenylephrine at a dose of 2 mcg/kg/min. How many mg of phenylephrine does the patient receive over 2 hours?

    (A) 0.30 mg
    (B) 9.1 mg
    (C) 18.2 mg
    (D) 40 mg
    (E) 5,060 mg

12. A formula for 2,000 levothyroxine tablets contains 274 mg of levothyroxine. How many mcg of levothyroxine are in each tablet?

    (A) 0.137 mcg
    (B) 1.37 mcg
    (C) 13.7 mcg
    (D) 137 mcg
    (E) 1,370 mcg

13. The formula for an analgesic ointment is 10 g menthol, 95 g benzocaine, 5 g camphor, 40 g mineral oil, and 850 g petrolatum. How many grams of benzocaine are needed to prepare 5 lbs. of this product?

    (A) 0.22 g
    (B) 215.7 g
    (C) 238.3 g
    (D) 253.7 g
    (E) 1,045 g

14. A solution of iodine in chloroform has a strength of 1.4% (w/v). How many mL of chloroform must be evaporated from the original 180 mL to adjust the iodine concentration to 2.4%?

    (A) 50 mL
    (B) 75 mL
    (C) 105 mL
    (D) 125 mL
    (E) 155 mL

15. How many grams of zinc oxide should be mixed with 8% zinc oxide ointment to make 250 g of a 12% zinc oxide ointment? Round your answer to one decimal place.

    (A) 10.9 g
    (B) 18.5 g
    (C) 37.9 g
    (D) 100 g
    (E) 239.1 g

16. A patient is to receive 2 mEq of sodium chloride per kilogram of body weight. If the patient weighs 186 lbs., how many milliliters of a 0.9% solution of sodium chloride (MW = 58.5) should be administered?

    (A)   11 mL
    (B)   321 mL
    (C)   550 mL
    (D)   1,099 mL
    (E)   5,320 mL

17. How many milliosmoles of calcium chloride (MW = 147) are represented in 200 mL of a 10% (w/v) calcium chloride solution?

    (A)   8.8 mOsm
    (B)   136 mOsm
    (C)   272 mOsm
    (D)   408 mOsm
    (E)   816 mOsm

18. If an ointment contains 60% (w/w) of polyethylene glycol 400 (specific gravity = 1.13), how many mL of polyethylene glycol are needed to prepare 1 kg of ointment?

    (A)   53 mL
    (B)   68 mL
    (C)   354 mL
    (D)   531 mL
    (E)   678 mL

19. How many mL of water should be added to 50 mL of zephiran chloride 1:750 solution to obtain a 1:10,000 strength solution?

    (A)   100 mL
    (B)   200 mL
    (C)   250 mL
    (D)   617 mL
    (E)   667 mL

20. You receive a prescription for fluticasone HFA 440 mcg BID with instructions to dispense a 90-day supply. Fluticasone HFA is available commercially as 220 mcg/metered dose with 120 doses per inhaler. How many inhalers should be dispensed for a 90-day supply?

    (A)   1 inhaler
    (B)   2 inhalers
    (C)   3 inhalers
    (D)   4 inhalers
    (E)   6 inhalers

21. You receive a prescription for insulin glargine 65 units once daily with instructions to dispense a 30-day supply. Insulin glargine is available commercially as 100 units/mL in 10-mL vials. How many vials should be dispensed for a 30-day supply?

    (A) 1 vial
    (B) 2 vials
    (C) 3 vials
    (D) 4 vials
    (E) 5 vials

22. You receive a prescription for oxycodone/acetaminophen 5/500 mg 1–2 tablets every 4–6 hours PRN pain. Based upon a maximum daily acetaminophen dose of 4 grams, how many tablets should be dispensed for a 30-day supply?

    (A) 60 tablets
    (B) 120 tablets
    (C) 240 tablets
    (D) 360 tablets
    (E) 480 tablets

23. An elixir contains 250 mg of active ingredient per 5 mL. You receive a prescription for 500 mg PO twice daily with instructions to dispense 120 mL of the elixir. How many days would the elixir last if taken as prescribed?

    (A) 4 days
    (B) 6 days
    (C) 8 days
    (D) 10 days
    (E) 12 days

24. A pediatric ferrous sulfate suspension contains 75 mg/1.5 mL (20% elemental). What dose (in mL) would provide the patient with 30 mg of elemental iron?

    (A) 0.3 mL
    (B) 0.6 mL
    (C) 1.5 mL
    (D) 3 mL
    (E) 6 mL

25. You are asked to compound a prescription for 120 mL of calamine lotion. The following formula is available.

Rx	Calamine	80 g
	Zinc oxide	80 g
	Glycerin	20 g
	Bentonite magma	250 mL
	Calcium hydroxide topical solution to make	1,000 mL

How many grams of calamine should be used to prepare the quantity specified?

(A) 0.96 g
(B) 8 g
(C) 9.6 g
(D) 80 g
(E) 96 g

26. You receive a prescription for 60 g of zinc oxide ointment. The following formula is available.

Rx	Zinc oxide	1 part
	Starch	1 part
	Petrolatum	2 parts

How many grams of zinc oxide should be used to prepare the quantity specified?

(A) 1 g
(B) 10 g
(C) 15 g
(D) 30 g
(E) 45 g

27. Approximately how many liters of a 0.9% aqueous solution can be made from 30 grams of sodium chloride?

(A) 1 L
(B) 2 L
(C) 3 L
(D) 4 L
(E) 5 L

28. You receive a prescription for 500 mL of a 0.5% w/v solution of drug A. You have on hand 10% w/v solution of drug A. What volume of your available solution should be diluted with water to make the 500 mL prescription?

    (A) 5 mL
    (B) 10 mL
    (C) 15 mL
    (D) 20 mL
    (E) 25 mL

29. A prescription is written for a total quantity of 100 mEq of NaCl. You have normal saline (0.9%) solution on hand. What volume should be dispensed? (MW NaCl = 58.5)

    (A) 58.5 mL
    (B) 65 mL
    (C) 527 mL
    (D) 585 mL
    (E) 650 mL

30. A medication order calls for 75 mL of a 0.8 mEq potassium/mL solution. How many grams of potassium chloride should be used to prepare the quantity specified? (MW KCl = 74.5)

    (A) 4.5 g
    (B) 7.5 g
    (C) 45 g
    (D) 75 g
    (E) 450 g

31. A medication order calls for 10 mL of a 1% tobramycin (E = 0.07) ophthalmic solution. You have on hand tobramycin 40 mg/mL solution. How much NaCl should be added to make the solution isotonic with tears?

    (A) 7 mg
    (B) 33 mg
    (C) 83 mg
    (D) 100 mg
    (E) 400 mg

32. You receive a prescription for amoxicillin 100 mg/5 mL. You have on hand amoxicillin 125 mg/5 mL powder for reconstitution. The label calls for the addition of 63 mL of water to make 80 mL of the 125 mg/5 mL suspension. What volume of water should be added to prepare the concentration specified?

    (A) 68 mL
    (B) 70 mL
    (C) 83 mL
    (D) 88 mL
    (E) 100 mL

33. What volume of a 10% w/v stock solution should be diluted with water to make 500 mL of a 0.25% w/v solution?

    (A) 12.5 mL
    (B) 25 mL
    (C) 50 mL
    (D) 125 mL
    (E) 200 mL

34. A prescription for lansoprazole suspension is written as follows.

Rx	Lansoprazole	3 mg/mL
	Sodium bicarbonate 8.4% ad	50 mL

    Sig. 5 mL BID

    How many lansoprazole 30 mg capsules are needed to compound the prescription?

    (A) 10 capsules
    (B) 15 capsules
    (C) 30 capsules
    (D) 45 capsules
    (E) 60 capsules

ANSWERS

1. B

$$240\,\text{mL} \times \frac{85\,\text{g sucrose}}{100\,\text{mL}} = 204\,\text{g sucrose}$$

$$204\,\text{g sucrose} \times \frac{100\,\text{mL}}{60\,\text{g sucrose}} = 340\,\text{mL total volume}$$

340 mL total volume − 240 mL 85% w/v sucrose syrup = 100 mL of water to add

2. D

$$250\,\text{mL} \times \frac{3\,\text{mEq Na}^+}{10\,\text{mL}} \times \frac{1\,\text{mmol Na}^+}{1\,\text{mEq Na}^+} \times \frac{1\,\text{mmol NaCl}}{1\,\text{mmol Na}^+} \times \frac{58.5\,\text{mg NaCl}}{1\,\text{mmol NaCl}} \times$$

$$\frac{1\,\text{g}}{1000\,\text{mg}} \times \frac{1\,\text{tablet}}{1\,\text{g}} = 4.4\,\text{tabs} = 5\,\text{tabs}$$

If you are using a partial tablet, you must always round up. If you use 4.4 tablets, you will actually expend 5 tablets from inventory, use 4.4 for your product, and discard the remainder of the fifth tablet.

3. C

Final solution: 1 L of 1:1,470 BC $1{,}000\,\text{mL} \times \dfrac{1\,\text{g BC}}{1{,}470\,\text{mL}} = 0.68\,\text{g BC}$

This solution was produced by diluting 20 mL of the solution you made. Therefore, the solution you made has 0.68 g of BC in every 20 mL.

$$500\,\text{mL} \times \frac{0.68\,\text{g BC}}{20\,\text{mL}} = 17\,\text{g of BC}$$

You need 17 g of benzalkonium chloride. How many milliliters of a 17% w/v stock solution will be required to deliver 17 g?

$$17\,\text{g} \times \frac{100\,\text{mL}}{17\,\text{g}} = 100\,\text{mL stock solution}$$

4. D

$$75\,\text{g ung} \times \frac{3\,\text{g ZnO}}{100\,\text{g ung}} = 2.25\,\text{g ZnO}$$

$$\frac{(2.25 + 5)\,\text{g ZnO}}{(75 + 5)\,\text{g ung}} = \frac{7.25\,\text{g ZnO}}{80\,\text{g ung}} = \frac{9.0625\,\text{g ZnO}}{100\,\text{g ung}} = 9.0626\%\ w/w$$

5. **E**

Step 1: Determine the weight of all chemicals present in this prescription.

Zinc chloride: $\dfrac{0.2\ g}{100\ mL} = \dfrac{x}{60\ mL}$

$$x = 0.12\ g$$

Phenacaine: $\dfrac{1\ g}{100\ mL} = \dfrac{y}{60\ mL}$

$$y = 0.6\ g$$

Step 2: Multiply each weight by the listed E value of the chemical.

Zinc chloride: $0.12\ g \times 0.62 = 0.0744\ g$

Phenacaine: $\quad 0.6\ g \times 0.17 = 0.102\ g$

Step 3: Add the weights from Step 2. The sum is the amount of NaCl currently present in this prescription.

$$0.0744\ g + 0.102\ g = 0.1764\ g$$

Step 4: Determine the theoretical amount of NaCl that would be necessary to make this prescription isotonic if no other chemical were present.

$$\dfrac{0.9\ g}{100\ mL} = \dfrac{p}{60\ mL}$$

$$p = 0.54\ g$$

Step 5: Subtract the value in Step 3 from the value in Step 4 to determine the amount of NaCl that needs to be added to make this prescription isotonic.

$$0.54\ g - 0.1764\ g = 0.3636\ g$$

Step 6: Determine the amount of boric acid that would be used instead of NaCl to make this prescription isotonic.

$$\dfrac{0.3636\ g\ NaCl}{q} = \dfrac{0.52\ g\ NaCl}{1\ g\ boric\ acid}$$

$$q = 0.698\ g \times 1{,}000 = \textbf{698 mg}$$

6. **D**

Step 1: Determine the weight of all chemicals present in this prescription.

$$\text{Phenylephrine: } \frac{0.5 \text{ g}}{100 \text{ mL}} = \frac{x}{30 \text{ mL}}$$

$$x = 0.15 \text{ g}$$

Step 2: Multiply each weight by the listed E value of the chemical. The product is the amount of NaCl currently present in this prescription.

Phenylephrine: $0.15 \text{ g} \times 0.32 = 0.048 \text{ g}$

Step 3: Determine the theoretical amount of NaCl that would be necessary to make this prescription isotonic if no other chemical were present.

$$\frac{0.9 \text{ g}}{100 \text{ mL}} = \frac{y}{30 \text{ mL}}$$

$$y = 0.27 \text{ g}$$

Step 4: Subtract the value in Step 2 from the value in Step 3 to determine the amount of NaCl that needs to be added to make this prescription isotonic.

$$0.27 \text{ g} - 0.048 \text{ g} = 0.222 \text{ g} \times 1{,}000 = \textbf{222 mg}$$

7. **D**

The concentration of the epinephrine solution is presented as a ratio strength. A concentration of 1:500 translates into 1 g/500 mL. The first step in solving this problem is to determine the amount of epinephrine (in grams) that would be contained in 60 mL of the solution.

$$\frac{1 \text{ g}}{500 \text{ mL}} = \frac{x}{60 \text{ mL}}$$

$$x = 0.12 \text{ g epinephrine}$$

Next, set up a ratio-proportion to determine the volume of the 1% epinephrine stock solution needed to obtain the 0.12 grams of epinephrine.

1% stock solution:

$$\frac{1 \text{ g}}{100 \text{ mL}} = \frac{0.12 \text{ g}}{y}$$

$$y = \textbf{12 mL}$$

8. **D**

To determine the percentage of witch hazel, you must calculate the amount of witch hazel in 100 mL of the compound. According to the problem, there are 45 mL of witch hazel in 120 mL of calamine lotion in this prescription. To solve this problem, set up a ratio-proportion.

$$\frac{45 \text{ mL}}{120 \text{ mL}} = \frac{x}{100 \text{ mL}}$$

$$x = \textbf{37.5\%}$$

9. **D**

First, calculate the number of teaspoons to be administered on a daily basis.

$$1.5 \text{ tsp/dose} \times 3 \text{ doses/day} = 4.5 \text{ tsp/day}$$

Next, set up a ratio-proportion to determine the total volume (in mL) of penicillin suspension to be administered (assuming 1 teaspoon = 5 mL).

$$\frac{4.5 \text{ tsp}}{x} = \frac{1 \text{ tsp}}{5 \text{ mL}}$$

$$x = 22.5 \text{ mL}$$

Finally, multiply this daily volume by 12 days to determine the total volume of suspension (in mL) that should be dispensed.

$$22.5 \text{ mL/day} \times 12 \text{ days} = \textbf{270 mL}$$

10. **B**

Using dimensional analysis, multiply the weight-based dose by the weight of the child (being sure to convert the weight into kilograms), then by 2 (since the weight-based dose is being given twice daily), and then by 30 (to account for the 30-day supply). You can see below that all the units cancel out except for mg. The answer in this first step is the total number of milligrams of Dilantin that will be dispensed for this child for a 30-day supply.

$$\frac{2.5 \text{ mg}}{\text{kg dose}} \times 40 \text{ lb} \times \frac{1 \text{ kg}}{2.2 \text{ lb}} \times \frac{2 \text{ doses}}{\text{day}} \times 30 \text{ days} = 2{,}727.27 \text{ mg}$$

Next, using the concentration of Dilantin suspension of 125 mg/5 mL given in the problem, set up a ratio-proportion to determine the volume of this suspension to be dispensed that will contain 2,727.27 mg.

$$\frac{125 \text{ mg}}{5 \text{ mL}} = \frac{2{,}727.27 \text{ mg}}{x}$$

$$x = \textbf{109 mL}$$

11. **C**

Set up the problem using dimensional analysis: Multiply the weight-based dose by the weight of the patient, being sure to convert into kilograms; convert the units of time to hours; and convert the dose from micrograms to milligrams, since that is what the question is asking. You can see below that all the units cancel out except for mg.

$$\frac{2 \text{ mcg}}{\text{kg/min}} \times 167 \text{ lb} \times \frac{1 \text{ kg}}{2.2 \text{ lb}} \times \frac{60 \text{ min}}{1 \text{ hr}} \times 2 \text{ hr} \times \frac{1 \text{ mg}}{1,000 \text{ mcg}} = \textbf{18.2 mg}$$

12. **D**

Given that there are 274 mg of levothyroxine in 2,000 tablets, set up a ratio-proportion to determine how many milligrams are in 1 tablet. Then multiply this answer (in milligrams) by 1,000 to arrive at the answer in micrograms.

$$\frac{274 \text{ mg}}{2,000 \text{ tablets}} = \frac{x}{1 \text{ tablet}}$$

$$x = 0.137 \text{ mg} \times 1,000 \text{ mcg/mg} = \textbf{137 mcg}$$

13. **B**

The first step is to determine the total amount of the analgesic ointment that will be made given the formula provided.

$$10 \text{ g} + 95 \text{ g} + 5 \text{ g} + 40 \text{ g} + 850 \text{ g} = 1,000 \text{ g ointment}$$

Next, convert the total amount of ointment to be prepared, 5 pounds, into grams.

$$5 \text{ lb} \times \frac{454 \text{ g}}{1 \text{ lb}} = 2,270 \text{ g}$$

Finally, set up a ratio-proportion to determine how much benzocaine is needed to prepare 2,270 g of ointment, given that 95 g of benzocaine is used to prepare 1,000 g of the same ointment.

$$\frac{95 \text{ g benzocaine}}{1,000 \text{ g ointment}} = \frac{x}{2,270 \text{ g ointment}}$$

$$x = \textbf{215.7 g}$$

14. **B**

In this problem, the solution of iodine in chloroform is being concentrated (rather than diluted). The $Q_1C_1 = Q_2C_2$ method can be used to solve the problem. The volume that is solved for x is the amount of the 2.4% solution that would be made.

$$(1.4\%)\,(180\text{ mL}) = (2.4\%)\,x$$

$$x = 105\text{ mL (this is the amount of 2.4\% solution)}$$

However, the question asks how much chloroform *must be evaporated from* the original 180 mL to adjust the iodine concentration to 2.4%. Therefore, this amount (105 mL) must be subtracted from the original amount (180 mL) to determine how much solution must be evaporated.

180 mL – 105 mL = **75 mL must be evaporated**

15. **A**

Alligation:

High Concentration [A]		Parts of High Concentration Ingredient [D]
	Desired Concentration [C]	
Low Concentration [B]		Parts of Low Concentration Ingredient [E]

Parts of high-concentration ingredient [D] = [C] – [B]

Parts of low-concentration ingredient [E] = [A] – [C]

Zinc Oxide Ointment:

Assume pure zinc oxide = 100%

100%		12 – 8 = 4 parts
	12%	
8%		100 – 12 = 88 parts
		Total = 92 parts

Quantity of 100% zinc oxide ointment needed:

$$\frac{4\text{ parts}}{92\text{ parts}} = \frac{x}{250\text{ g}}$$

$$x = \textbf{10.9 g}$$

16. **D**

The first step is to multiply the weight-based dose by the weight of the patient using dimensional analysis, being sure to convert the weight into kilograms.

$$\frac{186 \text{ lb}}{} \times \frac{1 \text{ kg}}{2.2 \text{ lb}} \times \frac{2 \text{ mEq}}{\text{kg}} = 169.1 \text{ mEq}$$

At this point, the milliequivalent formula below can be used to determine the weight of sodium chloride (in mg) present in 169.1 mEq. Remember that the valence of sodium chloride (NaCl) is 1. The molecular weight of sodium chloride was given to you in the problem (58.5).

$$\text{mEq} = \frac{(\text{mg of chemical}) (\text{valence})}{\text{molecular weight}}$$

$$169.1 = \frac{x\,(1)}{58.5}$$

$$x = 9,891.8 \text{ mg} / 1,000 = 9.89 \text{ g}$$

Once the weight of sodium chloride is known, a ratio-proportion can be used to determine the volume of 0.9% sodium chloride solution to be administered. Remember that a 0.9% solution of sodium chloride contains 0.9 g of sodium chloride in 100 mL of solution.

Volume of 0.9% NaCl needed:

$$\frac{0.9 \text{ g}}{100 \text{ mL}} = \frac{9.89 \text{ g}}{x}$$

$$x = \textbf{1,099 mL}$$

17. **D**

The first step is to determine how much calcium chloride (in grams) is contained in 200 mL of a 10% (w/v) solution. Set up a ratio-proportion to solve this step.

$$\frac{10 \text{ g}}{100 \text{ mL}} = \frac{x}{200 \text{ mL}}$$

$$x = 20 \text{ g CaCl}_2$$

At this point, the milliosmole formula below can be used to determine how many milliosmoles are represented by 20 grams of calcium chloride. Remember that calcium chloride dissociates into 3 species. The molecular weight of calcium chloride was given to you in the problem (147).

$$\text{mOsm} = \frac{\text{weight of substance (g)}}{\text{molecular weight}} \times 1{,}000 \times \text{\# of species}$$

$$\text{mOsm} = \frac{20 \text{ g}}{147} \times 1{,}000 \times 3$$

$$\text{mOsm} = \textbf{408 mOsm}$$

18. **D**

The first step is to determine how much of the polyethylene glycol 400 would be needed to prepare 1 kg (or 1,000 g) of ointment, starting with a 60% (w/w) polyethylene glycol 400 ointment. A ratio-proportion can be set up to solve this problem.

$$\frac{60 \text{ g}}{100 \text{ g}} = \frac{x}{1{,}000 \text{ g}}$$

$$x = 600 \text{ g of polyethylene glycol 400 needed}$$

Next, set up a ratio-proportion with this information to determine the volume of polyethylene glycol solution needed to prepare this compound. Remember that the specific gravity of a substance represents weight/volume.

Specific gravity (SG) = wt/vol

$$\frac{1.13 \text{ g}}{1 \text{ mL}} = \frac{600 \text{ g}}{y}$$

$$y = \textbf{531 mL}$$

19. **D**

This is a dilution problem that involves ratio strengths. The first step is to determine how much zephiran chloride (in grams) is contained in 50 mL of a 1:750 solution. This can be determined by setting up a ratio-proportion.

$$\frac{1 \text{ g}}{750 \text{ mL}} = \frac{x}{50 \text{ mL}}$$

$$x = 0.067 \text{ g}$$

Since the solution will be diluted to a 1:10,000 solution, the next step is to determine what volume of this solution would contain 0.067 g of zephiran chloride. Again, this can be determined by setting up a ratio-proportion.

$$\frac{1 \text{ g}}{10{,}000 \text{ mL}} = \frac{0.067 \text{ g}}{y}$$

$$y = 666.67 \text{ mL}$$

This dilution process involved going from 50 mL of a 1:750 solution to 666.67 mL of a 1:10,000 solution. However, 666.67 mL is not the final answer, as the question asked how many milliliters of water *should be added* to arrive at this amount. Thus, the final step of the problem is to subtract the initial volume from the total volume to arrive at the answer.

666.67 mL – 50 mL = 616.67 mL = **617 mL of water needs to be added**

20. **C**

Solve this problem using dimensional analysis: Multiply the number of doses per day (2) by the strength of each prescribed dose (440 mcg); by the strength per metered dose (220 mcg/dose) and the number of doses per inhaler (120) to factor in the available dosage form; and by the number of days needed (90). Each fraction should be set up such that all the units cancel out except for inhalers.

$$2 \times \frac{440 \text{ mcg}}{1 \text{ day}} \times \frac{1 \text{ dose}}{220 \text{ mcg}} \times \frac{1 \text{ inhaler}}{120 \text{ doses}} \times 90 \text{ days} = \textbf{3 inhalers}$$

21. **B**

Solve this problem using dimensional analysis: Multiply the number of units the patient will need each day (65) by the number of units in each milliliter of insulin (100); by the number of milliliters per vial (10); and by the number of days needed (30). Each fraction should be set up such that all the units cancel out except for vials.

$$\frac{65 \text{ units}}{1 \text{ day}} \times \frac{1 \text{ mL}}{100 \text{ units}} \times \frac{1 \text{ vial}}{10 \text{ mL}} \times 30 \text{ days} = 1.56 \text{ vials}$$

Therefore, **2 vials** should be dispensed.

22. **C**

Solve this problem using dimensional analysis: Convert the maximum daily dose (4 g/day) to milligrams, and multiply by the strength of each tablet (500 mg) and the number of days needed (30). Each fraction should be set up such that all the units cancel out except for tablets.

$$\frac{4 \text{ g}}{1 \text{ day}} \times \frac{1,000 \text{ mg}}{1 \text{ g}} \times \frac{1 \text{ tablet}}{500 \text{ mg}} \ 30 \text{ days} = \textbf{240 tablets}$$

23. **B**

Solve this problem using dimensional analysis: Multiply the strength of the elixir (250 mg/5 mL) by the desired dose (500 mg); by the number of doses per day (2); and by the quantity dispensed (120 mL). Each fraction should be set up such that all units cancel out except for days.

$$\frac{250 \text{ mg}}{5 \text{ mL}} \times \frac{1 \text{ dose}}{500 \text{ mg}} \times \frac{1 \text{ day}}{2 \text{ doses}} \times 120 \text{ mL} = \textbf{6 days}$$

24. **D**

First, use dimensional analysis to determine the amount of elemental iron per milliliter. Multiply the strength of the available suspension (75 mg/1.5 mL) by the percent of elemental iron (20%).

$$\frac{75 \text{ mg ferrous sulfate}}{1.5 \text{ mL suspension}} \times \frac{20 \text{ mg elemental iron}}{100 \text{ mg ferrous sulfate}} = 10 \text{ mg elemental iron/mL}$$

Then, set up a ratio-proportion to calculate the volume of the suspension needed to obtain the 30 mg of elemental iron, and cross-multiply to solve the problem.

$$\frac{10 \text{ mg elemental iron}}{1 \text{ mL}} = \frac{30 \text{ mg elemental iron}}{x}$$

$$10x = 30 \text{ mL}$$

$$x = 30 / 10 - \textbf{3 mL}$$

25. **C**

One approach to solving this problem is to identify the factor that represents the relationship between the desired quantity (120 mL) and the quantity specified in the compounding recipe (1,000 mL), then multiply by this factor to determine the appropriate amount of each ingredient. In this case, the relationship can be expressed by dividing 120 mL by 1,000 mL, yielding a factor of 0.12.

$$\frac{120 \text{ mL}}{1,000 \text{ mL}} = 0.12 \text{ (factor)}$$

Next, multiply the relevant ingredient—in this case, 80 g of calamine—by this factor to calculate the appropriate amount.

$$80 \text{ g calamine} \times 0.12 = \textbf{9.6 g}$$

26. **C**

First, determine the ratio of zinc oxide to the total recipe by finding the sum of the parts: 1 part + 1 part + 2 parts = 4 parts. So the ratio of parts zinc oxide to total parts is 1:4. Next, set up a ratio-proportion to calculate how much zinc oxide is contained in a total weight of 60 grams, and cross-multiply to solve.

$$\frac{1 \text{ part zinc oxide}}{4 \text{ parts total}} = \frac{x \text{ g zinc oxide}}{60 \text{ g total}}$$

$$4x = 60$$

$$x = 60 / 4 = \textbf{15 g}$$

27. **C**

The first step in solving this problem is to set up a ratio-proportion representing the relationship between the desired %w/v (0.9%) and the available weight of the product (30 g).

$$\frac{0.9\ g}{100\ mL} = \frac{30\ g}{x}$$

$$0.9x = 3{,}000\ mL$$

$$x = 3{,}000\ /\ 0.9\ mL$$

$$x = 3{,}333\ mL$$

The problem asks for liters, so convert from milliliters to liters to solve the problem.

$$3{,}333\ mL \times \frac{1\ L}{1{,}000\ mL} = \textbf{3.33 L}$$

28. **E**

The first step is to calculate how much of drug A (in grams) is contained in 500 mL of a 0.5% w/v solution. Solve this step using dimensional analysis.

$$\frac{0.5\ g\ drug\ A}{100\ mL} \times 500\ mL = 2.5\ g\ drug\ A$$

Next, set up a ratio-proportion to determine the volume of the available 10% w/v solution needed to obtain the desired weight of drug A (2.5 g), and cross-multiply to solve the problem.

$$\frac{10\ g}{100\ mL} = \frac{2.5\ g}{x\ mL} = \textbf{25 mL}$$

29. **E**

Sodium and chloride are monovalent ions, so 1 mol = 1 equivalent. The first step in solving this problem is to determine the number of grams of NaCl per mEq. Because there is 1 mol per equivalent, this is a simple calculation: Divide the molecular weight (which is equal to the EqW) by 1,000 to determine g/mEq.

MW NaCl = 58.5

$$EqW = \frac{58.5\ g}{1}$$

$$1\ mEq = \frac{58.5}{1{,}000} = 0.0585\ g$$

Next, multiply the weight by the desired number of mEq (100) to determine the total weight needed.

$$100 \text{ mEq} = 0.0585 \text{ g} \times 100 = 5.85 \text{ g NaCl needed}$$

Finally, set up a ratio-proportion indicating the relationship between the available concentration (0.9% for normal saline) and the desired weight of NaCl (5.85 g), and cross-multiply to solve the problem.

$$\frac{0.9 \text{ g}}{100 \text{ mL}} = \frac{5.85 \text{ g}}{x}$$

$$0.9x = 585$$

$$x = 585 / 0.9 = \textbf{650 mL}$$

30. **A**

Because KCl is made up of monovalent ions, the molecular weight is equal to the EqW. Divide the number by 1,000 to determine the weight/mEq.

$$MW \text{ KCl} = 74.5$$

$$EqW = \frac{74.5 \text{ g}}{1}$$

$$1 \text{ mEq} = \frac{74.5}{1,000} = 0.0745 \text{ g}$$

From here, the problem can be solved using dimensional analysis: Multiply the desired concentration (0.8 mEq/mL) by the weight/mEq (74.5 g/mEq) and by the total quantity desired (75 mL). Each fraction should be set up such that units cancel out except for grams.

$$\frac{0.8 \text{ mEq}}{1 \text{ mL}} \times \frac{0.0745 \text{ g}}{1 \text{ mEq}} \times 75 \text{ mL} = \textbf{4.5 g}$$

31. **C**

First, calculate the total amount of tobramycin in the desired product by multiplying the %w/v by the given volume.

$$1\% \text{ solution} = \frac{1 \text{ g tobramycin}}{100 \text{ mL}} \times 10 \text{ mL} = 0.1 \text{ g tobramycin}$$

Then, multiply the weight of the active ingredient by the E value of the active ingredient (0.07) to determine the weight of NaCl required to exert the tonic effect represented in the solution.

$$0.1 \text{ g tobramycin} \times \frac{0.07 \text{ g NaCl(eq)}}{1 \text{ g tobramycin}} = 0.007 \text{ g NaCl(eq)}$$

Next, use the %w/v of normal saline (0.9%) to calculate the total amount of NaCl needed to make the solution isotonic if this were the sole tonicity agent.

$$\frac{0.9 \text{ g NaCl}}{100 \text{ mL}} \times 10 \text{ mL} = 0.09 \text{ g NaCl}$$

Finally, subtract the amount of NaCl already present in the tobramycin (0.007 g) from this total amount (0.09 g) to determine how much should be added.

$$0.09 \text{ g} - 0.007 \text{ g} = 0.083 \text{ g NaCl} \times \frac{1,000 \text{ mg}}{1 \text{ g}} = \textbf{83 mg}$$

32. **C**

First, set up a ratio-proportion to calculate the total weight of medication in the bottle.

$$\frac{125 \text{ mg}}{5 \text{ mL}} = \frac{x}{80 \text{ mL}}$$

$$5 \text{ mL} \times x \text{ mg} = 125 \text{ mg} \times 80 \text{ mL}$$

$$x = 2,000 \text{ mg amoxicillin}$$

Then, set up another ratio-proportion to determine the total volume needed to provide the desired concentration.

$$\frac{100 \text{ mg}}{5 \text{ mL}} = \frac{2,000 \text{ mg}}{y}$$

$$100 \text{ mg} \times y = 2,000 \text{ mg} \times 5 \text{ mL}$$

$$y = 100 \text{ mL}$$

Next, calculate the volume of the dry powder to be used in this prescription by subtracting the amount of water added from the total end volume.

volume of dry powder = 80 mL − 63 mL = 17 mL

Finally, determine the amount of water to add for reconstitution by subtracting the volume of dry powder calculated in the previous step from the total volume needed.

100 mL − volume of dry powder (17 mL) = water to add = **83 mL**

33. **A**

This problem can be solved by setting up a simple ratio-proportion indicating the relationship between the available stock solution and the desired volume and concentration of the new solution.

$$(10\%) \times (x \text{ mL}) = (0.25\%) \times (500 \text{ mL})$$

$$10x = 125$$

$$x = 125 / 10 = \textbf{12.5 mL}$$

34. **B**

First, determine the total weight of drug needed by multiplying the concentration (3 mg/mL) by the given volume (150 mL).

$$\frac{3 \text{ mg}}{1 \text{ mL}} \times 150 \text{ mL} = 450 \text{ mg lansoprazole needed}$$

Next, divide the total weight needed by the available capsule strength (30 mg) to determine the number of capsules needed.

$$450 \text{ mg} / 30 \text{ mg capsules} = \text{total number of capsules needed} = \textbf{15 capsules}$$

Biostatistics

22

 Suggested Study Time: **15 minutes**

Statistics play an important role in the development and interpretation of clinical trials. The following section covers the most important definitions in biostatistics, and discusses various statistical tests, when to use them, and how to interpret them.

GENERAL STATISTICAL DEFINITIONS

The table below lists several general statistical definitions with which you should be familiar.

General Statistical Definitions

Measures of central tendency	Mean	Average value of a sample distribution
	Median	Value that lies closest to the center of a sample distribution
	Mode	Most commonly occurring number in a sample distribution
Estimates of variability	Range	Difference between the smallest and largest values in a sample distribution
	Standard deviation	Average of the distances between each value in a distribution and the mean of the distribution Most widely used estimate of variability
Hypotheses	Hypothesis	Theoretical statement that the study is intended to test
	Null hypothesis	States that there is no difference between the study and control groups
	Alternative hypothesis	States that the null hypothesis is incorrect; there is a difference between the study and control groups

Variables	Independent variable	Known variable(s)
	Dependent variable	Variable with a value dependent upon the value of an independent variable
Error	Type I Error	Rejecting a true null hypothesis: Finding a difference between the study and control groups that does not exist
	Type II Error	Accepting a false null hypothesis: Failing to detect a difference between the study and control groups that does exist
Tests	Parametric	Requires prior knowledge of the nature of the data under examination; data must fall under a normal (Gaussian) distribution and be measured on an interval or a ratio scale
	Nonparametric	Does not require prior knowledge of the distribution of the observations; data need not follow a normal or Gaussian distribution
Miscellaneous definitions	Accuracy	Measure of how close a measured value is to the expected value
	Precision	Measure of how close a particular measured value is to the other values in a set of measurements; does not imply proximity between measured values and the expected value
	Sample	Data set taken under homogenous conditions; a subset of a population
	Population	Entire group from which a sample is taken
	Gaussian (or normal) distribution	A bell-shaped distribution Given a large enough sample size, the Central Limit Theorem states that the distribution of means will follow this type of distribution even if the population is not Gaussian. • 69% of values fall within $\pm$ 1 SD of the mean • 95% of values fall within $\pm$ 2 SD of the mean • 98% of values fall within $\pm$ 3 SD of the mean

Several additional statistical concepts are included below, in slightly greater detail. Many of these concepts apply regardless of the statistical test chosen.

P-value and Statistical Significance

The p-value is the probability that the difference measured between your study group and the control group is the result of random chance rather than a true difference. The p-value is expressed as a value between 0 and 1.

The null hypothesis may be rejected if there is a sufficiently small probability that it is true. A significance level (or α) of 0.05 is most commonly chosen, although it should be chosen based on the relative consequences of making a Type I or Type II error in the particular study setting. When a 0.05 significance level is chosen, if $p \leq 0.05$, a statistically significant difference in treatment effect exists between the control and treatment groups. If $p > 0.05$, the results of the study are considered to be not statistically significant, meaning no difference exists between the treatment and control groups. Choosing a larger significance level, like $p = 0.1$, gives a higher probability of rejecting a true null hypothesis (Type I error, or false positive test).

Confidence Intervals

A confidence interval (CI) is the interval, computed from sample data, such that there is a given probability that the population mean value of the unknown parameter is contained within the interval. Ninety-five percent CI is the most common interval seen, but others may be calculated as well. Wider intervals (such as 99% CI) have a higher probability of containing the population mean; however, they also span more values.

Power

No discussion of statistical significance is complete without a discussion of statistical power. Two factors affect power:

- Sample size
- Amount of variation within the groups (i.e., standard deviation)

Low power may result in Type II errors, where a "not statistically significant" result is obtained even though there truly is a difference between the treatment and control groups. If necessary, the power of a study may be increased by studying more subjects, although there are practical and economic limits on study size. It is not appropriate to conclude that a treatment is ineffective based only on a study with insufficient power.

Correlation

Correlation measures the degree of a linear relationship between two variables. Correlation is often represented by the correlation coefficient (r), which can range in value from −1 to +1. A correlation coefficient of 0 indicates no linear relationship between variables. A coefficient of −1 reflects a perfect inverse relationship between variables, while a value of +1 reflects a perfect direct relationship. A key point to remember is that an observed correlation between two variables does not imply that there is a causal link between the two variables. For example, warm weather causes an increase in both the crime rate and the incidence of sunburn. Crime rate and sunburn incidence will therefore be positively correlated; however, crime does not cause sunburn and sunburn does not cause crime.

Another important point to consider is that correlation coefficient assumes a normal distribution of measured values; if this assumption is incorrect, the coefficient is not relevant.

STATISTICAL TEST SELECTION

The first thing that must be done when determining what statistical test should be employed is to identify the dependent variable and the scale of measurement that will be used for this variable. The scale of measurement may be numeric, ordinal, or nominal.

Tests Appropriate for Numerical Scales of Measurement

Numeric scales (also called interval or ratio scales) of measurement are used when the measured values are numbers. Examples include height, weight, or blood pressure level. When the data follows a Gaussian distribution, parametric statistical tests should be used.

- Two independent groups: T test
- Two dependent groups: Paired t-test
- Three or more independent groups: Analysis of variance (ANOVA)
- Three or more dependent groups: Repeated measures ANOVA

When the data does not follow a Gaussian distribution, the same tests used for ordinal data should be employed.

Tests Appropriate for Ordinal Scales of Measurement

Ordinal scales of measurement are used when characteristics have an underlying order to their values but the numbers used are arbitrary (such as Likert scales). Various non-parametric tests (such as Mann-Whitney U and Wilcoxon Signed-Rank) are used for analyzing such data.

Tests Appropriate for Nominal Scales of Measurement

Nominal scales are used for characteristics that do not have numerical value (such as gender or race). The Chi-square test and its variants are used to test the null hypothesis that proportions are equal, or that factors or characteristics are not associated with each other.

Finally, Kaplan-Meier is a frequently used statistical test that analyzes patient survival time. Probability of death is recalculated every time a trial subject dies. This method is similar to actuarial analysis in the insurance industry; although, unlike actuarial analysis, Kaplan-Meier gives exact survival proportions because it uses exact survival times instead of group approximations.

LEARNING POINTS

- Smaller p-values associated with a statement reflect a greater likelihood that the statement accurately reflects a difference between groups. Larger p-values mean that the difference detected between groups is more likely to have been due to random chance.

- Power is the ability of a study to detect an actual effect. Power can be increased by increasing the number of patients enrolled in a study. Inadequate power may result in a study failing to detect a difference that actually exists between groups.

- The mean is the numerical average of the entire range of data; the mode is the central point in the data distribution. In a pure Gaussian distribution, the median will be equal or very close to the mode; large variance between median and mode may reflect non-Gaussian distribution or significant outlying data.

- ANOVA and t-tests are appropriate only for numeric data in a Gaussian distribution. Nonparametric tests are appropriate for numeric data in a non-Gaussian distribution, as well as for ordinal data. Chi-square tests should be used for nominal data.

PRACTICE QUESTIONS

1. The median value of a data set is the

   (A) mathematical average of all the values in the data set.
   (B) value equidistant from the extremes of a distribution.
   (C) average of the difference between each value in the set and the mean.
   (D) most commonly occurring value in the data set.
   (E) distance between the smallest and largest values in the data set.

ANSWERS

1. **B**

The median value is the value equidistant from the extremes of the data set. The mathematical average of the values in the data set (A) is the mean. The average of the difference between each value and the mean (C) is the standard deviation. The most commonly occurring value in the data set (D) is the mode. The distance between the smallest and largest values in the data set (E) is the range.

Part Four

Resources and Policy

Drug Information

23

This chapter provides an overview of common tertiary literature resources that can be used as drug information resources for pharmacists.

 Suggested Study Time: **30 minutes**

GENERAL DRUG INFORMATION RESOURCES

American Hospital Formulary Service (AHFS) Drug Information (published by the American Society of Health-System Pharmacists [ASHP])

- Provides Food and Drug Administration (FDA)-approved and off-label uses
- Each monograph contains general drug information (e.g., pharmacology, pharmacokinetics, side effects, toxicology, drug interactions, dosing, administration, available preparations)

Drug Facts and Comparisons

- Provides information on:
  » Prescription/over-the-counter (OTC) drugs
  » Investigational/orphan drugs
- Each monograph contains general drug information
- Also provides helpful comparison tables

United States Pharmacopeia Drug Information (USP DI)

- Volume I: Drug Information for the Healthcare Professional
  » Provides general drug information
  » Various appendices (poison control centers, drug-induced side effects, selected therapeutic guidelines, drug identification color inserts)

- Volume II: Advice for the Patient: Drug Information in Lay Language
  - » Provides supplemental information for patient counseling
- Volume III: Approved Drug Products and Legal Requirements
  - » Provides information on therapeutic equivalence (contains FDA Orange Book), labeling/storage/packaging requirements, and pharmacy law

Physicians' Desk Reference (PDR)

- Contains FDA-approved package insert information
  - » Does not provide unlabeled drug uses
- Also contains a colored insert (for drug identification) and manufacturer information

Drug Information Handbook (Lexi-Comp)

- Provides general drug information
- Contains useful charts, tables, and treatment algorithms
- Also available in specialty versions (pediatrics, geriatrics, psychiatric, oncology)

Red Book

- Provides the following information on prescription and OTC drugs:
  - » Cost data (average wholesale price [AWP])
  - » National Drug Code (NDC) numbers
  - » Formulations available (dosage forms, sugar-free/alcohol-free preparations)
  - » Drug identification (colored inserts)
  - » Manufacturer

PHARMACOTHERAPY RESOURCES

Pharmacotherapy: A Pathophysiologic Approach (DiPiro)

- Provides the following information regarding various disease states: Pathophysiology, etiology, clinical presentation, diagnosis, treatment

Applied Therapeutics: The Clinical Use of Drugs (Koda-Kimble)

- Focuses on treatment of disease states
- Case-based format

INTERNAL MEDICINE RESOURCES

Harrison's Principles of Internal Medicine

- Focuses on pathophysiology, etiology, clinical presentation, and diagnosis
- Provides an overview of treatment; does not provide detailed information on drugs or dosing recommendations

Cecil Textbook of Medicine

- Not as comprehensive as Harrison's

Washington Manual of Medical Therapeutics

- Provides a general overview of disease states and treatment

Merck Manual of Diagnosis and Therapy

- Provides a quick summary of disease-state information (etiology, pathophysiology, clinical presentation, diagnosis, prognosis, treatment)

DRUG INTERACTION RESOURCES

Hansten and Horn's Drug Interaction Analysis and Management

- Provides the following information on drug interactions: Summary of interaction, proposed mechanism, significance, risk factors, treatment options

Drug Interaction Facts (published by Facts and Comparisons)

- Provides similar information as *Hansten and Horn's*

ADVERSE DRUG REACTION RESOURCES

Meyler's Side Effects of Drugs

- Provides critical review of literature regarding drugs' side effects: Effects on organ systems, interference with lab/diagnostic tests, withdrawal, and overdose
- Provides 2 indexes for ease of reference:
  - » Drugs
  - » Side effects

PARENTERAL DRUG COMPATIBILITY/STABILITY RESOURCES

Handbook on Injectable Drugs (published by ASHP)

- Previously known as Trissel's
- Provides information regarding compatibility/stability of parenteral drugs
- Also provides information on commercially available dosages, volumes, and sizes

King Guide to Parenteral Admixtures

- Provides similar information as *Handbook on Injectable Drugs*

PHARMACOLOGY RESOURCES

Goodman & Gilman's: The Pharmacological Basis of Therapeutics

- "Gold standard" pharmacology reference
- Provides very thorough discussion of the pharmacology of drugs; also provides information on the drugs' pharmacokinetics, pharmacodynamics, and toxicology

COMPOUNDING AND PHARMACEUTICS RESOURCES

Merck Index

- Different from the *Merck Manual*
- Provides chemical and pharmacologic information on drugs (e.g., chemical name, molecular formula, structure, molecular weight, solubility, drug class, toxicity, data, manufacturer)

Remington: The Science and Practice of Pharmacy

- Provides information on numerous issues concerning pharmacy practice (e.g., pharmaceutical calculations, chemistry, radioisotopes, compounding techniques/ingredients)

DRUG IDENTIFICATION RESOURCES

American Drug Index

- Cross-referenced by brand, generic, and chemical names
- Also provides available dosage forms/strengths and manufacturer information

IDENTIDEX (available through MICROMEDEX)

- Identifies drug after entering in imprint on tablet/capsule

Other useful resources are the color inserts in the following guides:

- *USP DI Volume I*
- *PDR*
- *Red Book*

FOREIGN DRUG INFORMATION RESOURCES

Martindale: The Complete Drug Reference

- Provides information on drugs used throughout the world

Index Nominum: International Drug Directory

- Provides similar information as *Martindale*

PEDIATRIC DRUG INFORMATION RESOURCES

The Harriet Lane Handbook

- Pocket guide that provides brief overview (especially diagnosis and treatment) of common disease states in children

Pediatric Dosage Handbook (Lexi-Comp)

- Provides drug information specific to the pediatric population

General drug information resources (e.g., MICROMEDEX, AHFS) also provide general pediatric dosing information.

PREGNANCY AND LACTATION RESOURCES

Drugs in Pregnancy and Lactation (Briggs)

- "Gold standard"
- Focuses on safety of drugs in pregnancy and lactation

La Leche League (www.llli.org)

- Provides practitioners and patients with clinical and practical information on all aspects of breastfeeding

OTC DRUG RESOURCES

Handbook of Nonprescription Drugs: An Interactive Approach to Self-Care (published by the American Pharmacists Association)

- Provides etiology, pathophysiology, clinical presentation, and treatment of disease states that may be amenable to self-care
- Provides comprehensive information on OTC products (e.g., side effects, drug interactions, dosing, dosage forms, patient counseling)

PDR for Nonprescription Drugs

NATURAL PRODUCTS RESOURCES

Natural Standard

- "Gold standard"
- Comprehensive database

PDR for Herbal Medicines

Complete German Commission E Monographs

PDR for Nonprescription Drugs, Dietary Supplements, and Herbs

Comparison of Tertiary Drug Information Resources

Reference	Monograph: Basic Info	Approved Uses	Unapproved Uses	Drug Interactions	Language for Patients	Manufacturer Contact Information	Product ID	Cost	Dosage Form Availability	Pathophysiology	Disease State Management	Treatment of Drug Overdoses	Foreign Drug Identification	IV Drug Compatibility	Chemical Properties	Generic Availability	Compounding Information	Lactation Information	Mechanism of Action
American Hospital Formulary Service Drug Information (AHFS)	X	X	X	X					X			X			X	X		X	X
Physicians' Desk Reference (PDR)	X	X		X		X	X		X			X			X			X	X
Drug Information Handbook (Lexi-Comp)	X	X	X	X					X			X			X			X	X
Facts and Comparisons	X	X	X	X					X			X			X			X	X
Martindale: The Complete Drug Reference													X						
USP DI Drug Information for the Healthcare Provider (Vol I)	X	X	X	X			X		X			X						X	X
USP DI Advice for the Patient: Drug Information in Lay Language (Vol II)					X														
USP DI Approved Drug Products and Legal Requirements (Vol III)		X																	
Pharmacotherapy: A Pathophysiologic Approach (DiPiro's)										X	X	X							X
Remington: The Science and Practice of Pharmacy															X		X		
Handbook on Injectable Drugs (Trissel's)									X					X					
King Guide to Parenteral Admixtures														X					

Reference	Monograph Basic Info	Approved Uses	Unapproved Uses	Drug Interactions	Language for Patients	Manufacturer Contact Information	Product ID	Cost	Dosage Form Availability	Pathophysiology	Disease State Management	Treatment of Drug Overdoses	Foreign Drug Identification	IV Drug Compatibility	Chemical Properties	Generic Availability	Compounding Information	Lactation Information	Mechanism of Action
Goodman and Gilman's: The Pharmacological Basis of Therapeutics																			X
Harrison's Principles of Internal Medicine										X	X	X							
Drug Interactions Analysis and Management (Hansten and Horn's)				X															
Drug Interaction Facts				X															
Harriet Lane Handbook	X	X		X							X							X	
Drugs in Pregnancy and Lactation (Briggs)																		X	
Red Book						X	X	X	X										

LEARNING POINTS

- Learn drug information resources by various categories. Once you know the kind of information that you need, you can select the most appropriate reference.
- Do not memorize the table above; it can be used to assess your general knowledge of tertiary literature sources.
- Remember the differences between primary, secondary, and tertiary literature:
  - Primary literature: Original journal articles (research reports, case reports, editorials); serves as information for development of secondary and tertiary literature resources
  - Secondary literature: Indexing and abstracting services (e.g., MEDLINE, IPA, EMBASE, Cochrane)
  - Tertiary literature: Textbooks and review articles; summarize and interpret primary literature

PRACTICE QUESTIONS

1. A physician calls to ask the pharmacist about the mechanism of action of a new drug that has been approved for hypercholesterolemia. Which of the following references is/are most appropriate for obtaining this information?

    I. AHFS Drug Information
    II. Facts and Comparisons
    III. USP DI Volume III

    (A) I only
    (B) III only
    (C) I and II only
    (D) II and III only
    (E) I, II, and III

2. A patient comes to your pharmacy and gives you a prescription for an ointment that needs to be compounded. Which of the following references would be most appropriate to obtain information regarding the preparation of this ointment?

    (A) *Martindale: The Complete Drug Reference*
    (B) *Pharmacotherapy: A Pathophysiologic Approach*
    (C) *Physicians' Desk Reference*
    (D) *Remington: The Science and Practice of Pharmacy*
    (E) *Harriet Lane Handbook*

ANSWERS

1. **C**

AHFS Drug Information (I) and Facts and Comparisons (II) both contain general drug information in monograph format, so choice (C) is correct. USP DI Volume III (III) contains information on approved drug products (generic availability) and legal requirements.

2. **D**

Remington would be the most appropriate reference to obtain information regarding compounding of an ointment, so choice (D) is correct. *Martindale* (A) provides information on foreign drugs. *Pharmacotherapy: A Pathophysiologic Approach* (B) is a general pharmacotherapy resource. *Physicians' Desk Reference* (C) is a general drug information resource. *Harriet Lane Handbook* (E) is a pediatric drug information resource.

Health Policy

24

This chapter covers three key areas of health policy:

- **HIPAA**
- **FDA regulatory process**
- **The Joint Commission accreditation process**

 Suggested Study Time: **30 minutes**

HIPAA

What is HIPAA? The Health Insurance Portability and Accountability Act of 1996 (HIPAA) required the U.S. Department of Health and Human Services (HHS) to issue regulations governing healthcare entities that engage in electronic healthcare transactions. HIPAA regulations apply both to the form of electronic healthcare transactions and the privacy of patient information. At the time they were enacted, the regulations were expected to have far-reaching consequences. Compliance with patient privacy regulations was mandated for April 2003.

The purpose of HIPAA is to improve the Medicare program under title XVIII of the Social Security Act, the Medicaid program under title XIX of that act, and the efficiency and effectiveness of the healthcare system, by encouraging the development of a health information system through the establishment of standards and requirements for the electronic transmission of certain health information.

The Office for Civil Rights (OCR) is responsible for enforcing the HIPAA Privacy Rule. One of the ways that OCR carries out this responsibility is to investigate complaints filed with it. OCR may also conduct compliance reviews to determine whether covered entities are in compliance, and OCR performs education and outreach to foster compliance with the requirements of the Privacy Rule.

If OCR accepts a complaint for investigation, OCR will notify the person who filed the complaint and the covered entity named in it. Then the complainant and the covered entity are asked to present information about the incident or problem described in the complaint. OCR may request specific information from each to get an understanding of the facts. Covered entities are required by law to cooperate with complaint investigations.

OCR reviews the information, or evidence, that it gathers in each case. In some cases, it may determine that the covered entity did not violate the requirements of the Privacy Rule. If the evidence indicates that the covered entity was not in compliance, OCR will attempt to resolve the case with the covered entity.

Most Privacy Rule investigations are concluded to the satisfaction of OCR through these types of resolutions. OCR provides written notice of the resolution result to the person who filed the complaint and to the covered entity.

If the covered entity does not take action to resolve the matter in a way that is satisfactory, OCR may decide to impose civil monetary penalties (CMPs) on the covered entity. If CMPs are imposed, the covered entity may request a hearing in which an HHS administrative law judge decides if the penalties are supported by the evidence in the case. Complainants do not receive a portion of CMPs collected from covered entities; the penalties are deposited in the U.S. Treasury.

Every pharmacy, regardless of size, is considered a covered entity under the regulations and, as such, each one is required to comply with the HIPAA regulations. Entities (pharmacies) may be fined for noncompliance (civil fines of up to $25,000 per violation and criminal penalties of up to $250,000 and 10 years imprisonment).

HIPAA protects the information found in your medical record from disclosure (being made available to other persons or organizations) without your authorization. The information protected by HIPAA includes:

- Any information related to your past, present, or future physical or mental health
- The past, present, or future payment for health services you have received
- The specific care that you have received, are receiving, or will receive
- Any information that identifies you as the individual receiving the care
- Any information that another person could reasonably use to identify you as the individual receiving the care

As a covered entity, a pharmacy is required to inform patients of how it may use your protected health information. In providing treatment to patients, a pharmacy should use patients' protected health information only for the purposes of treatment, payment, and healthcare operations.

Other general rules include the requirement that the pharmacy must provide a paper copy of the Notice to patients and the public in general about how the pharmacy will be protecting their privacy.

1. The Pharmacy must make the Notice available upon request to any person, even if that person is not a current pharmacy patient.

2. The Pharmacy must provide the Notice to the patient no later than the date that the Pharmacy first provides service to the patient, including service delivered electronically.

    In emergency treatment situations, the Notice will be provided as soon after the emergency as is reasonably practicable. The Pharmacy may send the Notice to all of its patients at once, give the notice to each patient as s/he comes into the Pharmacy or contacts the Pharmacy electronically, or by any combination of these approaches.

3. The Pharmacy must have the Notice available at the store for individuals who request a copy to take with them.

4. The Pharmacy must post the Notice in a clear and prominent location in the store where patients will be able to read it.

FDA REGULATORY PROCESS

For decades, the regulation and control of new drugs in the United States has been based on the New Drug Application (NDA). Since 1938, every new drug has been the subject of an approval process by the NDA before that drug can be sold commercially in the United States. The NDA application is the vehicle through which drug sponsors formally propose that the FDA approve a new pharmaceutical for sale and marketing in the United States. The data gathered during the animal studies and human clinical trials of an Investigation New Drug (IND) become part of the NDA.

During a new drug's early preclinical development, the sponsor's primary goal is to determine whether the product is reasonably safe for initial use in humans, and if the compound exhibits pharmacological activity that justifies commercial development. When a product is identified as a viable candidate for further development, the sponsor then focuses on collecting the data and information necessary to establish that the product will not expose humans to unreasonable risks when used in limited, early-stage clinical studies.

The FDA's role in the development of a new drug begins when the drug's sponsor (usually the manufacturer or potential marketer), having screened the new molecule for pharmacological activity and acute toxicity potential in animals, wants to test its diagnostic or therapeutic potential in humans. At that point, the molecule changes in legal status under the Federal Food, Drug, and Cosmetic Act and becomes a new drug subject to specific requirements of the drug regulatory system.

There are three IND types:

- Investigator IND is submitted by a physician who both initiates and conducts an investigation, and under whose immediate direction the investigational drug is administered or dispensed. A physician might submit a research IND to propose studying an unapproved drug, or an approved product for a new indication or in a new patient population.

- Emergency Use IND allows the FDA to authorize use of an experimental drug in an emergency situation that does not allow time for submission of an IND in accordance with FDA regulations. It is also used for patients who do not meet the criteria of an existing study protocol, or if an approved study protocol does not exist.

- Treatment IND is submitted for experimental drugs showing promise in clinical testing for serious or immediately life-threatening conditions while the final clinical work is conducted and the FDA review takes place.

There are two IND categories:

- Commercial
- Research (noncommercial)

The IND application must contain information in three broad areas:

- Animal Pharmacology and Toxicology Studies: Preclinical data to permit an assessment as to whether the product is reasonably safe for initial testing in humans. Also included is any previous experience with the drug in humans (often foreign use).

- Manufacturing Information: Information pertaining to the composition, manufacturer, stability, and controls used for manufacturing the drug substance and the drug product. This information is assessed to ensure that the company can adequately produce and supply consistent batches of the drug.

- Clinical Protocols and Investigator Information: Detailed protocols for proposed clinical studies to assess whether the initial-phase trials will expose subjects to unnecessary risks. Also, information on the qualifications of clinical investigators—professionals (generally physicians) who oversee the administration of the experimental compound—to assess whether they are qualified to fulfill their clinical trial duties. Finally, commitments to obtain informed consent from the research subjects, to obtain review of the study by an institutional review board (IRB), and to adhere to the investigational new drug regulations.

Once the IND is submitted, the sponsor must wait 30 calendar days before initiating any clinical trials. During this time, the FDA has an opportunity to review the IND for safety to assure that research subjects will not be subjected to unreasonable risk.

Once the IND data is gathered, the sponsor can then submit an NDA. The goals of the NDA are to provide enough information to permit the FDA reviewer to reach the following key decisions:

- Whether the drug is safe and effective in its proposed use(s), and whether the benefits of the drug outweigh the risks
- Whether the drug's proposed labeling (package insert) is appropriate, and what it should contain
- Whether the methods used in manufacturing the drug and the controls used to maintain the drug's quality are adequate to preserve the drug's identity, strength, quality, and purity

The documentation required in an NDA is supposed to tell the drug's whole story, including what happened during the clinical tests; what the ingredients of the drug are; the results of the animal studies; how the drug behaves in the body; and how it is manufactured, processed, and packaged.

Current Federal law requires that a drug be the subject of an approved marketing application before it is transported or distributed across state lines. Because a sponsor will probably want to ship the investigational drug to clinical investigators in many states, it must seek an exemption from that legal requirement.

Types of Clinical Trials

This section describes the different types of clinical trials used during the IDA and NDA application process following a chemotherapy drug.

Phase 1 (phase I)

These are the earliest trials in the life of a new drug or treatment. They are usually small trials, recruiting anywhere up to about 30 patients, although often a lot less. The trial may be open to people with any type of cancer.

For example, when laboratory testing shows that a new treatment might help treat cancer, phase 1 trials are done to find out:

- The safe dose range
- The side effects
- How the body copes with the drug
- If the treatment shrinks cancer

Patients are recruited very slowly onto phase 1 trials. So, although these trials do not recruit many patients, they can take a long time to complete. The first few patients to take part (called a "cohort," or group) will be given a very small dose of the drug. If all goes well, the next group will receive a slightly higher dose. The dose will be gradually increased with each group. The researchers will monitor the effect until they find the best dose to give. This is called a "dose escalation study."

In a phase 1 trial, patients may have many blood tests, as the researchers look at how the drug is affecting the patient and at how the body copes with and gets rid of the drug. Researchers will also record any side effects.

People entering phase 1 trials often have advanced cancer and have usually had all the treatment available to them. This is because they may benefit from the new treatment in the trial, but many will not. The aim of the trial is to study doses and side effects. This work must be done first before the potential new treatment can be tested to see if it works. Phase 1 trials are important because they are the first step in finding new treatments for the future.

Phase 2 (phase II)

Not all treatments tested in a phase 1 trial make it to a phase 2 trial. These trials may include people who all have the same type of cancer, or people who have different types of cancer. Phase 2 trials seek to determine:

- If the new treatment works well enough to test in a larger phase 3 trial
- On which types of cancer the treatment works
- More about side effects and how to manage them
- More about the best dose to use

Although these treatments have been tested at phase 1, patients may still have side effects that the doctors do not yet know about. Drugs can affect people in different ways.

Phase 2 trials are often larger than phase 1; there may be up to 50 or so people taking part. If the results of phase 2 trials show that a new treatment may be as good as (or better than) existing treatment, the drug then moves to phase 3.

Phase 3 (phase III)

Phase 3 trials compare new treatments with the best currently available treatment (the standard treatment). They may compare:

- A completely new treatment with the standard treatment
- Different doses or ways of giving a standard treatment
- A new radiotherapy schedule with the standard one

Phase 3 trials are usually much larger than phases 1 and 2. This is because differences in success rates may be small, so the trial would need to include many patients to show the difference.

For example, 6 out of 100 (6%) more people get a remission with a new treatment than with standard treatment. If there were 50 people in the new treatment group and 50 people in the standard treatment group, there may be 3 more people in remission in the new treatment group. The two groups would not look that different. But if each treatment were given to 5,000 people, there could be 300 more remissions in the new treatment group.

Sometimes phase 3 trials involve thousands of patients in many different hospitals, and even in different countries.

Randomization

Phase 3 trials are usually randomized. This means the researchers randomly place the people taking part into two groups. One group receives the new treatment and the other receives the standard treatment.

Overviews

Trial overviews are studies that combine all the results from phase 3 trials of a new treatment. They are sometimes called meta-analyses. The idea is to get a broader picture of how well a treatment works. The more data (information) we have, the more accurate the results are likely to be.

Phase 4 (phase IV)

Phase 4 trials are done after a drug has been shown to work and has been granted a license, so they are looking at drugs that are already available for doctors to prescribe, rather than new drugs that are still being developed.

The main reasons pharmaceutical companies run phase 4 trials are to:

- Find out more about the side effects and safety of the drug
- Identify the long-term risks and benefits
- Determine how well the drug works when it is used more widely than in clinical trials

Orphan Drugs Products

Since its inception in 1982, the Office of Orphan Products Development (OOPD) has been dedicated to promoting the development of products that demonstrate promise for the diagnosis and/or treatment of rare diseases or conditions. OOPD interacts with the medical and research communities, professional organizations, academia, and the pharmaceutical industry, as well as rare-disease groups. The OOPD administers the major provisions of the Orphan Drug Act (ODA), which provide incentives for sponsors to develop products for rare diseases. The ODA has been very successful—more than 200 drugs and biological products for rare diseases have been brought to market since 1983. In contrast, the decade prior to 1983 saw fewer than 10 such products come to market. In addition, the OOPD administers the Orphan Product Grants Program, which provides funding for clinical research in rare diseases.

THE JOINT COMMISSION ACCREDITATION PROCESS

TJC stands for the Joint Commission. It is a private, nonprofit organization that evaluates medical facility compliance based on a focused set of "requirements" that have long been known as essential to the delivery of good patient care.

TJC sets standards by which healthcare quality is measured. TJC accreditation means that healthcare facilities have demonstrated compliance with the standards of performance in meeting the needs of people they serve. To maintain accreditation, healthcare facilities undergo an extensive on-site review by TJC professionals. The review evaluates the facilities' performance in all areas that affect patient care. Each facility is evaluated and scored. Accreditation may then be awarded based on how well the facility met TJC standards.

LEARNING POINTS

- HIPAA was established due to the advent of electronic healthcare record-keeping and to ensure that patient information remains private.

- All pharmacies, regardless of size, are considered covered entities under the regulations and, as such, they are required to comply with the HIPAA regulations.

- During a new drug's early preclinical development, the sponsor's primary goal is to determine if the product is reasonably safe for initial use in humans, and if the compound exhibits pharmacological activity that justifies commercial development.

- Current Federal law requires that a drug be the subject of an approved marketing application before it is transported or distributed across state lines.

- The OOPD administers the major provisions of the Orphan Drug Act, which provides incentives for sponsors to develop products for rare diseases.

PRACTICE QUESTIONS

1. Which of the following does NOT serve the purpose of HIPAA?

    (A) To improve the Medical program
    (B) To improve the efficiency and effectiveness of the healthcare system
    (C) To encourage the development of health information standards
    (D) To ensure fair prices for procedures
    (E) To ensure safe and private electronic transmission of health information

ANSWERS

1. **D**

HIPAA was not established to ensure fair prices. The purpose of HIPAA is to improve the Medicare program under title XVIII of the Social Security Act, the Medicaid program under title XIX of such Act, and the efficiency and effectiveness of the healthcare system by encouraging the development of a health information system through the establishment of standards and requirements for the electronic transmission of certain health information.

Part Five

Full-Length Practice Test

Full-Length Practice Test

To mimic the realistic conditions of the NAPLEX, allow yourself a total of **4 hours and 15 minutes** to complete all 185 questions. Take a 10-minute break at the 2-hour time point.

While every test-taker is different, the average candidate takes 2.5 to 3 hours to complete the exam. There are no bonus points for finishing early.

The computer-adaptive format of the exam requires that you **answer all questions in the order in which they are presented**. You cannot skip a question or return to a previous question to review your answer. Again, to make this practice test as realistic as possible, **do not** return to the previous question to change your answer.

ANSWER GRID

1. Ⓐ Ⓑ Ⓒ Ⓓ Ⓔ
2. Ⓐ Ⓑ Ⓒ Ⓓ Ⓔ
3. Ⓐ Ⓑ Ⓒ Ⓓ Ⓔ
4. Ⓐ Ⓑ Ⓒ Ⓓ Ⓔ
5. Ⓐ Ⓑ Ⓒ Ⓓ Ⓔ
6. Ⓐ Ⓑ Ⓒ Ⓓ Ⓔ
7. Ⓐ Ⓑ Ⓒ Ⓓ Ⓔ
8. Ⓐ Ⓑ Ⓒ Ⓓ Ⓔ
9. Ⓐ Ⓑ Ⓒ Ⓓ Ⓔ
10. Ⓐ Ⓑ Ⓒ Ⓓ Ⓔ
11. Ⓐ Ⓑ Ⓒ Ⓓ Ⓔ
12. Ⓐ Ⓑ Ⓒ Ⓓ Ⓔ
13. Ⓐ Ⓑ Ⓒ Ⓓ Ⓔ
14. Ⓐ Ⓑ Ⓒ Ⓓ Ⓔ
15. Ⓐ Ⓑ Ⓒ Ⓓ Ⓔ
16. Ⓐ Ⓑ Ⓒ Ⓓ Ⓔ
17. Ⓐ Ⓑ Ⓒ Ⓓ Ⓔ
18. Ⓐ Ⓑ Ⓒ Ⓓ Ⓔ
19. Ⓐ Ⓑ Ⓒ Ⓓ Ⓔ
20. Ⓐ Ⓑ Ⓒ Ⓓ Ⓔ
21. Ⓐ Ⓑ Ⓒ Ⓓ Ⓔ
22. Ⓐ Ⓑ Ⓒ Ⓓ Ⓔ
23. Ⓐ Ⓑ Ⓒ Ⓓ Ⓔ
24. Ⓐ Ⓑ Ⓒ Ⓓ Ⓔ
25. Ⓐ Ⓑ Ⓒ Ⓓ Ⓔ
26. Ⓐ Ⓑ Ⓒ Ⓓ Ⓔ
27. Ⓐ Ⓑ Ⓒ Ⓓ Ⓔ
28. Ⓐ Ⓑ Ⓒ Ⓓ Ⓔ
29. Ⓐ Ⓑ Ⓒ Ⓓ Ⓔ
30. Ⓐ Ⓑ Ⓒ Ⓓ Ⓔ
31. Ⓐ Ⓑ Ⓒ Ⓓ Ⓔ
32. Ⓐ Ⓑ Ⓒ Ⓓ Ⓔ
33. Ⓐ Ⓑ Ⓒ Ⓓ Ⓔ
34. Ⓐ Ⓑ Ⓒ Ⓓ Ⓔ
35. Ⓐ Ⓑ Ⓒ Ⓓ Ⓔ
36. Ⓐ Ⓑ Ⓒ Ⓓ Ⓔ
37. Ⓐ Ⓑ Ⓒ Ⓓ Ⓔ
38. Ⓐ Ⓑ Ⓒ Ⓓ Ⓔ
39. Ⓐ Ⓑ Ⓒ Ⓓ Ⓔ
40. Ⓐ Ⓑ Ⓒ Ⓓ Ⓔ

41. Ⓐ Ⓑ Ⓒ Ⓓ Ⓔ
42. Ⓐ Ⓑ Ⓒ Ⓓ Ⓔ
43. Ⓐ Ⓑ Ⓒ Ⓓ Ⓔ
44. Ⓐ Ⓑ Ⓒ Ⓓ Ⓔ
45. Ⓐ Ⓑ Ⓒ Ⓓ Ⓕ
46. Ⓐ Ⓑ Ⓒ Ⓓ Ⓔ
47. Ⓐ Ⓑ Ⓒ Ⓓ Ⓔ
48. Ⓐ Ⓑ Ⓒ Ⓓ Ⓔ
49. Ⓐ Ⓑ Ⓒ Ⓓ Ⓔ
50. Ⓐ Ⓑ Ⓒ Ⓓ Ⓔ
51. Ⓐ Ⓑ Ⓒ Ⓓ Ⓔ
52. Ⓐ Ⓑ Ⓒ Ⓓ Ⓔ
53. Ⓐ Ⓑ Ⓒ Ⓓ Ⓔ
54. Ⓐ Ⓑ Ⓒ Ⓓ Ⓔ
55. Ⓐ Ⓑ Ⓒ Ⓓ Ⓔ
56. Ⓐ Ⓑ Ⓒ Ⓓ Ⓔ
57. Ⓐ Ⓑ Ⓒ Ⓓ Ⓔ
58. Ⓐ Ⓑ Ⓒ Ⓓ Ⓔ
59. Ⓐ Ⓑ Ⓒ Ⓓ Ⓔ
60. Ⓐ Ⓑ Ⓒ Ⓓ Ⓔ
61. Ⓐ Ⓑ Ⓒ Ⓓ Ⓔ
62. Ⓐ Ⓑ Ⓒ Ⓓ Ⓔ
63. Ⓐ Ⓑ Ⓒ Ⓓ Ⓔ
64. Ⓐ Ⓑ Ⓒ Ⓓ Ⓔ
65. Ⓐ Ⓑ Ⓒ Ⓓ Ⓔ
66. Ⓐ Ⓑ Ⓒ Ⓓ Ⓔ
67. Ⓐ Ⓑ Ⓒ Ⓓ Ⓔ
68. Ⓐ Ⓑ Ⓒ Ⓓ Ⓔ
69. Ⓐ Ⓑ Ⓒ Ⓓ Ⓔ
70. Ⓐ Ⓑ Ⓒ Ⓓ Ⓔ
71. Ⓐ Ⓑ Ⓒ Ⓓ Ⓔ
72. Ⓐ Ⓑ Ⓒ Ⓓ Ⓔ
73. Ⓐ Ⓑ Ⓒ Ⓓ Ⓔ
74. Ⓐ Ⓑ Ⓒ Ⓓ Ⓔ
75. Ⓐ Ⓑ Ⓒ Ⓓ Ⓔ
76. Ⓐ Ⓑ Ⓒ Ⓓ Ⓔ
77. Ⓐ Ⓑ Ⓒ Ⓓ Ⓔ
78. Ⓐ Ⓑ Ⓒ Ⓓ Ⓔ
79. Ⓐ Ⓑ Ⓒ Ⓓ Ⓔ
80. Ⓐ Ⓑ Ⓒ Ⓓ Ⓔ

81. Ⓐ Ⓑ Ⓒ Ⓓ Ⓔ
82. Ⓐ Ⓑ Ⓒ Ⓓ Ⓔ
83. Ⓐ Ⓑ Ⓒ Ⓓ Ⓔ
84. Ⓐ Ⓑ Ⓒ Ⓓ Ⓔ
85. Ⓐ Ⓑ Ⓒ Ⓓ Ⓔ
86. Ⓐ Ⓑ Ⓒ Ⓓ Ⓔ
87. Ⓐ Ⓑ Ⓒ Ⓓ Ⓔ
88. Ⓐ Ⓑ Ⓒ Ⓓ Ⓔ
89. Ⓐ Ⓑ Ⓒ Ⓓ Ⓕ
90. Ⓐ Ⓑ Ⓞ Ⓓ Ⓔ
91. Ⓐ Ⓑ Ⓒ Ⓓ Ⓔ
92. Ⓐ Ⓑ Ⓒ Ⓓ Ⓔ
93. Ⓐ Ⓑ Ⓒ Ⓓ Ⓔ
94. Ⓐ Ⓑ Ⓒ Ⓓ Ⓔ
95. Ⓐ Ⓑ Ⓒ Ⓓ Ⓔ
96. Ⓐ Ⓑ Ⓒ Ⓓ Ⓔ
97. Ⓐ Ⓑ Ⓒ Ⓓ Ⓔ
98. Ⓐ Ⓑ Ⓒ Ⓓ Ⓔ
99. Ⓐ Ⓑ Ⓒ Ⓓ Ⓔ
100. Ⓐ Ⓑ Ⓒ Ⓓ Ⓔ
101. Ⓐ Ⓑ Ⓒ Ⓓ Ⓔ
102. Ⓐ Ⓑ Ⓒ Ⓓ Ⓔ
103. Ⓐ Ⓑ Ⓒ Ⓓ Ⓔ
104. Ⓐ Ⓑ Ⓒ Ⓓ Ⓔ
105. Ⓐ Ⓑ Ⓒ Ⓓ Ⓔ
106. Ⓐ Ⓑ Ⓒ Ⓓ Ⓔ
107. Ⓐ Ⓑ Ⓒ Ⓓ Ⓔ
108. Ⓐ Ⓑ Ⓒ Ⓓ Ⓔ
109. Ⓐ Ⓑ Ⓒ Ⓓ Ⓔ
110. Ⓐ Ⓑ Ⓒ Ⓓ Ⓔ
111. Ⓐ Ⓑ Ⓒ Ⓓ Ⓔ
112. Ⓐ Ⓑ Ⓒ Ⓓ Ⓔ
113. Ⓐ Ⓑ Ⓒ Ⓓ Ⓔ
114. Ⓐ Ⓑ Ⓒ Ⓓ Ⓔ
115. Ⓐ Ⓑ Ⓒ Ⓓ Ⓔ
116. Ⓐ Ⓑ Ⓒ Ⓓ Ⓔ
117. Ⓐ Ⓑ Ⓒ Ⓓ Ⓔ
118. Ⓐ Ⓑ Ⓒ Ⓓ Ⓔ
119. Ⓐ Ⓑ Ⓒ Ⓓ Ⓔ
120. Ⓐ Ⓑ Ⓒ Ⓓ Ⓔ

ANSWER GRID

121. Ⓐ Ⓑ Ⓒ Ⓓ Ⓔ	146. Ⓐ Ⓑ Ⓒ Ⓓ Ⓔ	171. Ⓐ Ⓑ Ⓒ Ⓓ Ⓔ
122. Ⓐ Ⓑ Ⓒ Ⓓ Ⓔ	147. Ⓐ Ⓑ Ⓒ Ⓓ Ⓔ	172. Ⓐ Ⓑ Ⓒ Ⓓ Ⓔ
123. Ⓐ Ⓑ Ⓒ Ⓓ Ⓔ	148. Ⓐ Ⓑ Ⓒ Ⓓ Ⓔ	173. Ⓐ Ⓑ Ⓒ Ⓓ Ⓔ
124. Ⓐ Ⓑ Ⓒ Ⓓ Ⓔ	149. Ⓐ Ⓑ Ⓒ Ⓓ Ⓔ	174. Ⓐ Ⓑ Ⓒ Ⓓ Ⓔ
125. Ⓐ Ⓑ Ⓒ Ⓓ Ⓔ	150. Ⓐ Ⓑ Ⓒ Ⓓ Ⓔ	175. Ⓐ Ⓑ Ⓒ Ⓓ Ⓔ
126. Ⓐ Ⓑ Ⓒ Ⓓ Ⓔ	151. Ⓐ Ⓑ Ⓒ Ⓓ Ⓔ	176. Ⓐ Ⓑ Ⓒ Ⓓ Ⓔ
127. Ⓐ Ⓑ Ⓒ Ⓓ Ⓔ	152. Ⓐ Ⓑ Ⓒ Ⓓ Ⓔ	177. Ⓐ Ⓑ Ⓒ Ⓓ Ⓔ
128. Ⓐ Ⓑ Ⓒ Ⓓ Ⓔ	153. Ⓐ Ⓑ Ⓒ Ⓓ Ⓔ	178. Ⓐ Ⓑ Ⓒ Ⓓ Ⓔ
129. Ⓐ Ⓑ Ⓒ Ⓓ Ⓔ	154. Ⓐ Ⓑ Ⓒ Ⓓ Ⓔ	179. Ⓐ Ⓑ Ⓒ Ⓓ Ⓔ
130. Ⓐ Ⓑ Ⓒ Ⓓ Ⓔ	155. Ⓐ Ⓑ Ⓒ Ⓓ Ⓔ	180. Ⓐ Ⓑ Ⓒ Ⓓ Ⓔ
131. Ⓐ Ⓑ Ⓒ Ⓓ Ⓔ	156. Ⓐ Ⓑ Ⓒ Ⓓ Ⓔ	181. Ⓐ Ⓑ Ⓒ Ⓓ Ⓔ
132. Ⓐ Ⓑ Ⓒ Ⓓ Ⓔ	157. Ⓐ Ⓑ Ⓒ Ⓓ Ⓔ	182. Ⓐ Ⓑ Ⓒ Ⓓ Ⓔ
133. Ⓐ Ⓑ Ⓒ Ⓓ Ⓔ	158. Ⓐ Ⓑ Ⓒ Ⓓ Ⓔ	183. Ⓐ Ⓑ Ⓒ Ⓓ Ⓔ
134. Ⓐ Ⓑ Ⓒ Ⓓ Ⓔ	159. Ⓐ Ⓑ Ⓒ Ⓓ Ⓔ	184. Ⓐ Ⓑ Ⓒ Ⓓ Ⓔ
135. Ⓐ Ⓑ Ⓒ Ⓓ Ⓔ	160. Ⓐ Ⓑ Ⓒ Ⓓ Ⓔ	185. Ⓐ Ⓑ Ⓒ Ⓓ Ⓔ
136. Ⓐ Ⓑ Ⓒ Ⓓ Ⓔ	161. Ⓐ Ⓑ Ⓒ Ⓓ Ⓔ	
137. Ⓐ Ⓑ Ⓒ Ⓓ Ⓔ	162. Ⓐ Ⓑ Ⓒ Ⓓ Ⓔ	
138. Ⓐ Ⓑ Ⓒ Ⓓ Ⓔ	163. Ⓐ Ⓑ Ⓒ Ⓓ Ⓔ	
139. Ⓐ Ⓑ Ⓒ Ⓓ Ⓔ	164. Ⓐ Ⓑ Ⓒ Ⓓ Ⓔ	
140. Ⓐ Ⓑ Ⓒ Ⓓ Ⓔ	165. Ⓐ Ⓑ Ⓒ Ⓓ Ⓔ	
141. Ⓐ Ⓑ Ⓒ Ⓓ Ⓔ	166. Ⓐ Ⓑ Ⓒ Ⓓ Ⓔ	
142. Ⓐ Ⓑ Ⓒ Ⓓ Ⓔ	167. Ⓐ Ⓑ Ⓒ Ⓓ Ⓔ	
143. Ⓐ Ⓑ Ⓒ Ⓓ Ⓔ	168. Ⓐ Ⓑ Ⓒ Ⓓ Ⓔ	
144. Ⓐ Ⓑ Ⓒ Ⓓ Ⓔ	169. Ⓐ Ⓑ Ⓒ Ⓓ Ⓔ	
145. Ⓐ Ⓑ Ⓒ Ⓓ Ⓔ	170. Ⓐ Ⓑ Ⓒ Ⓓ Ⓔ	

Directions: Complete each of the following questions with the best possible answer.

1. Diarrhea is most common with which of the following medications?

   (A) Allopurinol
   (B) Probenecid
   (C) Indomethacin
   (D) Acetaminophen
   (E) Colchicine

2. Which of the following is NOT true regarding A1c?

   (A) It is used to evaluate glycemic control in patients with diabetes.
   (B) It represents a time frame of approximately 30–45 days.
   (C) It can be inaccurate in cases of severe anemia.
   (D) The most commonly used normal reference range is 4–6%.
   (E) An A1c of 10% would indicate average blood sugar over 200 mg/dL.

3. Which of the following atypical antipsychotics requires rigorous monitoring of WBC and ANC?

   (A) Olanzapine
   (B) Risperidone
   (C) Quetiapine
   (D) Ziprasidone
   (E) Clozapine

4. What information should the doctor consider prior to initiating Mirapex in a patient with Parkinson's disease?

   I. Decrease the levodopa dose by 20–30% when initiating Mirapex.
   II. Patient must wear patch for 24 hours for efficacy.
   III. Monitor for serious cardiac side effects.

   (A) I only
   (B) III only
   (C) I and II only
   (D) II and III only
   (E) I, II, and III

5. A patient has been diagnosed with depression and will begin antidepressant therapy today. Which of the following is MOST appropriate, assuming the patient has no other health conditions?

   (A) Venlafaxine 37.5 mg PO BID
   (B) Lexapro 10 mg PO BID
   (C) Fluvoxamine 80 mg PO weekly
   (D) Nortriptyline 300 mg PO daily
   (E) Mirtazapine 10 mg PO Q a.m.

6. Which of the following counseling points is/are TRUE?

   I. NuvaRing should be inserted once every month.
   II. Ortho-Evra should be applied once every week for 3 weeks/month.
   III. Seasonale should result in menses approximately every 3 months.

   (A) I only
   (B) III only
   (C) I and II only
   (D) II and III only
   (E) I, II, and III

7. Which of the following key monitoring parameters is NOT correctly matched to its corresponding medication?

   (A) Blood glucose – prednisone
   (B) CBC – methotrexate
   (C) Ocular exam – hydroxychloroquine
   (D) Serum creatinine – Enbrel
   (E) Hepatic enzymes – leflunomide

8. Which of the following statements regarding serum creatinine is TRUE?

   (A) Serum creatinine is most commonly used to assess hepatic disease.
   (B) Serum creatinine is dependent upon the amount of iron consumed in the diet.
   (C) Serum creatinine is a more accurate measure in the very elderly than in young adults.
   (D) Serum creatinine is used in the Cockroft-Gault equation.
   (E) Serum creatinine is synonymous with microalbumin.

9. Which of the following statements regarding the use of natalizumab in multiple sclerosis is/are TRUE?

   I. Patients must enroll in the TOUCH program prior to receiving.
   II. It should be reserved for those unresponsive to other medications.
   III. It should be added to other disease-modifying drugs when relapse occurs.

   (A) I only
   (B) III only
   (C) I and II only
   (D) II and III only
   (E) I, II, and III

10. Allopurinol is indicated for which of the following gout presentations?

    (A) Prophylaxis in patients with slightly elevated uric acid levels
    (B) Prophylaxis in patients with moderately elevated uric acid and uric acid overproduction
    (C) Prophylaxis in patients with uric acid excretion indicative of underexcretion
    (D) Treatment of acute gout
    (E) Treatment of asymptomatic hyperuricemia

11. Which of the following medication(s) require monitoring of serum drug concentrations?

       I. Lamotrigine
      II. Valproic acid
     III. Lithium

    (A) I only
    (B) III only
    (C) I and II only
    (D) II and III only
    (E) I, II, and III

12. Which of the following trade names is NOT correctly matched with its generic name?

    (A) Zyprexa – olanzapine
    (B) Risperdal – risperidone
    (C) Geodon – ziprasidone
    (D) Abilify – aripiprazole
    (E) Haldol – clozapine

13. Migraine prophylaxis could be achieved with which of the following medication classes?

    (A) ACE inhibitors
    (B) Acetaminophen
    (C) Antidepressants
    (D) H$_2$ antagonist
    (E) Anticholinergics

14. What is the MOST appropriate recommendation for a patient with osteoarthritis and stomach ulcers?

    (A) Aspirin 325 mg PO every 4–6 hours
    (B) Tramadol 25 mg PO every 4–6 hours
    (C) Diclofenac 50 mg PO BID
    (D) Daypro 600 mg PO daily
    (E) Mobic 7.5 mg PO daily

Questions 15–19 refer to the following patient profile.

Patient Name: Tamara Yates

Age: 40   **Height:** 5'2"

Sex: F   **Weight:** 90 lb

Allergies: Geodon

Diagnosis

  Primary:

    Hypertension

    Depression

    Schizophrenia

  Chief Complaint: tardive dyskinesia, dystonia

Lab/Diagnostic Tests

Date	Test/Result	
03/02	Sodium	133 mEq/L
(last week)	Potassium	3.5 mEq/L
	Serum creatinine	1.0 mg/dL
	Blood pressure	166/98 mmHg
	Heart rate	80 bpm

Medications

Date	Name and Strength	Route	Directions
02/20	HCTZ 25 mg	PO	1 tablet in the morning
	Citalopram 20 mg	PO	1 tablet daily
	Haloperidol 2 mg	PO	1 tablet BID

Additional Information

Date	Comment
03/02	Patient has been suspected of bulimia by her primary physician and dentist.

---

15. Which of the following is likely causing Ms. Yates's chief complaint?

    (A) Hydrochlorothiazide
    (B) Citalopram
    (C) Haloperidol
    (D) Hyponatremia
    (E) Uncontrolled blood pressure

16. What additional monitoring is needed to evaluate haloperidol?

    (A) Serum drug levels
    (B) A1c
    (C) Ejection fraction
    (D) Bone mineral density
    (E) CBC

17. Which of the following recommendations is/are appropriate to address Ms. Yates's chief complaint?

      I. Switch to the liquid formulation of haloperidol.
     II. Switch the haloperidol to ziprasidone.
    III. Switch the haloperidol to Risperdal.

(A) I only
(B) III only
(C) I and II only
(D) II and III only
(E) I, II, and III

18. What education should be provided to Ms. Yates concerning her antipsychotic medications?

(A) Medications for schizophrenia are absorbed better in an acidic environment and should be taken with orange juice or vitamin C.
(B) Medications for schizophrenia work quickly and should start to take effect within two to three doses.
(C) If side effects are bothersome, stop taking the medication.
(D) Alcohol should be avoided.
(E) If side effects are bothersome, cut the dose in half.

19. Ms. Yates was told by a friend that her citalopram is bad for her. Although you have tried to talk with her about it, she wants another antidepressant. Which of the following is the MOST appropriate recommendation?

(A) Bupropion 100 mg PO BID
(B) Alprazolam 1 mg PO TID
(C) Lexapro 10 mg PO daily
(D) Venlafaxine 37.5 mg PO BID
(E) Propranolol 80 mg PO daily

20. What is the purpose of adding carbidopa to levodopa in the treatment of Parkinson's disease?

      I. It prevents the peripheral degradation of levodopa.
     II. It allows for extended dosing intervals.
    III. It prevents some of the side effects of levodopa from occurring.

(A) I only
(B) III only
(C) I and II only
(D) II and III only
(E) I, II, and III

21. Which of the following is first-line treatment for acute gout?

(A) Acetaminophen 1,000 mg PO PRN up to QID
(B) Colchicine 2 mg PO PRN
(C) Indomethacin 25 mg PO TID
(D) Allopurinol 100 mg PO daily
(E) Probenecid 250 mg PO BID

22. Which of the following agents is/are correctly matched with common side effects?

      I. Mirtazapine – somnolence
     II. Paroxetine – disorder of ejaculation/impotence
    III. Amitriptyline – weight gain

(A) I only
(B) III only
(C) I and II only
(D) II and III only
(E) I, II, and III

23. Phenytoin is available in which of the following dosage forms?

      I. Chewable tablets
     II. Oral suspension
    III. Parenteral solution

(A) I only
(B) III only
(C) I and II only
(D) II and III only
(E) I, II, and III

24. What is the role of NSAIDs in rheumatoid arthritis?

(A) NSAIDs function as a disease-modifying antirheumatic drug (DMARD).
(B) NSAIDs are used for PRN symptomatic relief.
(C) NSAIDs are used as adjunctive therapy in patients with refractory symptoms.
(D) NSAIDs can prevent the flushing associated with biological injections.
(E) NSAIDs must be given in combination with infliximab.

25. What abortive therapy would be appropriate for a patient who experiences severe nausea and vomiting every time a migraine occurs?

      I. Amerge oral tablets
     II. Relpax oral tablets
    III. Maxalt MLT

(A) I only
(B) III only
(C) I and II only
(D) II and III only
(E) I, II, and III

26. Which of the following statements is TRUE?

(A) Oxcarbazepine and lamotrigine both have a possibility of causing Stevens-Johnson syndrome.
(B) Oxcarbazepine is the generic name for Tegretol.
(C) Lithium has a significant drug interaction with beta-blockers.
(D) Valproic acid is contraindicated in renal disease.
(E) Lithium works by increasing GABA concentration in the brain.

27. Which of the following is/are contraindications to using bupropion?

      I. Current smoker
     II. Bulimia
    III. Seizure disorder

(A) I only
(B) III only
(C) I and II only
(D) II and III only
(E) I, II, and III

28. Which of the following is NOT true of methotrexate?

(A) It may cause folate deficiency.
(B) It should be taken with food.
(C) It is the first-line DMARD for treatment of rheumatoid arthritis.
(D) The usual dose is 7.5 mg PO once weekly.
(E) It requires ophthalmic exams every 3 months.

29. Which of the following is/are TRUE regarding oxybutynin?

I. It is available in oral and transdermal patch formulations.
II. It is an anticholinergic medication.
III. Common side effects include dry mouth and dry eyes.

(A) I only
(B) III only
(C) I and II only
(D) II and III only
(E) I, II, and III

30. Which of the following can be used for both treatment and prevention of gout?

I. NSAIDs
II. Corticosteroids
III. Colchicine

(A) I only
(B) III only
(C) I and II only
(D) II and III only
(E) I, II, and III

Questions 31–35 apply to the following case.

Patient Name: Janelle Brown

Age: 21   **Height:** 5'2"
Sex: F   **Weight:** 120 lb

Allergies: Pollen

Diagnosis

Primary:

1. Acne vulgaris
2. Migraine headaches

Chief Complaint: Acne lesions and frequent migraine headaches

Lab/Diagnostic Tests

Date	Test/Result	
03/02	Sodium	134 mEq/L
(last week)	Potassium	3.5 mEq/L
	Serum creatinine	1.0 mg/dL
	Blood pressure	116/82 mmHg
	Heart rate	78 bpm

Medications

Date	Name and Strength	Route	Directions
02/20	Ovcon-50	PO	1 tablet daily utd
	Maxalt MLT 10 mg	PO	Take PRN

---

31. Which of the following side effects is MOST common with Ms. Brown's oral contraceptive?

    (A) Hot flushes
    (B) Decreased libido
    (C) Breast tenderness
    (D) Spotting
    (E) Dyspareunia

32. After talking with Ms. Brown, it seems she may be experiencing some side effects from her Ovcon-50. You call her physician, who provides you with a new prescription for Seasonale. Which of the following is/are the MOST appropriate counseling points for this medication?

    I. Take one tablet by mouth daily.
    II. Smoking while on this medication will increase your risk of serious side effects.
    III. Apply one patch each week.

    (A) I only
    (B) III only
    (C) I and II only
    (D) II and III only
    (E) I, II, and III

33. Ms. Brown is prescribed amoxicillin 500 mg PO TID for 1 week. Which of the following is the MOST appropriate counseling information for her?

   (A) There is no drug interaction present. Take the antibiotic three times daily as prescribed.
   (B) There is a drug interaction between the antibiotic and oral contraceptive, which renders the antibiotic less effective. Hold the contraceptive until the antibiotic regimen is complete.
   (C) There is a drug interaction between the antibiotic and oral contraceptive, which renders the oral contraceptive less effective. Do not take the antibiotics.
   (D) There is a drug interaction between the antibiotic and oral contraceptive, which renders the oral contraceptive less effective. Take two extra Seasonale tablets daily during the week of antibiotic therapy.
   (E) There is a drug interaction between the antibiotic and oral contraceptive, which renders the oral contraceptive less effective. Take both medications as prescribed and use a backup method of contraception for at least 7 days after finishing the antibiotic therapy.

34. Ms. Brown has several noninflammatory comedones on her face. She states that she has never tried therapy for her acne and requests a recommendation for a medication. Which of the following would be the MOST appropriate initial recommendation?

   (A) Tetracycline 500 mg PO QID
   (B) Isotretinoin 20 mg PO daily
   (C) Benzoyl peroxide 5% topical cream daily
   (D) Benzoyl peroxide 5% topical cream and tretinoin 0.1% gel applied daily
   (E) Isotretinoin 20 mg PO daily and tretinoin 0.1% gel applied daily

35. Ms. Brown asks for information about prophylactic migraine medications. She states that she is currently experiencing about four migraine headaches per week. Which of the following would be the MOST appropriate recommendation for migraine prophylaxis?

   (A) She is not a good candidate for migraine prophylaxis because she does not have headaches frequently enough.
   (B) Imitrex
   (C) Topiramate
   (D) Propranolol
   (E) Hydrocodone

36. Which of the following has no known drug interaction with oral contraceptives?

   (A) Neurontin
   (B) Carbamazepine
   (C) Valproic acid
   (D) Phenytoin
   (E) Phenobarbital

37. Which of the following trade names is correctly matched with its generic name?

   (A) Detrol – oxybutynin
   (B) Vesicare – tolterodine
   (C) Enablex – darifenacin
   (D) Ditropan – imipramine
   (E) Tofranil – solifenacin

38. When should biologics be initiated in rheumatoid arthritis?

   I. Within 3 months of a diagnosis
   II. For PRN symptom relief
   III. When DMARDs have been ineffective

   (A) I only
   (B) III only
   (C) I and II only
   (D) II and III only
   (E) I, II, and III

39. Which of the following is/are TRUE of tricyclic antidepressants?

   I. They may exhibit anticholinergic side effects.
   II. They are very dangerous and often fatal in overdosage.
   III. They have a significant drug–food interaction with aged cheese.

   (A) I only
   (B) III only
   (C) I and II only
   (D) II and III only
   (E) I, II, and III

40. A patient was started on a selegiline patch 3 days ago for major depression. The family states that it is not working. Which of the following is the MOST appropriate action to take at this time?

   (A) Add fluoxetine if the selegiline is still not working in 2 weeks.
   (B) Add duloxetine if he/she is not feeling better in 6–8 weeks.
   (C) Have the patient start a high caffeine intake so that the selegiline will be absorbed better.
   (D) Inform the family that the selegiline has not had time to work yet and may take 1–2 months.
   (E) Switch the patient to oral selegiline for better efficacy.

41. Which of the following products contains aspirin with butalbital and caffeine?

   (A) Fiorinal
   (B) Fioricet
   (C) Excedrin Migraine
   (D) Migranal
   (E) Amerge

42. A 15-year-old female patient is given a new prescription for Retin-A. Which of the following would be an appropriate counseling point?

   (A) This medication works best if combined with an astringent or abrasive soap.
   (B) This medication should result in rapid improvement within 1–2 days.
   (C) This medication should be used only as a "spot treatment" for blemishes.
   (D) It is important to use sunblock prior to sun exposure due to the risk of photosensitivity.
   (E) It is important to apply this product to wet skin immediately after washing the face.

43. Which of the following is/are alternative treatment(s) for osteoporosis in patients who are unable to tolerate bisphosphonates?

    I. Zoledronic acid
    II. Calcitonin
    III. Raloxifene

(A) I only
(B) III only
(C) I and II only
(D) II and III only
(E) I, II, and III

44. Which of the following antianxiety medications takes 2–3 weeks to reach maximal efficacy?

(A) Xanax
(B) Librium
(C) Buspar
(D) Valium
(E) Vistaril

45. Common side effects of isotretinoin include which of the following?

    I. Cheilitis
    II. Pruritus
    III. Hypertrichosis

(A) I only
(B) III only
(C) I and II only
(D) II and III only
(E) I, II, and III

46. Which of the following is NOT a treatment option for psoriasis?

(A) Methotrexate
(B) Prednisone
(C) Coal tar
(D) Benzoyl peroxide
(E) Anthralin

47. In the TNM classification of cancer staging, N represents which of the following?

(A) The size of the tumor in centimeters
(B) The number of tumors
(C) The number of involved lymph nodes
(D) The number of involved organs
(E) The presence of distant metastases

48. Which of the following is/are TRUE regarding neoadjuvant chemotherapy?

    I. It is given prior to surgery.
    II. The goal is to reduce tumor burden.
    III. It is given to relieve symptoms and has no effect on survival.

(A) I only
(B) III only
(C) I and II only
(D) II and III only
(E) I, II, and III

49. Leucovorin should be given as rescue therapy to patients receiving _____, but will increase both the toxicity and the chemotherapeutic activity of _____.

(A) fluorouracil; methotrexate
(B) doxorubicin; fluorouracil
(C) fluorouracil; cytarabine
(D) methotrexate; fluorouracil
(E) methotrexate; doxorubicin

50. Which of the following is/are TRUE regarding cytarabine?

    I. Its main mechanism of action is inhibition of DNA polymerase.

    II. Patients should be monitored for neurotoxicity at each office visit.

    III. Pre- and posttreatment corticosteroid eye drops should be given to prevent conjunctivitis.

(A) I only
(B) III only
(C) I and II only
(D) II and III only
(E) I, II, and III

51. Which of the following is the MOST significant adverse drug effect of anthracyclines?

(A) Ototoxicity
(B) Infusion-related reactions
(C) Folate deficiency
(D) Cardiotoxicity
(E) Hand and foot syndrome

52. Which of the following is the trade name for bevacizumab?

(A) Gleevec
(B) Herceptin
(C) Avastin
(D) Tarceva
(E) Platinol

Questions 53–56 refer to the following patient profile.

Patient Name: Mary Jefferson

Age: 42   **Height:** 5'6"
Sex: F   **Weight:** 125 lb

Allergies: None known

Diagnosis

  Primary:
    1. Adenocarcinoma
    2. Asthma

Lab/Diagnostic Tests

  WBC 1×10^3 cells/mm^3; 50% segs
    10% bands 30% lymphs
    10% monos
  Hgb: 14.5 g/dL
  Blood pressure: 134/85 mmHg
  Heart rate: 75 bpm

53. What is Ms. Jefferson's absolute neutrophil count?

(A) 3,000
(B) 750
(C) 600
(D) 300
(E) 50

54. Ms. Jefferson's neutropenia would be considered

(A) transient.
(B) mild.
(C) moderate.
(D) severe.
(E) absent. This patient is not neutropenic, as the ANC is within normal range.

55. Which of the following will put patients with neutropenia at risk for developing infection?

   (A) Severe neutropenia (ANC <100/mm³)
   (B) A rapid fall in ANC
   (C) Invasive procedures such as enemas, catheter placement, or dental procedures
   (D) Neutropenia lasting more than 7 days
   (E) All of the above

56. Which of the following drugs would be appropriate for Ms. Jefferson?

   (A) Neupogen
   (B) Epogen
   (C) Procrit
   (D) Aranesp
   (E) None of the above

57. Gender and race are considered which of the following types of data?

   (A) Nominal
   (B) Ordinal
   (C) Interval
   (D) Ratio
   (E) Frequency

58. To increase the power of a study, the researchers could

   (A) decrease the sample size.
   (B) lengthen the duration of the study.
   (C) decrease the duration of the study.
   (D) increase the number of dependent variables being studied.
   (E) increase the sample size.

59. Which of the following is FALSE regarding Type II errors?

   (A) A Type II error occurs when a study fails to detect a difference between study groups but in fact a difference does exist.
   (B) Not achieving power in a study may increase the likelihood of Type II errors.
   (C) A Type II error means that the null hypothesis was accepted when it actually is false.
   (D) A Type II error occurs when researchers find a difference between study groups when no difference actually exists.
   (E) All of the above are true regarding Type II errors.

60. A clinical trial is evaluating whether there is a difference in the mean LDL cholesterol levels between adults in three different treatment groups. The data collected follows a normal distribution. Which of the following would be the MOST appropriate statistical test for this analysis?

   (A) Student's t-test
   (B) Paired t-test
   (C) Chi-square test
   (D) ANOVA
   (E) Mann-Whitney U test

61. You need to make 30 g of 0.4% w/w hydrocortisone ointment. You have 2.5% w/w hydrocortisone ointment in stock. How much of the 2.5% ointment must you mix with white petrolatum to make the appropriate quantity of 0.4% ointment?

   (A) 2.4 g
   (B) 2.5 g
   (C) 4.8 g
   (D) 9.6 g
   (E) 30 g

$30 \times 0.4 = 2.5 \times c_2$

$c_2 = \dfrac{30 \times 0.4}{2.5}$

4.8

62. The formula for hydrophilic petrolatum USP is given below. How much white wax do you need to weigh out to compound 70 g of hydrophilic petrolatum?

Hydrophilic petrolatum:

3% w/w cholesterol

3% w/w stearyl alcohol

8% w/w white wax

86% w/w white petrolatum

(A) 2.1 g
(B) 8 g
(C) 5.6 g
(D) 60.2 g
(E) 70 g

63. How many 4-mg tablets of chlorpheniramine maleate would be required to compound 4 fluid ounces of a syrup containing 2 mg of chlorpheniramine maleate in every tablespoonful dose?

(A) 1
(B) 2
(C) 4
(D) 8
(E) 12

64. A 60-kg patient is to receive a constant IV infusion of dobutamine at a rate of 5 mcg/kg/min. The available solution has a concentration of 0.5 mg/mL. For what rate should the infusion pump be set?

(A) 0.6 mL/hr
(B) 3.6 mL/hr
(C) 18 mL/hr
(D) 36 mL/hr
(E) 600 mL/hr

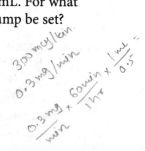

65. A patient is given an IV bolus dose of 1 g of Drug A. The plasma level is measured shortly after administration and is found to be 0.2 mg/mL. The same patient is later given an IV bolus dose of Drug B. The plasma level of Drug B shortly after administration is 83 mcg/mL. On the basis of this data, which of the following statements is/are TRUE?

I. Drug A has a smaller volume of distribution than Drug B.
II. Drug A is better absorbed than Drug B.
III. Drug A induced the metabolism of Drug B.

(A) I only
(B) III only
(C) I and II only
(D) II and III only
(E) I, II, and III

66. To treat preeclampsia, a patient receives an IV infusion of 40 mL of a 10% w/v solution of magnesium sulfate for injection. How many mEq of magnesium did she receive?
(MW $MgSO_4 \cdot (H_2O)_7$ = 246.36)

(A) 8.63 mEq Mg^{2+}
(B) 16.25 mEq Mg^{2+}
(C) 32.5 mEq Mg^{2+}
(D) 65 mEq Mg^{2+}
(E) 130 mEq Mg^{2+}

67. You receive a prescription for 240 mL of a potassium citrate solution with a concentration of 15 mEq/15 mL. How much potassium citrate must you weigh out to compound this prescription? (MW $C_6H_5K_3O_7$ = 306)

    (A) 2.72 g
    (B) 8.16 g
    (C) 24.40 g
    (D) 73.44 g
    (E) 367.2 g

68. You are considering adding HgbA1c monitoring services to your clinical pharmacy offerings and are evaluating an HgbA1c monitor to decide if it sufficiently precise and accurate to be used in your clinic. Using a test solution that produces a value of 7.5% on standardized laboratory tests, you perform 10 sample tests on the monitor. The values you obtain are:

    7.9
    8.1
    7.9
    8.0
    7.9
    7.9
    8.0
    8.1
    7.9
    8.0

    You would say that the monitor being evaluated produces readings that are

    (A) accurate but not precise.
    (B) precise but not accurate.
    (C) both precise and accurate.
    (D) neither precise nor accurate.
    (E) You do not have enough information to answer this question.

69. How much sodium chloride must be added to the prescription to make the solution isotonic?

    Rx: Tetracaine hydrochloride   0.5% w/v
              (E = 0.18)
           NaCl (0.9%)   qs
           Sterile water   add 30 mL

    M et ft isotonic eye drops

    (A) 0.027 g NaCl
    (B) 0.243 g NaCl
    (C) 0.27 g NaCl
    (D) 0.83 g NaCl
    (E) 0.9 g NaCl

70. Given the capsule recipe provided below, how much diphenhydramine must you weigh out to compound 60 capsules?

    Diphenhydramine hydrochloride: 0.5 g
    Acetaminophen: 6.5 g
    Lactose qs: M et div caps #10

    (A) 0.5 g
    (B) 3 g
    (C) 7 g
    (D) 30 g
    (E) 42 g

Questions 71–74 refer to the following patient information:

AJ is a 70-kg male with a creatinine clearance of 100 mL/min. You have the following information about the behavior of a particular drug in this patient:

CL = 400 mL/min;
    CLr = 25 mL/min

V_d = 140 L

95% bound to plasma proteins

---

71. What is the filtration clearance of this drug?

(A) 0 mL/min
(B) 1.25 mL/min
(C) 5 mL/min
(D) 20 mL/min
(E) 95 mL/min

72. You can conclude that this drug is

(A) only filtered.
(B) both filtered and reabsorbed.
(C) both filtered and secreted.
(D) secreted and reabsorbed but not filtered.
(E) You do not have enough information to answer this question.

73. The half-life of this drug in this patient is

(A) 4 hours.
(B) 12 hours.
(C) 24 hours.
(D) 48 hours.
(E) 60 hours.

74. What blood level would you expect after a single IV bolus dose of 250 mg of this drug?

(A) 0.1 mg/dL
(B) 0.13 mg/dL
(C) 0.15 mg/dL
(D) 0.18 mg/dL
(E) 0.2 mg/dL

75. MT is being treated for a serious infection with *Pseudomonas aeruginosa*. After obtaining culture and sensitivity data, her physician starts her on tobramycin 70 mg IV q8h. During her hospital stay, MT's serum creatinine increased from 0.8 to 1.6 mg/dL. What pharmacokinetic parameters have been affected, and what modification should be made to MT's tobramycin therapy?

(A) The bioavailability for tobramycin is increased, resulting in kidney impairment. The tobramycin should be discontinued.
(B) The clearance for tobramycin has decreased, resulting in a longer half-life. MT may experience drug accumulation, so the tobramycin dose should be decreased.
(C) The clearance for tobramycin has increased, resulting in a shorter half-life. MT may experience subtherapeutic drug concentrations, so the tobramycin dose should be increased.
(D) The clearance for tobramycin has decreased, resulting in a longer half-life. MT may experience subtherapeutic drug concentrations, so the tobramycin dose should be increased.
(E) The V_d of tobramycin has increased, resulting in a longer half-life. MT may experience drug accumulation, so the tobramycin dose should be decreased.

76. Penicillin is a weakly acidic drug that is secreted by the kidney. Probenecid, also a weakly acidic drug, competes for the carrier system that is responsible for the secretion of penicillin. When penicillin and probenecid are administered together, what do you expect will happen to penicillin's clearance and steady-state plasma concentrations?

    (A) Clearance decreases and steady-state concentrations increase.
    (B) Clearance increases and steady-state concentrations increase.
    (C) Clearance increases and steady-state concentrations decrease.
    (D) Clearance decreases and steady-state concentrations decrease.
    (E) Clearance and steady-state concentrations are nearly unchanged.

77. Which of the following modifications to a drug will increase its aqueous solubility?

    (A) Convert anhydrous to trihydrate form.
    (B) Convert crystalline to amorphous form.
    (C) Add a lipophilic group.
    (D) Remove a hydroxyl group.
    (E) All of the above will increase aqueous solubility.

78. The pKa of a weak base is 8.4. What form will the drug be in at an intestinal pH of 7.4?

    (A) 75% un-ionized
    (B) Greater than 90% un-ionized
    (C) 75% ionized
    (D) Greater than 90% ionized
    (E) Approximately equal amounts ionized/un-ionized

79. Which dosage form would be the BEST option for a drug that is prone to first-pass metabolism?

    (A) Tablet
    (B) Syrup
    (C) Capsule
    (D) Rapid-dissolve strip
    (E) Transdermal patch

80. Structured vehicles form suspensions by what means?

    (A) Promoting loose aggregation of suspended particles
    (B) Increasing viscosity, thereby slowing sedimentation
    (C) Maximizing sedimentation volume
    (D) Reducing repulsive forces between particles
    (E) All of the above

81. Phenytoin is formulated in a cosolvent system. IV administration of this drug should occur slowly because

    (A) the onset of drug action will be faster.
    (B) slow injection will prevent precipitation of the drug from solution.
    (C) rapid infusion will lead to hemolysis.
    (D) it will prevent the drug from being metabolized too quickly.
    (E) the cosolvent system is too viscous for rapid administration.

82. Which of the following ophthalmic products must contain a preservative?

    I. Saline in a multiple-dose container

    II. Saline in a single-dose container

    III. Single-use rinse solution used in eye surgery

(A) I only
(B) III only
(C) I and II only
(D) II and III only
(E) I, II, and III

83. Drug(s) may be administered rectally to provide local treatment for

(A) nausea.
(B) chronic pain.
(C) ulcerative colitis.
(D) hormone replacement.
(E) migraine headache.

84. Metronidazole leads to a disulfiram reaction when taken with alcohol. Which of the following liquid dosage forms would be the MOST appropriate way of delivering metronidazole?

(A) Spirit
(B) Elixir USP
(C) Tincture
(D) Suspension
(E) Fluid extract

85. A bottle of drug solution was left open in a dark room. After one day, the solution had changed from colorless to pink. An identical bottle, left capped, remained unchanged. The solution has undergone what type of degradation?

(A) Hydrolysis
(B) Photolysis
(C) Oxidation
(D) Sedimentation
(E) Polymorphism

86. Calamine lotion remains thick when sitting on the shelf, yet pours easily when shaken. What type of flow is calamine lotion exhibiting?

(A) Dilatant
(B) Newtonian
(C) Plastic
(D) Pseudoplastic
(E) Thixotropic

87. How many 50-mg phenytoin tablets should a 5-year-old child receive per day, given the following information?

V_{max} = 300 mg/day
K_M = 6.5 mg/L
C_{SS} (desired) = 14 mg/L
Salt factor for phenytoin tablets = 1

(A) 1 tablet
(B) 4 tablets
(C) 5 tablets
(D) 6 tablets
(E) 7 tablets

88. Which of the following tablet excipients would be most expected to decrease product bioavailability?

    (A) Starch
    (B) Microcrystalline cellulose
    (C) Lactose
    (D) Magnesium stearate
    (E) Mannitol

89. Poor metabolizers of CYP2D6 are most likely to receive therapeutic benefit from which of the following opioids?

    (A) Codeine
    (B) Morphine
    (C) Hydrocodone
    (D) Oxycodone
    (E) Dextromethorphan

90. Patients taking protease inhibitors should avoid drinking grapefruit juice because it

    (A) inhibits CYP3A, leading to toxic levels of the drug.
    (B) inhibits CYP3A, leading to subtherapeutic levels of the drug.
    (C) induces CYP3A, leading to toxic levels of the drug.
    (D) induces CYP3A, leading to subtherapeutic levels of the drug.
    (E) binds to the drug, preventing absorption.

91. You receive an order for 10 mL of epinephrine 1:10,000 solution. What is another way to express this concentration?

    (A) 10% w/v
    (B) 1% w/v
    (C) 0.1% w/v
    (D) 0.01% w/v
    (E) 0.001% w/v

92. You need to measure out 100 g of methyl salicylate to use in a compound. The specific gravity of methyl salicylate is 1.18. How much methyl salicylate should you measure, by volume, to deliver the appropriate amount?

    (A) 69.5 mL
    (B) 84.75 mL
    (C) 100 mL
    (D) 115.25 mL
    (E) 130.5 mL

Questions 93–97 refer to the following patient profile.

Patient Name: John Marx

Age: 70   **Height:** 5'10"

Sex: M   **Weight:** 198 lb

Race: Black

Allergies: NKDA

Diagnosis

Primary:

1. Hypertension
2. Dyslipidemia
3. Heart failure

Secondary:

1. MI (5 years ago)

Chief Complaint: Swelling in legs

Medications

Date	Name and Strength	Route	Directions
10/25	Aspirin 81 mg	PO	1 tablet daily
	Digoxin 0.125 mg	PO	1 tablet daily
	Furosemide 20 mg	PO	1 tablet in the morning
	Lisinopril 20 mg	PO	1 tablet daily
	Toprol XL 25 mg	PO	1 tablet daily
	Vytorin 40/10 mg	PO	1 tablet at bedtime

Lab/Diagnostic Tests

Date	Test/Result	
11/10	Sodium	145 mEq/L
	Potassium	3.9 mEq/L
	Serum creatinine	1.1 mg/dL
	Digoxin	0.8 ng/mL
	Blood pressure	122/80 mmHg
	Heart rate	70 bpm
	LVEF	35%

Additional Information

Date	Comment
11/10	Patient has gained 3 lb in the past week.

93. Vytorin is the brand name for which of the following combinations?

   (A) Atorvastatin and amlodipine
   (B) Atorvastatin and ezetimibe
   (C) Lovastatin and niacin
   (D) Simvastatin and ezetimibe
   (E) Simvastatin and lisinopril

94. Which of the following is/are appropriate nonpharmacological recommendations for Mr. Marx?

   I. Restrict fluid intake.
   II. Restrict sodium intake.
   III. Restrict vitamin K intake.

   (A) I only
   (B) III only
   (C) I and II only
   (D) II and III only
   (E) I, II, and III

95. Which of the following signs/symptoms is/are associated with digoxin toxicity?

   I. Anorexia
   II. Arrhythmias
   III. Visual disturbances

   (A) I only
   (B) III only
   (C) I and II only
   (D) II and III only
   (E) I, II, and III

96. Which of the following medications is contraindicated in Mr. Marx?

   (A) Aldactone
   (B) BiDil
   (C) Diovan
   (D) Calan SR
   (E) Inspra

97. Mr. Marx's furosemide is increased to 40 mg PO BID. The pharmacist should counsel the patient on which of the following?

   (A) He should separate both doses of furosemide from other medications by 2 hours.
   (B) He should take the second dose of furosemide before 5 p.m. each day.
   (C) He should take both doses of furosemide with food or milk.
   (D) He should take the second dose of furosemide at bedtime.
   (E) He should take both doses of furosemide on an empty stomach.

Questions 98–101 refer to the following patient profile.

Patient Name: Susan Brown

Age: 42   **Height:** 5'4"

Sex: F   **Weight:** 162 lb

Allergies: NKDA

Diagnosis

  Primary:

    1. UTI

    2. DVT (secondary to oral contraceptive use)

    3. Hypertension

  Chief Complaint: Pain with urination

Medications

Date	Name and Strength	Route	Directions
3/3	Depo-Provera 150 mg	IM	Every 3 months
5/5	Coumadin 5 mg	PO	1 tablet daily
	HCTZ 25 mg	PO	1 tablet daily
	Lisinopril 10 mg	PO	1 tablet daily

Lab/Diagnostic Tests

Date	Test/Result	
5/22	Urinalysis	pyuria, nitrite (+)
	Sodium	145 mEq/L
	Potassium	3.9 mEq/L
	Serum creatinine	0.9 mg/dL
	INR	2.3
	Blood pressure	125/72 mmHg
	Heart rate	71 bpm

Additional Information

Date	Comment
5/5	Patient contemplating smoking cessation
5/22	Patient prescribed Bactrim DS 1 tablet PO BID × 3 days, #6

---

98. Bactrim DS is MOST likely being used to treat which of the following microorganisms?

(A) *Chlamydia pneumoniae*
(B) *Clostridium difficile*
(C) *Enterococcus faecalis*
(D) *Escherichia coli*
(E) *Pseudomonas aeruginosa*

99. Which of the following lab alterations would you expect to see in Ms. Brown as a result of starting the Bactrim DS?

(A) Increased INR
(B) Decreased INR
(C) Increased potassium
(D) Decreased potassium
(E) Increased sodium

100. Bactrim DS is the brand name for which of the following medications?

(A) Amoxicillin and clavulanic acid
(B) Ciprofloxacin and doxycycline
(C) Imipenem and cilastatin
(D) Isoniazid and rifampin
(E) Trimethoprim and sulfamethoxazole

101. Lisinopril belongs to which of the following classes of drugs?

(A) Angiotensin-converting enzyme inhibitor
(B) Angiotensin II receptor blocker
(C) Aldosterone receptor antagonist
(D) Calcium channel blocker
(E) Potassium-sparing diuretic

102. A patient recently moved to the United States from England. She brings in her prescription bottle and asks the pharmacist if he carries the antibiotic that she has been taking for a UTI. Which of the following references could be used by the pharmacist to determine if there is an equivalent antibiotic available in the United States?

(A) Facts and Comparisons
(B) Martindale
(C) Merck Index
(D) PDR
(E) Red Book

103. A patient presents with a prescription for Xalatan. Xalatan is probably being used to treat which of the following disease states?

(A) Anxiety
(B) Asthma
(C) Depression
(D) Glaucoma
(E) Sepsis

104. Which of the following drugs is/are classified as macrolide(s)?

I. Keflex
II. Keppra
III. Ketek

(A) I only
(B) III only
(C) I and II only
(D) II and III only
(E) I, II, and III

105. Patients taking sulfasalazine for inflammatory bowel disease should be counseled on which of the following?

       I. Take on an empty stomach.
     II. It may cause orange bodily fluids.
   III. Wear sunscreen and protective clothing.

  (A) I only
  (B) III only
  (C) I and II only
  (D) II and III only
  (E) I, II, and III

106. During a hospital stay for pneumonia, David Jones developed *Clostridium difficile*. Which of the following antibiotics would be the BEST treatment for Mr. Jones?

  (A) Amoxicillin
  (B) Azithromycin
  (C) Levofloxacin
  (D) Metronidazole
  (E) Tobramycin

107. A 22-year-old woman comes to the pharmacy to pick up her new prescription for oral contraceptives. Which of the following references would be the MOST appropriate source of important counseling advice for this patient?

  (A) Harriet Lane Handbook
  (B) Index Nominum
  (C) Merck Index
  (D) USP-DI Volume I
  (E) USP-DI Volume II

108. Cytotec is the brand name of which of the following medications?

  (A) Cimetidine
  (B) Metoclopramide
  (C) Misoprostol
  (D) Olsalazine
  (E) Sucralfate

109. Which of the following drugs would be an appropriate treatment for genital herpes?

  (A) Acyclovir
  (B) Indinavir
  (C) Lamivudine
  (D) Oseltamivir
  (E) Valganciclovir

110. Which of the following references is the BEST source for obtaining the cost information of drugs?

  (A) Facts and Comparisons
  (B) The Harriet Lane Handbook
  (C) PDR
  (D) Red Book
  (E) USP-DI Volume I

111. Which of the following is/are potential side effects of niacin?

       I. Flushing
     II. Hyperglycemia
   III. Hyperuricemia

  (A) I only
  (B) III only
  (C) I and II only
  (D) II and III only
  (E) I, II, and III

112. Cosopt is the brand name for which of the following combinations?

    (A) Timolol and brimonidine
    (B) Timolol and dorzolamide
    (C) Latanoprost and carbachol
    (D) Pilocarpine and brinzolamide
    (E) Pilocarpine and carbachol

113. Which of the following medications could be used intravenously to treat an invasive *Aspergillus* infection?

    I. Caspofungin
    II. Linezolid
    III. Miconazole

    (A) I only
    (B) III only
    (C) I and II only
    (D) II and III only
    (E) I, II, and III

114. Which of the following is/are appropriate nonpharmacological recommendations for a patient with gastroesophageal reflux disease?

    I. Avoid chocolate
    II. Stop smoking
    III. Lose weight

    (A) I only
    (B) III only
    (C) I and II only
    (D) II and III only
    (E) I, II, and III

115. Which of the following IV medications should be protected from light?

    (A) Enalaprilat
    (B) Esmolol
    (C) Fenoldopam
    (D) Nitroglycerin
    (E) Nitroprusside

116. A patient presents to the pharmacy with prescriptions for Biaxin, Amoxil, and Nexium. The patient is probably being treated for which of the following infections?

    (A) *Helicobacter pylori*
    (B) *Haemophilus influenzae*
    (C) *Klebsiella pneumoniae*
    (D) *Moraxella catarrhalis*
    (E) *Neisseria meningitidis*

117. Trusopt belongs to which of the following classes of drugs?

    (A) Antihistamine
    (B) Beta blocker
    (C) Carbonic anhydrase inhibitor
    (D) Cholinergic agonist
    (E) Prostaglandin analog

118. The Commission E Monographs provide information on which of the following?

    (A) Dietary supplements
    (B) Foreign drugs
    (C) Herbal products
    (D) Homeopathic products
    (E) Nonprescription drugs

119. Clotrimazole is available in which of the following dosage forms?

    I. Troche
    II. Capsule
    III. Powder

    (A) I only
    (B) III only
    (C) I and II only
    (D) II and III only
    (E) I, II, and III

120. Which of the following is/are the most appropriate monitoring recommendations for a patient receiving amiodarone?

    I. Chest x-ray should be performed every 6 months.
    II. Thyroid function tests should be performed annually.
    III. Liver function tests should be performed every 6 months.

(A) I only
(B) III only
(C) I and II only
(D) II and III only
(E) I, II, and III

121. A patient using ophthalmic preparations should be given which of the following counseling information?

(A) The preparations can be used safely with contact lenses.
(B) The dropper tip should be placed on the edge of the lower eyelid.
(C) The upper eyelid should be pulled outward to form a pocket in which the medication can be placed.
(D) The eyes should be rubbed after the eye drops are administered.
(E) The administration of different medications should be separated by intervals of at least 10 minutes.

122. Information on IV medication compatibility can be found in which of the following references?

    I. Facts and Comparisons
    II. Physician's Desk Reference
    III. Trissel's Handbook on Injectable Drugs

(A) I only
(B) III only
(C) I and II only
(D) II and III only
(E) I, II, and III

123. Tagamet belongs to which of the following classes of drugs?

(A) Aminosalicylate
(B) H_2 receptor antagonist
(C) Immunosuppressant
(D) Prostaglandin analog
(E) Proton pump inhibitor

124. A patient brings in a prescription for methotrexate for the treatment of Crohn's disease. Which of the following tests should be monitored in this patient?

    I. Electrocardiogram
    II. Complete blood count
    III. Liver function tests

(A) I only
(B) III only
(C) I and II only
(D) II and III only
(E) I, II, and III

125. Which of the following medications may result in hyperkalemia?

      I. Candesartan
     II. Eplerenone
    III. Triamterene

(A) I only
(B) III only
(C) I and II only
(D) II and III only
(E) I, II, and III

126. Which of the following medications can be administered via a nasogastric tube?

      I. Esomeprazole
     II. Lansoprazole
    III. Pantoprazole

(A) I only
(B) III only
(C) I and II only
(D) II and III only
(E) I, II, and III

127. A patient is prescribed felodipine for her hypertension. She should be counseled to do which of the following?

(A) Avoid drinking grapefruit juice.
(B) Avoid foods with tyramine.
(C) Take the felodipine with folic acid.
(D) Take the felodipine on an empty stomach.
(E) Take the felodipine 2 hours before taking other medications.

128. An otherwise healthy patient develops community-acquired pneumonia. Which of the following antibiotics would be the best empiric treatment option for this patient?

(A) Azithromycin
(B) Metronidazole
(C) Penicillin
(D) Rifampin
(E) Vancomycin

129. Amoxicillin is available in which of the following dosage forms?

      I. IV injection
     II. Oral suspension
    III. Capsule

(A) I only
(B) III only
(C) I and II only
(D) II and III only
(E) I, II, and III

130. Which of the following drugs would be MOST appropriate to use for the treatment of hypertension in a pregnant patient?

(A) Doxazosin
(B) Lisinopril
(C) Methyldopa
(D) Metolazone
(E) Valsartan

131. A patient is prescribed Prevacid for his peptic ulcer disease. He should be counseled to take it

(A) 15 to 30 minutes before breakfast.
(B) 30 minutes after breakfast.
(C) 2 hours before taking other medications.
(D) with the first bite of a meal.
(E) with a high-fat meal.

132. Sporanox is the brand name for which of the following medications?

    (A) Aripiprazole
    (B) Fluconazole
    (C) Itraconazole
    (D) Lansoprazole
    (E) Rabeprazole

133. A patient presents to the pharmacy with a prescription for simvastatin 40 mg PO at bedtime and gemfibrozil 600 mg PO BID. Which of the following adverse reactions is this patient likely to experience?

    (A) Dyspnea
    (B) Edema
    (C) Headache
    (D) Insomnia
    (E) Myopathy

134. A patient presents with a new prescription for Synthroid. Which of the following medications might have contributed to her recent diagnosis of hypothyroidism?

    (A) Amiodarone
    (B) Bisoprolol
    (C) Dofetilide
    (D) Hydralazine
    (E) Propafenone

135. Levaquin belongs to which of the following classes of drugs?

    (A) Aminoglycosides
    (B) Cephalosporins
    (C) Fluoroquinolones
    (D) Macrolides
    (E) Tetracyclines

136. Which of the following statements regarding amiodarone is/are CORRECT?

    I. It is only effective for the treatment of atrial arrhythmias.
    II. It does not undergo cytochrome P450 metabolism by the liver.
    III. If pulmonary fibrosis develops, the amiodarone should be discontinued.

    (A) I only
    (B) III only
    (C) I and II only
    (D) II and III only
    (E) I, II, and III

137. Which of the following drug classes is/are used in the treatment of inflammatory bowel disease?

    I. Aminosalicylates
    II. Corticosteroids
    III. Immunosuppressants

    (A) I only
    (B) III only
    (C) I and II
    (D) II and III
    (E) I, II, and III

138. Which of the following drugs can be used in an appropriate combination regimen to treat *H. pylori*?

    I. Amoxicillin
    II. Lansoprazole
    III. Clarithromycin

    (A) I only
    (B) III only
    (C) I and II
    (D) II and III
    (E) I, II, and III

Questions 139–143 refer to the following patient profile.

Patient Name: William Boyd

Age: 56   **Height:** 5'8"

Sex: M   **Weight:** 148 lb

Allergies: Codeine, PCN, Sulfa

Diagnosis

Primary
1. Hypertension
2. Hypothyroidism
3. Type 2 diabetes mellitus × 5 years

Secondary
1. Heartburn

Chief Complaint: Fatigue, tiredness, cold fingers, feeling down

Medications

Date	Name and Strength	Route	Directions
7/10	Prilosec OTC 10 mg	PO	3 tablets daily
	Synthroid 100 mcg	PO	1 tablet daily
	Metformin 1,000 mg	PO	1 tablet TID
	Lisinopril 10 mg	PO	1 tablet daily
	Ferrous sulfate 325 mg	PO	1 tablet daily

Lab/Diagnostic Tests

Date	Test/Result	
7/9	Sodium	141 mEq/L
	Potassium	3.5 mEq/L
	Serum creatinine	0.9 mg/dL
	TSH	10 mIU/L
	AST	18 IU/L
	ALT	16 IU/L
	A1c	5.5%
	Blood pressure	139/80 mmHg
	Heart rate	90 bpm
	GDS	4

Additional Information

Date	Comment
7/10	Patient complains of fatigue and lack of energy.
3/9	Pharmacist advised patient to start taking Prilosec OTC.
3/9	Pharmacist counseled patient to check blood sugars.

---

139. Which of the following statements regarding the metformin is TRUE?

    (A) It should be discontinued due to the patient's A1c level.
    (B) The pharmacist should contact the patient's physician because the dose is too high.
    (C) The pharmacist should recommend increasing the dose.
    (D) It is not indicated in this patient.
    (E) There is a significant drug interaction with lisinopril.

140. Which of the following is/are appropriate recommendations for Mr. Boyd?

    I. Continue taking all medications as prescribed.
    II. Start taking a multivitamin for energy.
    III. Call the doctor regarding the patient's heartburn.

    (A) I only
    (B) III only
    (C) I and II only
    (D) II and III only
    (E) I, II, and III

141. Which of the following is/are MOST likely associated with Mr. Boyd's chief complaints?

    I. Undertreated hypothyroidism
    II. Hypoglycemia
    III. Untreated depression

    (A) I only
    (B) III only
    (C) I and II only
    (D) II and III only
    (E) I, II, and III

142. Lisinopril helps to do which of the following for this patient?

    (A) Improve blood sugars by inhibiting ACE
    (B) Block renin to lower blood pressure
    (C) Inhibit ACE, which blocks the angiotensin II receptor
    (D) Block ACE to vasodilate
    (E) Protect his kidneys by lowering bradykinin

143. Mr. Boyd's Synthroid was increased to 125 mcg PO daily by the medical resident. The pharmacist should counsel Mr. Boyd to

    (A) monitor his blood sugar, as the Synthroid may cause hypoglycemia.
    (B) avoid taking the Synthroid with ferrous sulfate.
    (C) take the Synthroid only in the evening.
    (D) avoid taking the Synthroid with metformin.
    (E) take the Synthroid with milk.

144. Nevirapine is the generic name of which brand drug, and belongs in which drug class?

    (A) Viramune; non-nucleoside reverse transcriptase inhibitors
    (B) Ziagen; non-nucleoside reverse transcriptase inhibitors
    (C) Kaletra; protease inhibitors
    (D) Videx; nucleoside reverse transcriptase inhibitors
    (E) Fuzeon; fusion inhibitors

145. When should antiviral therapy for HIV be initiated?

    I. When diagnosis is confirmed by Western blot
    II. When the CD4 cell count is less than 500 cells/mm^3
    III. When the patient has a history of an opportunistic infection

(A) I only
(B) III only
(C) I and II only
(D) II and III only
(E) I, II, and III

146. Which of the following drugs is/are inhaled corticosteroids?

    I. Pulmicort Respules
    II. Tilade
    III. Zyflo

(A) I only
(B) III only
(C) I and II only
(D) II and III only
(E) I, II, and III

Questions 147–151 refer to the following patient profile.

Patient Name: Mary Christensen

Age: 75   **Height:** 5'4"
Sex: F   **Weight:** 183 lb

Allergies: NKDA

Diagnosis

  Primary

    1. Asthma
    2. Hypertension
    3. Osteoarthritis

  Chief Complaint: Thrush, dizziness, tachycardia,
                nausea, and vomiting

Lab/Diagnostic Tests

Date	Test/Result	
7/9	Sodium	140 mEq/L
	Potassium	3.5 mEq/L
	Serum creatinine	0.9 mg/dL
	Personal best FEV_1	325 L/sec
	FEV1	300 L/sec
	Blood pressure	90/70 mmHg
	Heart rate	60 bpm
	Theophylline level	23 mcg/mL

Medications

Date	Name and Strength	Route	Directions
7/20	Advair	PO	1 puff BID
	Theophylline XR 600 mg	PO	1 tablet daily
	Albuterol MDI	PO	1–2 puffs TID PRN
	Metoprolol 50 mg	PO	1 tablet BID
	Aspirin 325 mg	PO	1 tablet daily
	Fish oil 1,000 mg	PO	1 capsule daily
	Hydrocodone/ APAP 5/500 mg	PO	1–2 tablets q6h for pain
	Tylenol Arthritis 650 mg	PO	1 tablet TID

Additional Orders

Date	Comment
5/10	Pharmacist counseled patient on swish and spit after Advair use.
6/15	Pharmacist counseled patient on use of peak flow meter.
7/2	Patient stated she got a new cat.

---

147. The patient's chief complaints are likely caused by which of the following?

   I. Theophylline toxicity
   II. Lack of swishing and spitting after Advair use
   III. Excessive metoprolol dose

   (A) I only
   (B) III only
   (C) I and II only
   (D) II and III only
   (E) I, II, and III

148. Which of the following medications would you recommend discontinuing?

   (A) Advair because of thrush
   (B) Aspirin because of nausea
   (C) Albuterol due to excessive use
   (D) Theophylline because of toxicity
   (E) Metoprolol because of tachycardia

149. What is/are the generic ingredient(s) of Advair?

   (A) Fluticasone
   (B) Salmeterol
   (C) Fluticasone and salmeterol
   (D) Flunisolide
   (E) Flunisolide and salmeterol

150. What is the likely reason that this patient is taking fish oil?

   (A) To reduce total cholesterol
   (B) To reduce LDL cholesterol
   (C) To increase HDL cholesterol
   (D) To reduce HDL cholesterol
   (E) To reduce triglycerides

151. This patient is potentially taking excessive doses of acetaminophen. Which of the following is the MOST appropriate action to take?

   (A) Call her doctor.
   (B) Discuss how much acetaminophen is appropriate per day.
   (C) Discontinue the hydrocodone/APAP.
   (D) Discontinue the Tylenol Arthritis.
   (E) Consider switching the Tylenol Arthritis to an aspirin-containing product.

152. What is/are the major difference(s) between Spiriva and Atrovent?

   I. Atrovent has fewer side effects.
   II. Spiriva is taken once daily.
   III. Spiriva is a dry powder inhaler.

   (A) I only
   (B) III only
   (C) I and II only
   (D) II and III only
   (E) I, II, and III

153. Which of the following is the mechanism of action of Zyban?

   (A) It inhibits reuptake of serotonin.
   (B) It inhibits reuptake of norepinephrine.
   (C) It inhibits reuptake of dopamine.
   (D) It inhibits reuptake of dopamine and norepinephrine.
   (E) It inhibits reuptake of serotonin, norepinephrine, and dopamine.

154. Which of the following drugs is NOT commonly used in the treatment of nonresistant tuberculosis?

(A) Isoniazid
(B) Rifampin
(C) Pyrazinamide
(D) Ethambutol
(E) Streptomycin

155. Vitamin K can be used to reverse the effects of which of the following drugs?

(A) Unfractionated heparin
(B) Dabigatran
(C) Enoxaparin
(D) Warfarin
(E) Clopidogrel

156. Flumazenil is used to treat an overdose of which of the following medications?

(A) Benzodiazepines
(B) Opioids
(C) Ethanol
(D) Methotrexate
(E) Cisplatin

157. Cytomel is the brand name for which active ingredient?

(A) Liothyronine
(B) Levothyroxine
(C) Dessicated thyroid
(D) T4
(E) TSH

158. Which of the following drugs is/are considered pregnancy category X?

    I. Finasteride
    II. Isotretinoin
    III. Ramipril

(A) I only
(B) III only
(C) I and II only
(D) II and III only
(E) I, II, and III

159. When counseling a patient about medroxyprogesterone, which of the following is/are important factors to discuss?

    I. Weight gain
    II. Osteoporosis
    III. Risk of pulmonary embolism

(A) I only
(B) III only
(C) I and II only
(D) II and III only
(E) I, II, and III

160. How long does it take for the fentanyl patch to begin working?

(A) 12 hours
(B) 24 hours
(C) 48 hours
(D) 72 hours
(E) 84 hours

161. Which of the following is/are important points to discuss with a patient taking morphine for chronic pain?

   I.   The need for a stimulant laxative
   II. The importance of not driving a vehicle
   III. Compliance

   (A) I only
   (B) III only
   (C) I and II only
   (D) II and III only
   (E) I, II, and III

162. A woman comes into the pharmacy and requests an OTC medication for pain in her knee, though she can't remember what her physician told her to purchase. She informs you that she has kidney problems. Which of the following medications is acceptable?

   (A) Ibuprofen
   (B) Ketoprofen
   (C) Naprosyn
   (D) Acetaminophen
   (E) Aspirin

163. A PPD should be performed on which of the following individuals?

   I.   Healthcare worker
   II. HIV-infected patient
   III. Immigrant

   (A) I only
   (B) III only
   (C) I and II only
   (D) II and III only
   (E) I, II, and III

164. The doses of which of the following pain medications must be adjusted in patients with renal dysfunction?

   I.   Morphine
   II. Codeine
   III. Oxycodone

   (A) I only
   (B) III only
   (C) I and II only
   (D) II and III only
   (E) I, II, and III

165. Which NSAID has a maximum dose of 1,250 mg per day?

   (A) Naproxen
   (B) Ibuprofen
   (C) Relafen
   (D) Ketoprofen
   (E) Daypro

166. Which of the following is NOT a warning sign of stroke?

   (A) Numbness or weakness of the face, arm, or leg
   (B) Sudden confusion, trouble speaking or understanding
   (C) Sudden trouble seeing in one or both eyes
   (D) Sudden seizure for no known reason
   (E) Sudden trouble walking, dizziness, loss of balance

167. Folic acid is important in which of the following conditions?

   I.   Methotrexate treatment
   II. Neural tube defects
   III. Iron deficiency anemia

   (A) I only
   (B) III only
   (C) I and II only
   (D) II and III only
   (E) I, II, and III

168. Which of the following is/are the MOST common side effects of long-term treatment with ferrous sulfate?

    I. Constipation
    II. Dark stools
    III. Discoloration of urine

(A) I only
(B) III only
(C) I and II only
(D) II and III only
(E) I, II, and III

169. A patient with osteomalacia would BEST be given a nutritional supplement high in

(A) pyridoxine.
(B) ascorbic acid.
(C) beta-carotene.
(D) nicotinic acid.
(E) cholecalciferol.

170. Iron deficiency anemia requires a minimum of how many months of treatment?

(A) 1 month
(B) 3 months
(C) 6 months
(D) 9 months
(E) 12 months

171. What is the mechanism of epoetin alfa?

(A) It induces reticulocytes to create more iron stores.
(B) It induces erythropoiesis and the release of reticulocytes.
(C) It stimulates granulocyte colony-stimulating factor to generate more reticulocytes.
(D) It is a thrombopoietic growth factor, which stimulates iron absorption in the gut.
(E) It stimulates colony-stimulating factor to generate more iron absorption.

172. A patient taking chronic doses of isoniazid should be supplemented with which of the following?

(A) Beta-carotene
(B) Ascorbic acid
(C) Cyanocobalamin
(D) Thiamine
(E) Pyridoxine

173. The organization responsible for the enforcement of controlled substances is the

(A) Federal Drug Association.
(B) Food and Drug Administration.
(C) Drug Enforcement Administration.
(D) National Provider Indicators.
(E) State Patrol.

174. Which of the following statements regarding lifestyle modifications is NOT correct?

   (A) Smoking cessation for more than a year can lead to an improvement in lung function.
   (B) Avoidance of asthma triggers such as mold, pollen, dust, cockroaches, grass, and smoke can replace the need for a short-acting beta-2 agonist bronchodilator.
   (C) NCEP guidelines recommend 6 months of lifestyle modifications prior to starting medical therapy for the treatment of dyslipidemia in most cases.
   (D) Patients with heartburn may raise the head of the bed by 2–3 inches to relieve symptoms during sleeping hours.
   (E) Patients with hypertension should limit their salt intake to less than 2.4 g/day.

175. Which of the following statements regarding the Dietary Supplement Health and Education Act of 1994 is FALSE?

   (A) Manufacturers are not required to demonstrate safety, purity, or efficacy of supplements.
   (B) Labeling must include the FDA statement: "This drug is not evaluated by the FDA, and not intended to diagnose, treat, cure, or prevent disease."
   (C) Products cannot have specific claims on their labels or use phrases such as "helps boost/support/ enhance."
   (D) The FDA requires certain standards for manufacturing practices.
   (E) Manufacturers are not required to demonstrate safety.

176. Which of the following herbal products does NOT have the potential to interact with anticoagulant/antiplatelet agents?

   (A) Ginkgo biloba
   (B) Ginseng
   (C) Garlic
   (D) Saw palmetto
   (E) Feverfew

177. Which of the following is the best therapeutic substitution for Robitussin AC?

   (A) Robitussin
   (B) Robitussin CF
   (C) Robitussin DAC
   (D) Robitussin DM
   (E) Robitussin PE

178. Which of the following is NOT a setting within an insulin pump?

   (A) Basal insulin rate
   (B) Insulin to carbohydrate ratio
   (C) Insulin sensitivity factor
   (D) Rule of 1,800
   (E) Goal blood sugar

179. Doses of vitamin E over 400 IU are known to increase

   (A) cardiovascular events.
   (B) Alzheimer's disease.
   (C) hepatotoxicity.
   (D) kidney dysfunction.
   (E) gastrointestinal discomfort.

180. Compilations of information concerning parenteral drug solutions are found in

    (A) Goodman and Gilman.
    (B) Martindale.
    (C) Merck Index.
    (D) Remington.
    (E) Trissel's Handbook on Injectable Drugs.

181. Solubility data for potassium gluconate will be found in which of the following?

    I. Merck Index
    II. USP-NF
    III. Remington

    (A) I only
    (B) III only
    (C) I and II only
    (D) II and III only
    (E) I, II, and III

182. _____ are currently available on the market.

    (A) Metformin 1,250-mg tablets
    (B) Ferrous sulfate 5-grain tablets
    (C) Synthroid 212-mcg tablets
    (D) Boniva 3.5-mg tablets
    (E) Lisinopril 80-mg tablets

183. Which statin is equivalent to Lipitor 10 mg?

    (A) Rosuvastatin 10 mg
    (B) Simvastatin 20 mg
    (C) Pravastatin 20 mg
    (D) Simvastatin 80 mg
    (E) None of the above

184. St. John's wort interacts with which of the following medications?

    I. Pravachol
    II. Sertraline
    III. Warfarin

    (A) I only
    (B) III only
    (C) I and II only
    (D) II and III only
    (E) I, II, and III

185. A patient who is experiencing a runny nose, sneezing, headache, and watery eyes should be counseled to take which of the following OTC agents?

    I. Diphenhydramine
    II. Acetaminophen
    III. Pseudoephedrine

    (A) I only
    (B) III only
    (C) I and II only
    (D) II and III only
    (E) I, II, and III

Full-Length Practice Test
Answers & Explanations

1. E

Diarrhea is a possible side effect of nearly any medication including approximately 1–10% of patients taking allopurinol (A), indomethacin (C), and acetaminophen (D); and <5% of patients taking probenecid (B). However, up to 25% of patients taking colchicine will experience this common, limiting side effect.

2. B

A1c is the gold standard for monitoring glycemic control in patients with diabetes (A). Because A1c measures glycosylated hemoglobin, the time frame it represents correlates with the lifespan of a red blood cell (90–120 days). In patients with severe anemia, low hemoglobin (Hgb) values can make the A1c value inaccurate (C). The most common normal reference range is 4–6% (D) while an A1c of 10% correlates with blood sugar values averaging in excess of 200 mg/dL (E).

3. E

Clozapine requires rigorous monitoring of WBC and ANC due to the possibility of clozapine-induced agranulocytosis or severe granulocytopenia. Counts for both parameters should be obtained at baseline and at least weekly for the first 6 months of treatment with clozapine. If counts remain stable, then the WBC and ANC can be monitored every other week for the next 6 months and monthly thereafter. Due to these frequent monitoring requirements, clozapine is used less than other atypical antipsychotics and is often used for refractory cases of schizophrenia. Agranulocytosis is not associated with olanzapine (A), risperidone (B), quetiapine (C), or ziprasidone (D).

4. A

When initiating a dopamine agonist such as Mirapex, the levodopa dose should be decreased by 20–30%. II is incorrect because Mirapex does not come in a patch, which eliminates answer choices (C), (D), and (E). The ergot-derivative bromocriptine must be monitored for the cardiac side effects (III), which is why the nonergot derivatives such as Mirapex are much more commonly used.

5. A

Venlafaxine is an appropriate antidepressant medication to initiate and the initial dose should be 37.5 mg PO twice daily. Lexapro is dosed once daily (B). Fluvoxamine should be dosed once daily (C); fluoxetine can be dosed weekly. The maximum dose of nortriptyline is 150 mg/day (D). Mirtazapine does not come in a 10-mg formulation and should be dosed at bedtime due to somnolence (E).

6. E

NuvaRing should be inserted once per month and left in place for 3 weeks, then removed for 1 week (I); Ortho-Evra is applied once each week for 3 consecutive weeks followed by 1 patch-free week per month (II); and Seasonale is a continuous oral contraceptive that is taken as 84 active pills followed by 7 inactive pills, resulting in menses approximately once every 3 months (III).

7. D

Corticosteroids such as prednisone may increase blood glucose (A) and blood pressure. Methotrexate may cause a folate deficiency; therefore, a CBC must be monitored (B). Hydroxychloroquine may cause macular damage, corneal deposits, or retinopathy, so ocular exams must be performed every 3 months (C). The dose of Enbrel (etanercept) is not dependent on renal function and the drug does not cause nephrotoxicity; therefore, serum creatinine does not need to be monitored during therapy with this drug (D). Leflunomide is contraindicated in hepatic disease and may elevate liver enzymes, so alanine aminotransferase (ALT) must be monitored monthly for 6 months, then periodically (E).

8. D

Serum creatinine is most commonly used to assess renal function, not hepatic function (A). Serum creatinine is not dependent upon the amount of iron in the diet and is sometimes an inaccurate representation of renal function in the very elderly (B, C). Serum creatinine is commonly used in the Cockroft-Gault equation to calculate creatinine clearance (D). Microalbumin, a microscopic protein, is measured in the urine and is not synonymous with serum creatinine (E).

9. C

Natalizumab is reserved for patients that have not responded to other disease-modifying drugs (DMDs) (II). Natalizumab is available only through a restrictive prescribing program called TOUCH, in which both prescribers and patients must enroll (I), eliminating choices (A) and (D). Natalizumab should be used only as monotherapy and not in combination with other DMDs (III), eliminating choices (B), (D), and (E). Using natalizumab with DMDs increases the risk of progressive multifocal leukoencephalopathy.

10. B

Allopurinol is indicated for prophylaxis of gout exacerbations in patients with moderately elevated serum uric acid levels and a history of nephrolithiasis, tophi, serum creatinine >2 mg/dL, or urinary uric acid excretion indicative of overproduction (B). If the serum uric acid levels are only slightly elevated, colchicine is used for prophylaxis (A). In patients who have urinary uric acid excretion levels indicative of underexcretion, uricosuric drugs (e.g., probenecid) are used for prophylaxis (C). Acute gout is never treated with allopurinol and can actually worsen the symptoms (D). Asymptomatic hyperuricemia does not require therapy (E).

11. D

Lamotrigine (I) does not require monitoring of serum drug concentrations. Valproic acid (II) should be monitored to achieve serum drug concentrations of 50–100 mcg/mL. Therapeutic serum drug concentrations of lithium (III) are 0.6–1.5 mEq/L.

12. E

All of the trade/generic names are correctly matched except that Haldol is the trade name for haloperidol. Clozapine is the generic name for Clozaril.

13. C

Available prophylactic agents for migraines include beta-blockers (such as propranolol, atenolol, metoprolol), antidepressants (such as amitriptyline, paroxetine, fluoxetine, sertraline), and anticonvulsants (such as valproic acid, gabapentin, tiagabine, topiramate). Acetaminophen (B) is considered abortive treatment for migraines and is not taken for prophylaxis. Angiotensin-converting enzyme (ACE) inhibitors (A), H_2 antagonists (D), and anticholinergics (E) have no role in the prevention of migraines.

14. B

Tramadol (B) is an oral analgesic that does not cause GI upset or bleeding. Aspirin (A) is an NSAID that may cause GI bleeding. Diclofenac (C) and Daypro (oxaprozin; D) are both NSAIDs that may cause GI upset and bleeding. Although Mobic (meloxicam; E) is more COX-2–selective than traditional NSAIDs, it still possesses the potential to cause GI upset and stomach bleeding.

15. C

Haloperidol (C) is a first-generation antipsychotic. First-generation antipsychotics are known for the potential to cause extrapyramidal symptoms (EPS) such as tardive dyskinesia and dystonia. Hydrochlorothiazide (A) is a common antihypertensive that does not cause EPS. Citalopram (B) is a common antidepressant that does not cause EPS. Although low sodium (D) can be dangerous, it does not cause EPS. Uncontrolled blood pressure (E) may lead to organ damage but does not cause EPS.

16. E

Haloperidol (E) requires periodic monitoring of a CBC because of its potential to cause agranulo-cytosis. Serum drug levels (A) are not measured with haloperidol. Although a baseline electrocardiogram is recommended upon haloperidol initiation, monitoring of ejection fraction (C) is not necessary. A1c (B) could be monitored with atypical antipsychotics (such as olanzapine or ziprasidone) due to their likelihood of causing metabolic syndrome. Bone mineral density (D) is not routine monitoring for any antipsychotic.

17. B

Switching between formulations of haloperidol (I) would not provide any benefit with extrapyramidal side effects. Changing the patient to an atypical antipsychotic would be the best option since atypicals have fewer extrapyramidal side effects. This patient is allergic to Geodon (ziprasidone) so (II) would not be appropriate. This leaves the atypical Risperdal (risperidone; III), which would be appropriate.

18. D

Alcohol should be avoided in combination with antipsychotics due to the excessive CNS depression it may cause. An acidic environment is not required with antipsychotic medications and patients may take most of the medications with food if GI upset occurs (A). Medications for schizophrenia may take 2–4 weeks to work, so (B) is not correct. It is also important that these medications not be abruptly stopped (C) or self-adjusted (E). If bothersome side effects occur, physicians should be contacted to make adjustments and changes in the medications.

19. C

Alprazolam (B) is not used for depression but may be used in anxiety disorders. Propranolol (E) is a beta-blocker which may actually worsen depression. Although not contraindicated, venlafaxine (D) may not be the best option for this patient considering her uncontrolled blood pressure. Venlafaxine can increase blood pressure and should be monitored closely. Bupropion (A) is contraindicated if the patient actually has an eating disorder. Since this woman is suspected of having an eating disorder, this is not the most appropriate recommendation. Lexapro (escitalopram; C) is an SSRI similar to her current citalopram and would be an appropriate substitution.

20. **A**

Carbidopa is a dopa-decarboxylase inhibitor, which must be combined with levodopa to prevent the peripheral degradation of levodopa (I). If the levodopa is degraded in the periphery, it does not enter into the blood-brain barrier for site of action. The carbidopa does not extend the dosing interval (II) or prevent side effects from occurring (III), therefore eliminating answer choices (B)–(E).

21. **C**

NSAIDs such as indomethacin are the first-line treatment for acute gout. If the patient is unable to take NSAIDs, the time course of the event must be evaluated. If the symptoms have been present for less than 48 hours, colchicine (B) is recommended. If the symptoms have been present for >48 hours, a corticosteroid is recommended. Allopurinol (D) should never be used in the treatment of acute gout and can worsen the symptoms. Probenecid (E) is not useful in an acute exacerbation of gout and should be avoided as it may precipitate attacks. Acetaminophen (A) plays no role in the treatment of acute gout.

22. **E**

All of the medications are correctly matched with their common side effects. Mirtazapine is typically dosed at bedtime because of the somnolence it causes (I). All of the SSRIs (par-oxetine) have the potential to cause ejaculation disorders or impotence (II). The tricyclic antidepressants (TCAs) (amitriptyline) have the potential to cause weight gain along with anticholinergic side effects (III).

23. **E**

Phenytoin is available in many dosage forms including chewable tablets (I), capsules, extended-release capsules, and oral suspension (II). Phenytoin can also be given IM or IV, as it comes in a parenteral solution (III).

24. **B**

NSAIDs are used for symptomatic relief during the onset of disease-modifying antirheumatic drug (DMARD) therapy and PRN symptomatic relief (B). NSAIDs do not alter the disease progression of rheumatoid arthritis; therefore, they are not considered DMARDs (A). Although NSAIDs can be given along with DMARDs for symptoms, they are not considered adjunctive therapy for patients with refractory symptoms (C); that is the role of corticosteroids. The biologics are not known to cause flushing, (D) although NSAIDs could be used for PRN symptom relief with the biologics. Methotrexate must be given in combination with infliximab, not NSAIDs (E).

25. **B**

If a patient is experiencing severe nausea and vomiting whenever a migraine occurs, most likely he/she will not receive maximum benefit from a regular oral tablet (I and II) due to the emesis. Many other dosage forms are available within the triptan class of abortive therapies. Maxalt MLT (rizatriptan) (III) is a rapidly disintegrating tablet that is one possible option for treatment in these patients. Other triptan options for patients experiencing severe nausea and vomiting include Imitrex (sumatriptan) injection or nasal spray and Zomig (zolmitriptan) orally disintegrating tablet or nasal spray.

26. **A**

Oxcarbazepine and lamotrigine both have the potential to cause Stevens-Johnson syndrome (A), especially when lamotrigine is used in combination with valproic acid. Oxcarbazepine is the generic name for Trileptal (B). Lithium does not interact with beta-blockers (C); however, it does have significant drug interactions with ACE inhibitors and diuretics. Lithium works by altering the sodium transport (E), which helps in understanding the interaction with ACE inhibitors and diuretics; while valproic acid is thought to affect GABA. Valproic acid is contraindicated in hepatic dysfunction and requires baseline and periodic liver function tests (D).

27. **D**

Bupropion can be used for smoking cessation (I). Bupropion is contraindicated in patients with seizure disorders due to an increased risk of seizures (III). Bupropion is also contraindicated in patients with eating disorders such as bulimia or anorexia (II). A patient's medical history must be obtained before initiation of bupropion.

28. **E**

Methotrexate is first-line DMARD therapy for patients with rheumatoid arthritis (C). Patients may be supplemented with folic acid during treatment with methotrexate to decrease adverse effects and prevent folate deficiency (A). To lessen GI upset, methotrexate should be taken with food (B). The usual dosing for rheumatoid arthritis is 7.5 mg PO once weekly (D). Methotrexate does not require frequent ophthalmic exams; that is a requirement of hydroxychloroquine.

29. **E**

Oxybutynin is available in an oral form (Ditropan and Ditropan XL) as well as a transdermal form (Oxytrol patch) (I). It is also available as a topical gel (Gelnique). It is an anticholinergic medication used to treat incontinence (II). Common anticholinergic side effects include dry mouth and dry eyes (III).

30. **B**

Colchicine can be used both for prophylaxis and treatment of gout (III). NSAIDs are used only for acute symptoms and do not prevent gout from occurring (I). Corticosteroids are used during acute attacks when symptoms have been present for >48 hours (II).

31. **C**

Hot flushes (A), decreased libido (B), spotting (D), and dyspareunia (E) are all common side effects of estrogen deficiency. Since Ovcon-50 is a high estrogen-containing oral contraceptive, side effects of estrogen excess (such as breast tenderness) would be more common.

32. **C**

Seasonale is an oral contraceptive and should be taken by mouth once daily (I). Smoking while on any oral contraceptive will increase the risk of thromboembolic events (II). Seasonale is not available in a transdermal patch formulation (III).

33. **E**

Oral antibiotics inhibit the efficacy of oral contraceptive medications, so (A) and (B) are inaccurate. It would be inappropriate to advise a patient not to take an antibiotic and it would also be inappropriate to advise a patient to double the dose of oral contraceptive during the use of the antibiotics; the safety and efficacy of this practice have not been established and this could pose harm to the patient. During the use of interacting antibiotics, it is important to advise a patient to adhere to a backup method of contraception during, for at least 7 days, and up to a full cycle after the completion of the antibiotic.

34. C

First-line therapy for comedonal acne is topical benzoyl peroxide (C). The use of oral antibiotics (A) would be recommended in pustular acne or in cases that were not responsive to topical therapy. Also, tetracycline would interact with Ms. Brown's oral contraceptive medication and would not be ideal. Isotretinoin (B and E) is reserved for severe cystic or refractory acne, and topical retinoid agents should not be initially combined with topical benzoyl peroxide (D) due to an increased risk of drying of the skin.

35. D

Ms. Brown's headaches are quite frequent, making her a candidate for prophylactic therapy (A). Imitrex (sumatriptan; B) is an abortive therapy medication and is not appropriate for prophylaxis. Topiramate (C) is used as prophylactic therapy, but would have a drug interaction with her oral contraceptive. Hydrocodone (E), an opiate analgesic, is used for the treatment of pain and would be inappropriate for migraine prophylaxis. Propranolol (D) is commonly used for migraine prophylaxis and would be the most appropriate of these options.

36. A

Patients taking oral contraceptives should be educated to consult their pharmacist or physician when starting any new medication because of the strong possibility of multiple drug interactions. Neurontin (gabapentin; A) does not have any known drug interactions. Carbam-

azepine (B), valproic acid (C), phenytoin (D), and phenobarbital (E) have a long list of drug interactions, decreasing the effectiveness of oral contraceptives.

37. C

Tolterodine is the generic name for Detrol, oxybutynin is the generic name for Ditropan, solifenacin is the generic name for Vesicare, and imipramine is the generic name for Tofranil.

38. B

When a diagnosis of rheumatoid arthritis is made, DMARDs should be initiated within 3 months to slow the progression of the disease (I, eliminating choices A, C, and E). Biologics should be initiated when methotrexate monotherapy has been ineffective and possibly other DMARDs have been tried and ineffective as well (III). Biologics would not provide PRN relief as they are given by injection at weekly or longer intervals, with the exception of anakinra, which is a daily injection (II, eliminating choice D). NSAIDs are used for PRN symptom relief.

39. C

Tricyclic antidepressants (TCAs) often exhibit anticholinergic side effects (I). In overdose situations, these agents are very dangerous and often fatal (II); therefore, in patients with high suicidality, they should be used with caution. There is no drug–food interaction between aged cheese and TCAs; this interaction is with the monoamine oxidase inhibitors (MAOIs; III).

40. D

Antidepressants may take several weeks to show maximum efficacy. Neither SSRIs such as fluoxetine (A) nor SNRIs such as duloxetine (B) should be used in combination with MAOIs (selegiline). Choice (C) is incorrect because caffeine should be avoided in combination with MAOIs. Although there is an oral formulation of selegiline (E), it is not indicated for depression (used for Parkinson's disease) and would not increase efficacy.

41. A

Fiorinal contains aspirin with butalbital and caffeine. Fioricet (B) contains acetaminophen with butalbital and caffeine. Exedrin Migraine (C) contains acetaminophen and aspirin with caffeine. Migranal (D) is a dihydroergotamine nasal spray. Amergen (E) is naratriptan.

42. D

Photosensitivity is a common side effect with Retin-A (tretinoin), and the use of sunblock prior to sun exposure is very important. Retinoids such as Retin-A should not be used with astringents or abrasive soaps due to the increased risk of excessive drying of the skin (A). Topical retinoids take significantly longer than 1–2 days to result in a benefit (B). Topical retinoids are not used as spot treatment (C) and should be applied sparingly over the face after the face has been allowed to dry fully (E) after cleansing.

43. B

Zoledronic acid (I) is an annual infusion for the treatment of osteoporosis but is a bisphosphonate, so it is not an alternative to bisphosphonate therapy. Calcitonin (II) is an endogenous hormone that is indicated for the treatment of osteoporosis; it is usually administered intranasally. Raloxifene (III) is a selective estrogen receptor modulator that is recommended as an alternative choice for the treatment of osteoporosis.

44. C

The benzodiazepines including Xanax (alprazolam; A), Librium (chlordiazepoxide; B), and Valium (diazepam; D) vary in their peak activity and duration of action, but all have an onset of effect of minutes to hours. Vistaril (hydroxyzine; E) also works within minutes to hours, while Buspar (buspirone; C) takes up to 2 to 3 weeks to reach maximal efficacy.

45. C

Cheilitis (chapped lips; I) is the most common side effect of isotretinoin therapy. Pruritus (itching; II) related to dry skin is also a very common side effect of isotretinoin therapy. Hypertrichosis, or excessive hair growth (III), is not a known side effect of this medication.

46. D

Topical agents such as coal tar (C) and anthralin (E) are commonly used in the treatment of psoriasis. Systemic agents such as antimetabolites (methotrexate; A) and corticosteroids (prednisone; B) are often used in combination with topical agents in the treatment of psoriasis. Benzoyl peroxide (D) is not an effective treatment option for psoriasis.

47. C

In the TNM classification, T represents the severity of the primary tumor, N represents the severity of lymph node involvement, and M represents the severity of distant metastases. Generally, N0 and M0 mean no nodal involvement and no metastases, respectively.

48. C

Adjuvant chemotherapy is chemotherapy given after surgical treatment to provide further reduction in tumor burden. Neoadjuvant chemotherapy is given prior to surgical treatment, to provide an initial decrease in tumor burden. Both adjuvant and neoadjuvant chemotherapy are expected to increase survival. Palliative chemotherapy is given to relieve symptoms without expectation of survival benefit. The answer, therefore, is (B).

49. D

Methotrexate inhibits dihydrofolate reductase. When administered at the appropriate time in a chemotherapy cycle, leucovorin permits healthy cells to continue DNA replication and RNA transcription by providing a folic acid source that is not dependent on the action of dihydrofolate reductase. 5-fluorouracil inhibits thymidylate synthase, as does leucovorin. The two agents therefore have a synergistic effect. Doxorubicin (B) is an anthracycline antibiotic that works as an intercalating agent, interrupting DNA synthesis. Cytarabine (C) inhibits DNA polymerase. Leucovorin does not interact with the mechanism of action of doxorubicin or cytarabine.

50. E

The primary mechanism of action of cytarabine is inhibition of DNA polymerase (I). Common side effects of cytarabine treatment include conjunctivitis and neurotoxicity (II). Corticosteroid eye drops are recommended as prophylaxis of conjunctivitis before and after cytarabine treatment (III).

51. D

The most clinically important side effect of anthracyclines is cardiac damage, including acute arrhythmias and cardiomyopathy following prolonged exposure. The risk of cardiotoxicity increases with cumulative lifetime dose. Hand and foot syndrome (E), or palmar-plan-

tar erythrodysesthesia, is more common with 5-fluorouracil. Ototoxicity (A) is rarely seen with anthracyclines, and is more commonly a side effect of platinum compounds and nitrogen mustards. Methotrexate can cause symptoms of folate deficiency (C). Infusion reactions (B) are more common with etoposide, platinum compounds, and mustard compounds.

52. C

Avastin is the brand name for bevacizumab (C). Gleevec (A) is imatinib, Herceptin (B) is trastuzumab, Tarceva (D) is erlotinib, and Platinol (E) is cisplatin.

53. C

ANC = white blood cells × (% segs + % bands).

54. B

The ANC range for mild neutropenia is 500–1,000/mm³. Moderate neutropenia (C) is 100–500/mm³, while severe (D) is less than 100/mm³. A normal ANC is 3,000–7,000/mm³ (E).

55. E

Severe (A) or prolonged neutropenia (D) or a sudden drop in ANC (B) are all risk factors for infection. Invasive procedures, including dental procedures, catheter placement, and enemas, also increase the risk of infection (C).

56. E

None of the erythropoietin derivatives (Epogen, Procrit, and Aranesp) are indicated in this patient, as her hemoglobin level is normal at 14.5 g/dL. She is suffering mild neutropenia, which does not warrant treatment with a colony-stimulating factor (such as Neupogen [filgrastim]). Therefore, none of the listed drugs are appropriate and choice (E) is correct.

57. A

Nominal or categorical data are qualitative and have no implied order among the categories. These data can be answered by "yes" or "no" responses. Gender and race are considered nominal data. Ordinal data (B) are ordered categories where the differences between categories cannot be considered equal. Satisfaction surveys and pain scales are examples of ordinal data. With interval data (C), there is an equal distance between the numeric values; however, there is an arbitrary zero point. The Celsius temperature scale is an example of interval data. With ratio data (such as weight or blood pressure; D), there is an equal distance between values and the zero point is meaningful. Frequency (E) refers to a proportion and not a type of data.

58. E

Power depends on sample size and variation within groups. The easiest way to increase power is to increase the sample size of a study. Altering the duration of the study (B, C) or decreasing the sample size (A) will not increase power. Increasing the number of dependent variables being studied (D) will also not increase the power of the study.

59. D

Type II errors occur when it is stated that there is no difference when a difference actually exists. The null hypothesis is the hypothesis that there is no difference between study groups; not detecting a true difference between groups will lead to a Type II error. Insufficient study power may mean that a difference between groups will not be discovered or will not be found to be statistically significant. Therefore, choices (A), (B), and (C) are all true statements about Type II errors. Type I errors occur when a difference between groups is detected that does not

actually exist. Because the question is asking for which statement regarding Type II errors is false, the answer is (D).

60. D

ANOVA is the only test listed that is appropriate for such data (D). A student's T-test and a paired t-test are appropriate only when studying two groups. The Mann-Whitney U is a non-parametric test appropriate for ordinal data. Chi-square tests are used on nominal data.

61. C

$$0.12\,g \times \frac{100\,g\,ung}{2.5\,g\,HC} = 4.8\,g\,ung$$

$$30\,g\,ung \times \frac{0.4\,g\,HC}{100\,g\,ung} = 0.12\,g\,HC\,required$$

4.8 g of the 2.5% ointment is required to deliver the correct amount of hydrocortisone.

62. C

$$70\,g\,HPet \times \frac{8\,g\,WW}{100\,g\,HPet} = 5.6\,g\,WW$$

63. C

$$4\,floz \times \frac{30\,mL}{1\,floz} \times \frac{1\,tbsp}{15\,mL} \times \frac{2\,mg}{1\,tbsp} \times \frac{1\,tab}{4\,mg} = 4\,tabs$$

64. D

$$60\,kg \times \frac{5\,mcg}{kg\,x\,min} \times \frac{1\,mg}{1{,}000\,mcg} \times$$

$$\frac{1\,mL}{0.5\,mg} \times \frac{60\,min}{1\,hr} = 36\,mL/hr$$

65. A

The initial concentration (C_0) will be obtained by drawing blood very soon after administration. Using the equation $V_d = \dfrac{dose}{C_0}$, we can see that for equal doses, V_d will vary inversely with C_0. Drug A has a higher C_0 than Drug B

(0.2 mg/mL > 83 mcg/mL); therefore, Drug A has a smaller volume of distribution.

66. C

$$40\,mL\,soln \times \frac{10\,g\,MgSO_4}{100\,mL\,soln} \times \frac{1000\,mg}{1\,g} \times$$

$$\frac{1\,mmol\,MgSO_4}{246.36\,mg\,MgSO_4} \times \frac{1\,mmol\,Mg^{2+}}{1\,mmol\,MgSO_4} \times$$

$$\frac{2\,mEq\,Mg^{2+}}{1\,mmol\,Mg^{2+}} = 32.5\,mEq\,Mg^{2+}$$

67. C

$$240\,mL \times \frac{15\,mEq}{15\,mL} \times \frac{1\,mmol\,K^+}{1\,mEq\,K^+} \times$$

$$\frac{1\,mmol\,C_6H_5K_3O_7}{3\,mmol\,K^+} \times \frac{1\,mol}{1,000\,mmol} \times$$

$$\frac{306\,g\,C_6H_5K_3O_7}{1\,mol\,C_6H_5K_3O_7} = 24.48\,g\,C_6H_5K_3O_7$$

68. B

Accuracy refers to how closely test values approach the true value. Precision refers to how closely test values approach each other. Because the test values given are tightly grouped (8.0 ± 0.1) but differ significantly from the true value given (7.5), it can be said the values are precise but not accurate.

69. B

$$\frac{0.9\,g\,NaCl}{100\,mL} \times 30\,mL = 0.27\,g\,NaCl$$

needed to make volume isotonic

$$30\,mL \times \frac{0.5\,g\,TetHCl}{100\,mL} \times \frac{0.18\,g\,NaCl(Eq)}{1\,g\,TetHCl} = 0.027\,g$$

NaCl equivalent present

0.27 g – 0.027 g = 0.243 g NaCl needed to make the solution isotonic

70. B

The recipe makes 10 capsules (M et div caps #10). Therefore each capsule contains (0.5/10) or 0.05 g diphenhydramine. Then, 0.05 × 60 = 3 g.

71. C

fup = 1 – (fraction bound to proteins) = 0.05

Filtration clearance = fup × CLcr = 0.05 × 100 mL/min = 5 mL/min

72. C

CLr = amount filtered + amount secreted – amount reabsorbed

All molecules small enough to pass through the glomerular membrane, which includes most nonprotein-bound small molecule drugs, are filtered.

If CLr > filtration clearance, some drug must be secreted. (Some reabsorption may also occur, but less is reabsorbed than secreted.)

If CLr < filtration clearance, some drug must be reabsorbed. (Some secretion may also occur, but less is secreted than is reabsorbed.)

Because CLr = 25 mL/min, while filtration clearance is only 5 mL/min, the drug must be secreted as well as filtered.

73. A

$$k = \frac{CL}{V_d} = \frac{400\,mL/min}{140\,L} \times \frac{1\,L}{1,000\,mL} \times$$

$$\frac{60\,min}{hr} = 0.171\,hr^{-1}$$

$$t_{1/2} = \frac{0.693}{k} = \frac{0.693}{0.171\,hr^{-1}} = 4.04\,hr$$

74. D

$$C_{peak} = \frac{dose}{V_d} = \frac{250\,mg}{140\,L} = 1.79\,mg/L = 0.179\,mg/dL$$

75. B

Tobramycin is predominantly cleared by the kidneys. The increase in serum creatinine concentration indicates a decrease in creatinine clearance, which in turn implies a decrease in tobramycin clearance. Therefore, choices (C) and (E) are wrong. The bioavailability of any drug given IV is 1; therefore, choice (A) is wrong. When clearance decreases, the half-life and serum concentration will increase, leading to drug accumulation. Therefore, choice (D) is wrong and (B) is correct.

76. A

Because penicillin and probenecid compete for the same saturable excretion pathway, administration of probenecid will decrease the secretion and therefore the overall clearance of penicillin. Choices (B), (C), and (E) are incorrect. When clearance decreases, the steady-state plasma concentration of the drug will increase, so choice (D) is incorrect and (A) is the right answer.

77. B

Amorphous compounds are more soluble in water than their crystalline counterparts. Hydrates are less soluble in water than anhydrous drugs (A). Adding lipophilic groups (C) and removing hydroxyl groups (D) will also decrease water solubility.

78. D

For weak bases, when pH < pKa the drug will be mostly ionized. Therefore the answer is choice (D).

79. E

All medication given by mouth is subject to first-pass metabolism. Only medications given by routes that bypass the GI tract can escape first-pass metabolism. Syrups (B), tablets (A), and capsules (C) are all swallowed, and their contents undergo first-pass metabolism. The rapid-dissolve strip (D) is also an oral product: The strip dissolves in the mouth, and the resultant solution is swallowed. Do not confuse a rapid-dissolve strip with a sublingual or buccal tablet—in these latter two dosage forms, the drug is absorbed across the oral mucosa, escaping the first-pass effect. Of the choices listed, only the transdermal patch is given by a nonoral route. Therefore (E) is the only choice that is not subject to first-pass metabolism.

80. B

Maximizing sediment volume (C) and promoting loose aggregation of suspended particles (A) are functions of controlled flocculation, not structured vehicles. Reducing repulsion between particles (D) will lead to increased sediment density, causing caking. Only slowing sedimentation by increasing viscosity is a behavior of structured vehicles, so (B) is correct.

81. B

The cosolvent system for phenytoin injection contains water, propylene glycol, and alcohol. The cosolvent system is necessary to keep phenytoin in solution, as phenytoin has only limited aqueous solubility. Rapid infusion would dilute the cosolvents, creating a super-saturated concentration of drug in a primarily aqueous environment, leading to precipitation. Onset of action will not be faster as a result of slow injection (A). Rapid injection is unlikely to lead to hemolysis (C); this is a complication of hypertonic solutions. The cosolvent system would have no effect on drug metabolism (D). The viscosity of the solution is not high enough to prevent rapid injection (E).

82. A

Ophthalmic products must contain preservative if they are in multiple-use containers to limit the possibility of severe eye infections. They do not require preservative when packaged in single-dose containers (II), or when being used as rinse solutions in eye surgery or trauma (III).

83. C

Ulcerative colitis is a local condition of the intestinal tract; medications administered rectally are providing treatment at the site of action. Nausea (A), chronic pain (B), hormone deficiency (D), and migraine headaches (E) may be treated with medications administered rectally; however, these drugs are absorbed into the systemic circulation to act at distant sites of action.

84. D

The disulfiram reaction results from the inhibition of acetaldehyde dehydrogenase. Ethanol consumption leads to the buildup of acetaldehyde, causing nausea, vomiting, and severe discomfort. Tinctures (C), spirits (A), fluid extracts (E), and Elixir USP (B) all contain ethanol, and will trigger this reaction if taken in combination with metronidazole. Suspensions do not customarily contain ethanol and would be an appropriate way to deliver metronidazole.

85. C

Hydrolysis (A) results when the drug reacts with water in the dosage form. Because the reaction occurred in only one of the two bottles, this is unlikely. Photolysis (B) is chemical breakdown caused by light exposure; however, the drug was stored in a dark room. Sedimentation (D) and polymorphism (E) are physical changes, rather than chemical changes, and there was no difference in conditions between the capped and uncapped bottles that would explain a difference in the occurrence of these changes. Because only the open bottle was affected, while the capped bottle did not change color, the oxygen in the atmosphere likely caused the degradation.

86. E

Dilatant substances (A) become more viscous on agitation, and thin at rest. Newtonian substances (B) do not change viscosity when stirred or agitated. Plastic flow (C) occurs when a substance is thick at rest and remains thick until it receives sufficiently vigorous agitation, after which it behaves in a Newtonian manner. Pseudoplastic flow (D) is similar to plastic flow, but the material continues to thin if agitated more vigorously. Thixotropy is the property where a suspension remains thick until agitated, and then becomes easily pourable.

87. B

$$DR = \frac{V_{max} - C_{ss}}{K_m \cdot C_{ss}} = \frac{(300)(14)}{6.5 + 14} =$$

$205\ mg\ /\ day = 4\ tablets$

88. D

Magnesium stearate is a lubricant, and at high concentration has a tendency to waterproof particles, preventing them from dissolving. Starch (A), microcrystalline cellulose (B), lactose (C), and mannitol (E) would not be expected to affect bioavailability.

89. B

Morphine is the only one of these products not metabolized by CYP2D6. Codeine (A), hydrocodone (C), and oxycodone (D) require metabolism by CYP2D6 in order to be activated to a therapeutically useful form. While structurally related to codeine, dextromethorphan (E) is not considered an opioid. This cough suppressant also requires metabolism via CYP2D6 to produce its active form.

90. **A**

Grapefruit juice inhibits CYP3A, the enzyme that metabolizes protease inhibitors. Therefore, choices (C), (D), and (E) can be eliminated. Inhibition of CYP3A will decrease clearance of drugs metabolized by that enzyme, leading to increased serum concentrations. Increased serum concentration will lead to toxic, rather than subtherapeutic (B), levels.

91. **D**

$$1:10,000 = \frac{1\,g}{10,000\,mL} = \frac{0.01\,g}{100\,mL} = 0.01\%\,w/v$$

92. **B**

$$SG = \frac{density_{substance}}{density_{water}}$$

$$SG \times density_{water} = density_{substance}$$

$$1.18 \times 1\,g/mL = 1.18\,g/mL$$

$$100\,g \times \frac{1\,mL}{1.18\,g} = 84.75\,mL$$

93. **D**

Simvastatin and ezetimibe combined are called Vytorin. The combination of atorvastatin and amlodipine (A) is called Caduet; and the combination of lovastatin and niacin (C) is called Advicor. There are no combinations of atorvastatin and ezetimibe (B), or simvastatin and lisinopril (E).

94. **C**

Nonpharmacological therapies that can be recommended to patients with heart failure include restricting fluid intake (<2 L/day) (I) and restricting sodium intake (≤3 g/day) (II). There is no specific reason why a patient with heart failure needs to restrict vitamin K in the diet (III).

95. **E**

Anorexia (I), arrhythmias (II), and visual disturbances (III) are all associated with digoxin toxicity.

96. **D**

Calan SR (verapamil) is a nondihydropyridine calcium channel blocker that is contraindicated in systolic heart failure (LVEF <40%). Aldactone (spironolactone; A) and Inspra (eplerenone; E), which are both aldosterone receptor antagonists, as well as the angiotensin receptor blocker, Diovan (valsartan; C), would be safe to use in a patient with heart failure. In addition, BiDil (B), the combination of hydralazine and isosorbide dinitrate, would also be appropriate to use in a patient with heart failure.

97. **B**

The second dose of furosemide should be taken before 5 p.m. to minimize nocturia. Furosemide does not need to be separated from other medications (A), does not need to be taken with food or milk (C), and does not need to be taken on an empty stomach (E). The second dose should not be taken at bedtime, as this will likely result in increased nocturia (D).

98. **D**

Bactrim DS (sulfamethoxazole/trimethoprim) is most likely being used to treat *Escherichia coli*, a common cause of urinary tract infections (UTIs). Bactrim DS does not cover the other bacteria listed.

99. **A**

The combination of Bactrim DS and Coumadin (warfarin) may lead to a significant drug interaction that would result in an increase in Ms. Brown's INR.

100. E

The combination of trimethoprim and sulfamethoxazole is called Bactrim DS. The combination of amoxicillin and clavulanic acid (A) is called Augmentin, and the combination of imipenem and cilastatin (C) is called Primaxin. There are no combinations of ciprofloxacin and doxycycline (B), or of isoniazid and rifampin (D).

101. A

Lisinopril is an ACE inhibitor.

102. B

Martindale is the only reference that contains foreign drug information.

103. D

Xalatan (latanoprost) is an ophthalmic prostaglandin analog used to treat glaucoma.

104. B

Ketek (telithromycin; III) is a macrolide antibiotic. Keflex (cephalexin; I) is a cephalosporin antibiotic, and Keppra (levetiracetam; II) is an anticonvulsant.

105. D

Sulfasalazine may cause bodily fluids (e.g., urine, tears) to turn orange (II) and may cause photosensitivity (III). Sulfasalazine should be taken with food rather than on an empty stomach (I).

106. D

Metronidazole is the only option listed that can be used to treat *Clostridium difficile*.

107. E

USP-DI Volume II contains information for the patient in lay language. The other choices are all references for the healthcare professional.

108. C

Cytotec is the brand name for misoprostol. Cimetidine (A) is Tagamet. Metoclopramide (B) is Reglan. Olsalazine (D) is Dipentum. Sucralfate (E) is Carafate.

109. A

Acyclovir is an appropriate treatment for genital herpes. Indinavir (B) and lamivudine (C) are used to treat HIV. Oseltamivir (D) is used to treat influenza. Valganciclovir (E) is used to treat cytomegalovirus.

110. D

The Red Book is the only choice listed that contains cost information.

111. E

Potential side effects of niacin include flushing (I), hyperglycemia (II), and hyperuricemia (III).

112. B

The combination of timolol and dorzolamide is called Cosopt. The combination of timolol and brimonidine (A), is called Combigan. There are no combinations of latanoprost and carbachol (C), pilocarpine and brinzolamide (D), or pilocarpine and carbachol (E).

113. A

Caspofungin is an intravenous antifungal that could be used to treat an invasive *Aspergillus* infection. While miconazole (III) is also an antifungal drug, it is available only in topical formulations and as a buccal tablet and is used to treat superficial fungal infections. Linezolid (II) is used to treat gram-positive bacterial infections, such as methicillin-resistant *Staphylococcus aureus* or vancomycin-resistant *Enterococcus faecium*.

114. E

Avoiding chocolate (I), smoking cessation (II), and weight loss (III) are all appropriate non-pharmacological recommendations for a patient with GERD.

115. E

Nitroprusside should be protected from light. None of the other IV medications listed need to be protected from light.

116. A

The three-drug combination regimen of Biaxin (clarithromycin), Amoxil (amoxicillin), and Nexium (esomeprazole) would be used to treat a *Helicobacter pylori* infection.

117. C

Trusopt (dorzolamide) is an ophthalmic carbonic anhydrase inhibitor used in treating glaucoma.

118. C

The Commission E monographs provide information on herbal products.

119. A

Clotrimazole is available as a troche (I), topical cream, vaginal cream, and topical solution. However, it is not available as a capsule (II) or powder (III).

120. B

In patients receiving amiodarone, liver function tests should be performed every 6 months (III) to monitor for potential hepatotoxicity. A chest x-ray should be performed every 12 months to monitor for pulmonary toxicity. Thyroid function tests should be performed every 6 months to monitor for hyper- or hypothyroidism.

121. E

Patients should separate the administration of different ophthalmic preparations by intervals of at least 10 minutes. Contact lenses should be removed before using ophthalmic products (A). Patients should not touch the tip of the dropper to any part of the eye (B). Patients should pull out the lower eyelid (not the upper eyelid) to form a pocket for the medication to be placed (C). Patients should not rub their eyes after administration of ophthalmic preparations (D).

122. B

Trissel's (III) contains information on intravenous drug compatibility. Facts and Comparisons (I) and the Physician's Drug Reference (II) contain general drug information and do not contain IV drug compatibility information.

123. B

Tagamet (cimetidine) is an H_2 receptor antagonist.

124. D

Patients taking methotrexate should have a CBC (II) monitored for potential bone marrow suppression, and their liver function tests (III) monitored for potential hepatotoxicity. It is not necessary to have an electrocardiogram (I) while taking methotrexate.

125. E

Candesartan (angiotensin II receptor antagonist; I), eplerenone (aldosterone receptor antagonist; II), and triamterene (potassium-sparing diuretic; III) may all result in hyperkalemia.

126. E

For esomeprazole (I), the capsules can be opened and mixed with water or the granules for oral suspension can be mixed with water prior to administration via nasogastric tube. For lansoprazole (II), the capsules can be opened and mixed with apple juice or the orally disintegrating tablets can be mixed with water in a syringe prior to administration via nasogastric tube. The pantoprazole (III) granules for suspension can be mixed with apple juice prior to administration via nasogastric tube.

127. A

A patient who is taking felodipine should avoid drinking grapefruit juice because grapefruit juice inhibits CYP3A4, which would result in increased concentrations of felodipine. Tyramine-containing foods (B) should be avoided in patients taking monoamine oxidase inhibitors. Felodipine does not cause folate deficiency, and therefore does not to be administered with folic acid (C). Felodipine does not need to be taken on an empty stomach (D), and does not need to be separated from other medications (E).

128. A

Azithromycin is the best option, as it will cover the most likely bacteria that would cause community-acquired pneumonia in this patient (*Streptococcus pneumoniae*, *Mycoplasma pneumoniae*, *Haemophilus influenzae*). The other antibiotic choices would not cover the appropriate bacteria.

129. D

Amoxicillin is available as an oral suspension (II) or a capsule (III), but not as an IV injection. A related antibiotic, ampicillin, can be administered intravenously.

130. C

Antihypertensives that can be used safely in pregnancy are methyldopa, a calcium channel blocker, and labetalol. ACE inhibitors (such as lisinopril; B) and angiotensin II receptor blockers (such as valsartan; E) are contraindicated in pregnancy. Diuretics (ARBs, such as metolazone; D) and α_1-receptor antagonists (such as doxazosin; A) are not recommended in pregnant patients.

131. A

Proton pump inhibitors (PPIs) should be taken 15–30 minutes before breakfast.

132. C

Sporanox is the brand name for itraconazole. Abilify is the brand name of aripiprazole (A). Diflucan is the brand name of fluconazole (B). Prevacid is the brand name of lansoprazole (D). Aciphex is the brand name of rabeprazole (E).

133. E

Simvastatin plus gemfibrozil is likely to result in myopathy (and possibly rhabdomyolysis). In fact, if a fibric acid derivative must be used with a statin, gemfibrozil should be avoided and fenofibrate should be used alternatively.

134. A

Amiodarone contains iodine and may potentially cause hyper- or hypothyroidism. The other listed medications do not cause hypothyroidism.

135. C

Levaquin (levofloxacin) is a fluoroquinolone.

136. B

Amiodarone-induced pulmonary fibrosis is a potentially life-threatening condition. Therefore, if this adverse effects occurs in a patient taking amiodarone, this antiarrhythmic must be discontinued. Amiodarone undergoes significant

CYP450 metabolism (II) and is a substrate of the CYP3A4 isozyme. It is also an inhibitor of the CYP1A2, CYP2C9, CYP2D6, and CYP3A4 isozymes. Amiodarone is effective for the treatment of both ventricular and atrial arrhythmias (I).

137. E

Aminosalicylates (I), corticosteroids, and immunosuppressants (III) can all be used to treat inflammatory bowel disease. Other drug therapy includes biological agents, such as infliximab, adalimumab, certolizumab, or natalizumab.

138. E

All three of the drugs listed can be used in a 3-drug combination regimen to treat *H. pylori*. A 3-drug combination regimen for *H. pylori* consists of 2 antibiotics and a proton pump inhibitor.

139. B

The maximum daily dose of metformin is 2,550 mg/day. This patient's dose (3,000 mg/day) exceeds this, so the doctor should be contacted. Choice (A) is incorrect because this patient has controlled blood sugars based on A1c less than 7%. The dose of metformin should not be increased (C), because it already exceeds the maximum recommended daily dose. Choice (D) is incorrect because the American Diabetes Association recommends metformin as the drug of choice in newly diagnosed patients with type 2 diabetes and this patient has no contraindications such as heart failure, renal disease, or age greater than 80 years. Lisinopril does not interact with metformin, so choice (E) is incorrect. There truly are no major drug interactions with metformin.

140. B

Choice (B) is the best answer because this patient is taking more than the recommended daily dose of Prilosec OTC: 20 mg daily × 14 days, which can be repeated in 4 months. Mr. Boyd has continued the treatment longer than the recommended 14 days for Prilosec OTC. A multivitamin (II) is not a bad option for any patient in any circumstances; however, Mr. Boyd's complaint of fatigue that he is experiencing is likely due to the symptoms of hypothyroidism.

141. A

Hypothyroidism (I) is the best answer because Mr. Boyd's thyroid-stimulating hormone (TSH) concentration is well out of the normal range (0.3–6 mIU/L). His symptoms are very consistent with hypothyroidism: weakness, fatigue, depression, cold feeling, weight gain. Hypoglycemia (II) is incorrect because he is taking metformin only, which does not cause hypoglycemia in monotherapy. Depression (III) is incorrect because his general depression score (GDS) was not greater than 7 and the hypothyroidism must be ruled out first.

142. D

Choice (D), ACE inhibitors, is the best answer because inhibiting ACE blocks the conversion of angiotensin I to angiotensin II. Angiotensin II is the most potent vasoconstrictor in the body; therefore, decreasing concentrations of angiotensin II results in vasodilation. Choice (A) is incorrect because current literature does not support ACE inhibitors lowering blood sugars. Choice (B) is incorrect because ACE inhibitors do not inhibit renin. Choice (C) is incorrect because ARBs, not ACE inhibitors, block the angiotensin II receptor. Choice (E) is incorrect because ACE inhibitors lead to increased, not decreased, concentrations of bradykinin by preventing its breakdown.

143. B

Mr. Boyd should avoid taking the Synthroid (levothyroxine) with ferrous sulfate, which will bind to the levothyroxine and prevent it from being absorbed. Synthroid does not cause hypoglycemia (A). Taking Synthroid only in the evening (C) is possible, but the patient must be informed not to take it with the ferrous sulfate, so (B) is still the best option. There is no drug interaction with metformin (D), so Mr. Boyd could take the Synthroid at the same time as the metformin. Synthroid should not be taken with dairy products, as the calcium will bind to levothyroxine and prevent it from being absorbed (E).

144. A

There are only four drugs in the nonnucleoside reverse transcriptase inhibitor class, nevirapine, efavirenz, etravirine, and rilpivirine. The brand name of nevirapine is Viramune. Nearly all the protease inhibitors end in "-navir," which leaves the remaining drugs to be nucleoside reverse transcriptase inhibitors (NRTIs). Choice (B), Ziagen (abacavir), is an NRTI. Choice (C), Kaletra (lopinavir/ritonavir), is a protease inhibitor. Choice (D), Videx (didanosine), is an NRTI. Choice (E) Fuzeon (enfuvirtide) is the only fusion inhibitor.

145. D

Patients diagnosed with HIV will need to have a Western blot performed (I); however, starting highly active antiretroviral therapy is not recommended because of the long-term side effects and because some patients' viral load and CD4 rise and drop differently. However, when the CD4 cell count drops to less than 500 cells/mm^3 (II), it is recommended to start therapy. In addition,

if patients have a history of an opportunistic infection regardless of their CD4 cell count (III), antiviral therapy should be initiated as well as treatment for the opportunistic infection.

146. A

Pulmicort Respules (budesonide; I) is the only nebulized inhaled corticosteroid available on the market. Tilade (nedocromil; II) is a mast cell stabilizer and Zyflo (zileuton; III) is a 5-lipoxygenase inhibitor.

147. C

Thrush is a common side effect of inhaled corticosteroids (II). The classic toxicity symptoms for theophylline include tachycardia, nausea, and vomiting, along with a theophylline that exceeds the normal range of 5–15 mcg/mL (I). The metoprolol dose is well within the normal range (III).

148. D

The Advair does not need to be discontinued (A). Thrush must be treated with nystatin and the patient must be counseled to swish and spit after each use of Advair. The patient's nausea is likely due to the theophylline toxicity, and not the aspirin (B). There is not enough information to assess whether the patient is using the albuterol excessively (C). Theophylline should be discontinued due to toxicity symptoms. Metoprolol (E) does not cause tachycardia; it would cause bradycardia.

149. C

Fluticasone and salmeterol combined are called Advair. Fluticasone alone (A) is called Flovent or Flonase. Salmeterol alone (B) is called Serevent and is available only as a dry powder inhaler. Flunisolide alone (D) is the ingredient of Nasarel. There are no combinations of flunisolide and salmeterol (E).

150. E

Fish oil targets triglyceride reduction. It is available over-the-counter and as a prescription product called Lovaza. Lovaza is concentrated fish oil made through a distilling process. Fish oil is thought to inhibit acylCA:1,2 diacylglycerol acyltransferase and to increase hepatic beta-oxidation, causing a reduction in the hepatic synthesis of triglycerides or an increase in plasma lipoprotein lipase activity. Fish oils have only modest effects on the other lipid profiles, so choices (A), (B), (C), and (D) are incorrect.

151. B

The maximum daily dose of acetaminophen is 4,000 mg per day. The patient could potentially take 5,950 mg/day by taking 2 hydrocodone/acetaminophen tablets every 6 hours and the Tylenol 650 mg 3 times daily. Choice (B) is the best option because the pharmacist can easily educate the patient on the 4,000-mg guideline and help develop a plan of administration. There is no need to call the doctor (A); and the patient can have the flexibility to decide if she needs over-the-counter acetaminophen or the combination product with hydrocodone for more severe pain, so choices (C) and (D) are also incorrect. Aspirin is not a good option because she is already taking 325 mg/day of aspirin and this could increase her risk of bleeding.

152. D

Spiriva (tiotropium) and Atrovent (ipratropium) both block the action of acetylcholine at parasympathetic sites at the M3 receptor located on bronchial smooth muscle, causing bronchodilation. Ipratropium is a metered-dose inhaler used 4 times per day and tiotropium is a dry powder inhaler (DPI) administered with the HandiHaler device once daily. DPIs are breath-actuated, lessening the need for hand and breath coordination and allowing for better lung deposition. Tiotropium is longer-acting due to structural differences from ipratropium allowing for higher affinity to the M3 receptor. Ipratropium and tiotropium have virtually the same side effect profile, so (I) is incorrect.

153. D

The active ingredient in Zyban is bupropion. Bupropion is indicated both as an antidepressant and smoking cessation agent. It is not a serotonergic inhibitor (A); as a result, bupropion does not cause sexual dysfunction like most serotonergic antidepressants. Bupropion inhibits both norepinephrine and dopamine; therefore, choices (B) and (C) are incorrect. Effexor (venlafaxine) inhibits serotonin, norepinephrine, and dopamine (E).

154. E

Streptomycin is used only as a substitute for ethambutol and for drug-resistant tuberculosis. The other choices are commonly used in combination for treatment of tuberculosis.

155. D

Vitamin K is used to reverse the anticoagulant effects of warfarin. Protamine is used to reverse the effects of unfractionated heparin (A), and it may be used to partially reverse the effects of low molecular weight heparins, such as enoxaparin (C). Dabigatran (B) does not currently have an antidote. Clopidogrel (E) is an antiplatelet agent and does not have an antidote.

156. A

Flumazenil is the antidote for benzodiazepines. Choice (B) is incorrect because there are several antidotes for opioids, including naloxone, nalmefene, and naltrexone. With ethanol (C), the antidote is fomepizole. The antidote for an overdose of methotrexate (D) is leucovorin. Amifostine is used to prevent nephrotoxicity associated with repeated administration of cisplatin (E).

157. A

Liothyronine is called Cytomel. Levothyroxine (B) has multiple brand name products, including Levothyroid, Levoxyl, Synthroid, Tirosint, and Unithroid. Choice (C) is the natural animal thyroid which is desiccated from pig or cow and is called Armour Thyroid. T4 is the abbreviated name for levothyroxine. TSH (E) is not an active ingredient in any drug.

158. C

ACE inhibitors (ramipril; III) decrease placental blood flow, lower birth weight, cause fetal hypotension, and cause preterm delivery but as a class are not category X drugs. They are pregnancy category D. Finasteride (I) causes abnormalities of external male genitalia; and isotretinoin (II) causes major fetal abnormalities, both internal and external. Both drugs are pregnancy category X.

159. E

Weight gain (I), osteoporosis (II), and pulmonary embolism (III) are all potential side effects of medroxyprogesterone administration and should be discussed with the patient.

160. B

During the initial application, the absorption of transdermal fentanyl requires 12 to 24 hours to reach plateau. The transdermal fentanyl, then, is inappropriate for management of acute pain. Choice (D) is misleading, as the patch needs to be changed every 72 hours.

161. E

For a patient who is taking morphine, it is highly recommended that a stimulant laxative be started to minimize the risk of constipation. Due to possible sedation, it is not recommended that antihistamines or other pain medications be used, as these can add to morphine's sedative effects. Likewise, it is not recommended that the patient drive a motorized vehicle (II). Compliance (III) is important for the treatment of chronic pain so the patient is able to prevent and stay ahead of the pain.

162. D

This question is designed to assess whether you know that choices (A), (B), (C), and (E) are all forms of NSAIDs. NSAIDs inhibit prostaglandins, which normally help to keep the afferent arterioles of the kidneys open. As a result, a recommendation other than acetaminophen (D) could compromise the patient's kidney function.

163. E

A PPD is a tuberculin test for tuberculosis. Tuberculosis results in individuals becoming sensitized to certain antigenic components of the *M. tuberculosis* organism. Healthcare workers (I) are at risk for being exposed to patients with tuberculosis. HIV-infected patients (II) are immunocompromised, which allows for easier inoculation and growth of the organism. Immigrant workers (III) have a higher rate of infection and lack of access to healthcare.

164. C

The doses of morphine (I) and codeine (II) should be reduced to 75% of the normal dose in patients with a creatinine clearance of 10–50 mL/min. When the creatinine clearance is less than 10 mL/min, the doses of these drugs should be reduced by 50%. Morphine has a metabolite, morphine-6-glucuronide, which can accumulate in renal insufficiency. The dose of oxycodone should be adjusted in patients with hepatic dysfunction (III); however, the dose does not need to be adjusted in renal impairment.

165. A

Naproxen's maximum daily dose is 1,250 mg. Other maximum daily doses are: ibuprofen (B), 3,200 mg/day; Relafen (nabumetone; C), 2,000 mg/day; and ketoprofen (D), 300 mg/day. Daypro's (oxaprozin; E) maximum daily dose is 1,200 mg/day in patients who weigh less than 50 kg and 1,800 mg/day in patients who weigh more than 50 kg.

166. D

There are four warning signs for stroke. Of the five answer choices, only sudden seizure for no reason (D) is not considered common with stroke. Regardless, a patient should be rushed to the emergency room for care if a seizure occurred. The four warning signs for stroke (choices A, B, C, and E) are important in helping patients to receive treatment as soon as possible.

167. C

Folic acid is used with methotrexate treatment because methotrexate is a folate antimetabolite that inhibits DNA synthesis. Methotrexate irreversibly binds to dihydrofolate reductase and inhibits the formation of reduced folates. Use of folic acid is important in preparation for pregnancy to prevent neural tube defects. Iron deficiency anemia (III) is a deficiency of iron. Folate deficiency is found in megaloblastic (macrocytic) anemias.

168. E

All three of these side effects are common with ferrous sulfate. It is important to recommend a stool softener and to counsel patients regarding the dark stools and discoloration of urine.

169. E

Cholecalciferol is vitamin D3 and can be used for the treatment of vitamin D deficiency. Pyridoxine (A) is used for vitamin B6 deficiency or acute toxicity from isoniazid. Ascorbic acid (B) is used for prevention and treatment of scurvy and to acidify the urine. Beta-carotene (C) is used for prophylaxis and treatment of polymorphous light eruption, and for erythropoietic protoporphyria. Nicotinic acid (D) is used for dyslipidemias to lower the risk of recurrent myocardial infarction and slow the progression of coronary artery disease.

170. C

One of the problems with treating iron deficiency anemia (IDA) is the side effects associated with treatment. Patients are often unable to tolerate the side effects, which limits the length of therapy. The minimum length of therapy with the lowest rates of relapsing IDA is 6 months.

171. B

The mechanism of action of epoetin alfa is inducing erythropoiesis and releasing reticulocytes, which are immature red blood cells. Choices (A), (C), (D), and (E) are all combinations of other drug mechanisms of actions.

172. E

Pyridoxine is used to prevent neurological toxicities associated with isoniazid therapy. The other options are not used with isoniazid treatment.

173. C

The Drug Enforcement Administration is the organization that is ultimately responsible for controlling and regulating controlled substances. The Federal Drug Association (A) is not a known association. The Food and Drug Administration (B) is in charge of approving drugs for particular indications. The National Provider Indicators (D) is a group that assigns a national provider number to all healthcare professionals. The State Patrol (E) is often called on to arrest or investigate persons involved in drug diversion.

174. C

Choices (A), (B), (D), and (E) are all correct lifestyle modifications for their respective diseases. Choice (C) is incorrect (and thus the correct answer) because the most recent NCEP guidelines recommend only 3 months of lifestyle modifications for the treatment of dyslipidemia.

175. D

Choices (A), (B), and (C) are all correct statements within the Dietary Supplement Health and Education Act of 1994. Choice (D) is not written into that act and has created much debate and controversy; the FDA is considering making a change but, to date, has not.

176. D

Saw palmetto has very few drug interactions. This is important because its prescription counterparts finasteride and dutasteride do interact with warfarin. Choices (A), (B), (C), and (E) all interact with warfarin by increasing INR levels by inhibiting CYP450 enzymes 1A2, 2D6, and 3A4. These herbal products may also increase the risk of bleeding when used with antiplatelet drugs, such as aspirin.

177. D

Robitussin DM contains dextromethorphan and guaifenesin for suppressing cough and thinning mucus; this is the best answer, as it does not involve treating any other symptoms. Robitussin AC contains guaifenesin to enhance mucus thinning and codeine to suppress the cough. The active ingredient in Robitussin (A) is guaifenesin for thinning the mucus. In Robitussin CF (B), the active ingredients are guaifenesin, dextromethorphan, and phenylephrine for cough, mucus, and congestion, respectively. Robitussin DAC (C) contains guaifenesin, pseudoephedrine, and codeine for mucus, congestion, and cough, respectively. Robitussin PE (E) contains guaifenesin and pseudoephedrine for mucus and congestion.

178. D

The most modern insulin pumps have basal insulin rates that typically run for 24 hours per day, providing a small amount of continuous insulin. Insulin-to-carbohydrate ratio settings are used for bolus injections during carbohydrate intake, and insulin sensitivity factor settings are used for elevated blood sugars that are not related to food intake. The goal blood sugar setting is used to determine how tightly controlled the patient should be. The rule of 1,800 is used to determine the insulin sensitivity factor but is not within the insulin pump, so choice (D) is an incorrect statement and is thus the correct answer.

179. A

It has been suggested that vitamin E has several benefits, including serving as an antioxidant and preventing Alzheimer's disease. However, a recent meta-analysis suggests that doses greater than 400 IU can increase the risk for cardiovascular events.

180. E

Trissel's provides a compilation of all currently available stability information on drugs in compounded oral, enteral, topical, and ophthalmic formulations. Goodman and Gilman (A) focuses on drug pharmacology. Martindale (B) is a comprehensive drug list in which the first volume contains the preface and the drug monographs, and the second volume holds all proprietary preparations as well as manufacturer's contact information. It is also known to include foreign drugs. The Merck Index (C) focuses on precise, comprehensive information on chemicals, drugs, and biologicals, whereas the Merck Manual focuses on diseases. Remington (D) is considered the pharmacy encyclopedia for pharmacology, theoretical science, sterilization, and practical pharmacy practice.

181. E

All three options provide solubility data on potassium gluconate. USP-NF (II) has official monographs for drug structure, solubilities, assays, and therapeutic category, but provides limited information on dosage and dosage forms. The other two options are described in the previous question.

182. B

Ferrous sulfate 5 grain (B) is equivalent to 325 mg and is available on the market. The metformin dosage form in choice (A) does not exist. Synthroid's highest dosage form (C) is 300 mcg; however, a 212 mcg tablet is not available. Boniva 3.5 mg (D) is not available; however, Boniva is available in once-daily dosing at 2.5 mg/day. Lisinopril's highest dosage form (E) is 40 mg.

183. B

Simvastatin is half as potent as Lipitor (atorvastatin), so simvastatin 20 mg is the correct answer. Rosuvastatin (A) is twice as potent as Lipitor (atorvastatin). Pravastatin (C) is one-fourth as potent at atorvastatin and would require 40 mg to be equivalent.

184. D

St. John's wort is commonly used by patients for mild to moderate depression. However, it is associated with numerous drug interactions. It is a strong inducer of the CYP3A4 enzyme. Warfarin is metabolized by 3A4; therefore, concomitant use with St. John Wort may lead to a reduction in warfarin concentrations, which may place a patient at risk for thromboembolic events. Sertraline interacts with St. John's wort because both inhibit the reuptake of serotonin, which could result in serotonin syndrome. Pravachol is the only statin not metabolized by 3A4; in fact, pravastatin is not metabolized at all via the CYP450 enzyme system.

185. C

This is a classic NAPLEX question which guides you to assess each complaint of the patient. There is no need to overtreat with an unneeded medication such as pseudoephedrine (III); the patient is not experiencing any congestion. Diphenhydramine (I) is used for the runny nose and sneezing, and the acetaminophen (II) is for the pain of the headache. Thus, options (I) and (II) are appropriate, making choice (C) correct.

Part Six

Appendix

Appendix

As the number of prescription medications continues to grow, it becomes increasingly challenging for pharmacists to remain familiar with brand and generic names of medications. Although it is unrealistic to memorize ALL of the medication names, it is essential that a new graduate know both trade and generic names for the most commonly prescribed medicines, better known as the Top 200. These lists represent the 200 medications (brand name and generic) that have been prescribed the most in the previous year.

When studying for the NAPLEX, focusing on these drugs will best prepare you for passing the exam. You will also find references to the lists throughout the chapters in the drug charts.

TOP 200 GENERIC DRUGS BY RETAIL DOLLARS IN 2010

Rank	Product	Total $ (add 000)
1	Hydrocodone/APAP	1,905,254,710
2	Metoprolol succinate	1,340,685,817
3	Oxycodone	1,260,137,537
4	Pantoprazole	1,196,298,685
5	Omeprazole	1,179,816,419
6	Simvastatin	1,113,234,642
7	Amphetmn salt cmb SR	979,431,270
8	Fentanyl transdermal	940,979,500
9	Azithromycin	912,237,755
10	Valacyclovir HCl	886,255,653
11	Venlafaxine ER	860,082,136
12	Fexofenadine	824,482,761
13	Gabapentin	822,839,898
14	Oxycodone/APAP	797,300,459
15	Lisinopril	731,417,174
16	Amlodipine besy benz	714,057,509
17	Lansoprazole	694,089,570
18	Levothyroxine	668,318,209
19	Amoxicillin/pot clav	648,733,127
20	Amlodipine besylate	648,185,657
21	Fluticasone nasal	624,590,284
22	Alprazolam	601,961,332
23	Tamsulosin HCl	548,989,018
24	Budesonide	510,329,993
25	Metformin	487,759,686
26	Sertraline	474,677,637
27	Bupropion XL	442,339,222
28	Cefdinir	439,789,169
29	Losartan potassium	427,556,384
30	Risperidone	426,937,649
31	Pravastatin	415,350,309
32	Amoxicillin	415,108,501
33	Divalproex sodium	411,529,273
34	Claravis	404,570,166
35	Fluoxetine	399,936,629
36	Zolpidem tartrate	372,412,773
37	Lamotrigine	335,760,945
38	Topiramate	332,745,008
39	Lovastatin	324,822,601
40	Diltiazem CD	319,504,507
41	Tramadol	317,207,557
42	Levetiracetam	314,504,640
43	Lisinopril/HCTZ	306,352,972
44	Citalopram HBR	304,034,022
45	Lorazepam	302,154,620
46	Warfarin	298,115,197
47	Losartan pot/HCTZ	296,878,086
48	Ocella	295,060,506
49	Clonazepam	291,691,543
50	Alendronate	288,712,684
51	Hydrochlorothiazide	279,221,916
52	Sumatriptan oral	277,945,390
53	Pramipexole dihydroc	273,806,463
54	Carvedilol	273,201,303
55	Fentanyl citrate buc	272,968,602
56	Amphetmn salt cmb	272,442,314
57	Budeprion XL	269,290,045
58	Metoprolol tartrate	262,779,417
59	Atenolol	260,373,570
60	Enoxaparin sodium	258,771,534
61	Fenofibrate	256,917,818
62	Paroxetine	237,014,049
63	Cephalexin	229,749,016
64	Finasteride	226,400,919
65	Metaxalone	226,373,763
66	Imiquimod	224,879,615
67	Tacrolimus	224,362,039
68	Cyclobenzaprine	223,823,780
69	Oxcarbazepine	219,885,021
70	Furosemide oral	214,725,901

Rank	Product	Total $ (add 000)
71	Endocet	211,851,753
72	Bupropion SR	208,158,151
73	Ondansetron	207,624,430
74	Nifedipine ER	205,112,357
75	Ibuprofen	203,472,727
76	Albuterol ncb soln	198,381,136
77	Carisoprodol	196,949,818
78	Oxycodone HCl CR	194,180,431
79	Fexofenadine/pseudo	193,189,010
80	Oxybutynin chlor ER	191,413,895
81	Ranitidine HCl	186,176,175
82	Famciclovir	182,172,076
83	Ciprofloxacin HCl	181,746,681
84	Morphine sulfate ER	180,918,620
85	Clonidine	177,574,869
86	Potassium chloride ER	177,481,424
87	Propoxyphn-N/APAP	171,307,540
88	Meloxicam	171,259,657
89	Klor-Con	170,964,548
90	Ramipril	168,459,754
91	Phentermine	167,256,528
92	Venlafaxine	164,404,394
93	Trimethoprim/Sulfa	163,631,746
94	Gianvi	161,934,752
95	Spironolactone	161,175,844
96	Temazepam	160,675,553
97	Trazodone HCl	160,552,578
98	Dorzlmide HCl/timolol	159,752,720
99	Potassium chloride	158,051,496
100	Mycophenlt mofetil	152,522,252
101	Diclofenac sodium SR	150,496,459
102	Prednisone oral	147,999,196
103	Triamterene/HCTZ	144,428,614
104	Bupropion ER	142,767,101
105	Naproxen	142,146,043

Rank	Product	Total $ (add 000)
106	Verapamil SR	138,652,790
107	Polyethylene glycol	136,775,971
108	Hydroxyzine	136,297,885
109	Diazepam	135,729,840
110	Clindamycin systemic	135,328,948
111	Isosorbide mononitrt	134,716,417
112	Ropinirole HCl	130,990,993
113	Acetaminophen/cod	130,156,059
114	Paroxetine SR	129,367,553
115	Felodipine ER	128,196,910
116	Fluconazole	127,763,760
117	Clobetasol	127,541,918
118	Enalapril	125,921,689
119	Metformin HCl ER	125,219,280
120	Promethazine tabs	124,479,395
121	Gemfibrozil	124,200,848
122	Glyburide	122,512,299
123	Tri-Sprintec	119,544,940
124	Clozapine	119,370,755
125	Nabumetone	116,505,668
126	Dronabinol	115,489,173
127	Glimepiride	115,040,445
128	Morphine sulfate CR	113,134,785
129	Mirtazapine	112,982,564
130	Mupirocin	112,637,784
131	Doxycycline	109,345,186
132	Methadn HCl non-inj	108,627,673
133	Minocycline	108,018,438
134	Desoximetasone	108,014,040
135	Methylprednsln tabs	107,568,894
136	Albuterol sulfate/iprat	107,221,166
137	Allopurinol	105,860,532
138	Buspirone HCl	101,413,132
139	Desmopressin acetate	101,284,138
140	Tobramycin/dex ophth	100,681,493

Rank	Product	Total $ (add 000)
141	Tretinoin	99,198,822
142	Tramadol HCl/APAP	98,978,415
143	Phenytoin sodium ext	98,813,913
144	Tizanidine HCl	98,132,116
145	Acyclovir	97,124,649
146	Clarithromycin	96,973,448
147	Amitriptyline	96,716,554
148	Nitrofrntoin mono mcr	95,190,283
149	Glyburide/metfrm HCl	94,994,936
150	Carbidopa/levodopa	91,535,681
151	Hydralazine	90,330,872
152	Sumatriptan stat refill	89,887,484
153	Benazepril	89,865,072
154	Calcium acetate	89,817,705
155	Hydromorphone HCl	89,525,003
156	Aviane	88,730,876
157	Triamcinolone acet top	85,235,370
158	Clotrimazl/betamthsn	84,172,212
159	Dextroamphetmn sulf	83,451,462
160	Calcitriol	83,053,496
161	Nitroglycerin	82,306,630
162	Methotrexate	81,603,353
163	Meclizine HCl	81,296,929
164	Diltiazem	79,515,296
165	Quinapril	79,350,650
166	Ursodiol	78,315,826
167	Ketoconazole topical	77,028,101
168	Fluorouracil	76,157,984
169	Trinessa	75,785,304
170	Nystatin systemic	74,709,149
171	Nifedical XL	74,566,965
172	Glipizide ER	74,125,685
173	Terbinafine HCl	73,812,292
174	Cefprozil	73,403,080
175	Benzonatate	73,396,360

Rank	Product	Total $ (add 000)
176	Clindmycn/benz perox	73,026,312
177	Ondansetron ODT	72,467,758
178	Propranolol HCl	71,989,592
179	Famotidine	71,661,385
180	Nifedipine	70,911,933
181	Medrxyprgesterone inj	70,782,904
182	Colchicine	69,832,163
183	Penicillin VK	68,142,458
184	Digoxin	67,815,713
185	Hydrocodone/ibuprof	66,921,611
186	Promethazine/cod	66,704,399
187	Anastrozole	66,519,296
188	Folic acid	66,333,196
189	Butalbital/APAP/caf	66,039,254
190	Hydroxychloroquine	65,986,315
191	Galantmn hydrobrom	65,953,604
192	Terazosin	65,088,560
193	Labetalol	63,863,408
194	Glipizide	63,804,778
195	Clindamycin topical	63,148,011
196	Baclofen	62,082,676
197	Tramadol HCl ER	60,851,753
198	Etodolac	60,803,978
199	Donepezil	59,802,828
200	Testosterone cypionate	59,281,380

Source: Drug Topics, June 2011

TOP 200 NAME BRAND DRUGS BY UNITS IN 2010

Rank	Product	Total Rxs (add 000)
1	Lipitor	37,523,566
2	Nexium	25,872,311
3	Plavix	25,000,508
4	Singulair	24,666,972
5	Lexapro	23,000,456
6	Crestor	20,945,607
7	Synthroid	20,272,359
8	ProAir HFA	18,616,827
9	Advair Diskus	16,580,931
10	Cymbalta	14,591,949
11	Diovan	14,360,575
12	Ventolin HFA	13,523,514
13	Diovan HCT	11,480,540
14	Actos	11,193,068
15	Seroquel	10,260,420
16	Levaquin	9,322,197
17	Lantus	8,960,452
18	Nasonex	8,834,010
19	Viagra	8,829,457
20	Lyrica	8,714,215
21	Celebrex	8,643,515
22	Concerta	7,949,409
23	Spiriva	7,738,168
24	Premarin tabs	7,691,197
25	Effexor XR	7,603,949
26	Tricor	7,588,438
27	Zetia	7,398,986
28	Vytorin	7,165,747
29	OxyContin	6,869,557
30	Abilify	6,799,343
31	Loestrin 24 Fe	6,693,687
32	Vyvanse	6,604,632
33	Cialis	6,584,896
34	Suboxone	6,476,241
35	Aricept	6,252,862

Rank	Product	Total Rxs (add 000)
36	Benicar	6,098,994
37	Januvia	5,919,456
38	Lunesta	5,714,739
39	Ambien CR	5,687,633
40	Niaspan	5,618,908
41	Xalatan	5,516,848
42	Levoxyl	5,452,741
43	Benicar HCT	5,215,681
44	Flovent HFA	5,047,632
45	NuvaRing	4,756,490
46	Lovaza	4,583,660
47	Yaz	4,567,146
48	NovoLog	4,443,860
49	Combivent	4,270,924
50	Namenda	4,193,637
51	Detrol LA	4,160,847
52	Ortho Tri-Cyclen Lo	4,157,693
53	Lantus SoloSTAR	4,035,957
54	Proventil HFA	3,952,848
55	Aciphex	3,897,030
56	Avapro	3,811,895
57	Bystolic	3,666,287
58	Adderall XR	3,625,997
59	Symbicort	3,618,811
60	Zyprexa	3,616,933
61	Trilipix	3,608,974
62	Boniva	3,524,839
63	Avodart	3,466,894
64	Glipizide XL	3,423,438
65	Pristiq	3,412,354
66	Lidoderm	3,402,179
67	Humalog	3,343,036
68	Vigamox	3,327,763
69	Evista	3,296,079
70	Flomax	3,132,677

Rank	Product	Total Rxs (add 000)
71	Chantix	2,980,917
72	Avalide	2,879,195
73	Protonix	2,848,122
74	Cozaar	2,837,637
75	Vivelle-DOT	2,832,173
76	Vesicare	2,814,667
77	Prempro	2,702,035
78	Avelox	2,693,235
79	Dexilant/Kapidex	2,675,863
80	Focalin XR	2,667,245
81	Strattera	2,606,700
82	Xopenex HFA	2,584,196
83	Actonel	2,558,636
84	Travatan Z	2,543,583
85	Levemir	2,535,211
86	Lumigan	2,518,408
87	Apri	2,394,198
88	Levitra	2,359,725
89	Geodon oral	2,332,901
90	Micardis	2,324,180
91	Exforge	2,267,437
92	Coumadin tabs	2,248,254
93	Janumet	2,245,817
94	Ciprodex otic	2,204,258
95	Valtrex	2,180,482
96	Restasis	2,156,415
97	Seroquel XR	2,101,144
98	Micardis HCT	2,088,803
99	Actonel 150	2,045,479
100	Lotrel	2,041,615
101	Tussionex	2,024,442
102	Prometrium	1,989,773
103	AndroGel	1,969,279
104	Kariva	1,967,203
105	Patanol	1,960,988

Rank	Product	Total Rxs (add 000)
106	Voltaren gel	1,931,594
107	Hyzaar	1,899,131
108	Thyroid, Armour	1,893,236
109	Nasacort AQ	1,807,665
110	Coreg CR	1,782,976
111	Qvar	1,781,072
112	Pataday	1,755,473
113	Xyzal	1,747,745
114	Humulin N	1,715,002
115	Vagifem	1,650,317
116	Toprol XL	1,650,078
117	Byetta	1,638,475
118	NovoLog Mix 70/30	1,633,160
119	Veramyst	1,584,391
120	Azor	1,562,043
121	Caduet	1,561,704
122	Welchol	1,560,389
123	Actoplus Met	1,531,222
124	Provigil	1,517,573
125	EpiPen	1,512,146
126	Aggrenox	1,497,553
127	Dilantin	1,475,541
128	Enablex	1,466,634
129	Alphagan P	1,461,043
130	Premarin vaginal	1,452,843
131	Xopenex	1,444,380
132	Uroxatral	1,419,250
133	Asmanex	1,412,419
134	Prevacid SoluTab	1,393,708
135	Moviprep	1,363,832
136	Avandia	1,345,507
137	Tekturna	1,321,901
138	Propecia	1,319,959
139	Ortho Evra	1,312,634
140	Solodyn	1,311,733

Rank	Product	Total Rxs (add 000)
141	Humulin 70/30	1,298,395
142	Lanoxin	1,265,185
143	Asacol	1,258,480
144	Prevacid	1,248,021
145	Atacand	1,238,609
146	Nitrostat	1,220,125
147	Combigan	1,169,315
148	Halflytely bwl prep	1,128,414
149	Relpax	1,113,336
150	Novolin 70/30	1,106,168
151	Femara	1,098,445
152	Tamiflu	1,094,916
153	Zovirax topical	1,075,542
154	Lovenox	1,057,051
155	Zymar	1,055,235
156	Maxalt	1,028,658
157	Estrace vaginal	1,024,694
158	Exelon Patch	1,008,200
159	Intuniv	983,113
160	Allegra-D 24 Hour	975,833
161	Astepro 0.15%	955,880
162	Maxalt MLT	949,328
163	Arimidex	946,656
164	Amitiza	941,191
165	Doryx	939,008
166	Differin	913,676
167	Clarinex	906,614
168	Lotemax	905,561
169	Astelin	896,918
170	Transderm-Scop	883,269
171	Humulin R	878,274
172	Levothroid	869,398
173	Advair HFA	868,420
174	Truvada	866,743
175	Nuvigil	852,695

Rank	Product	Total Rxs (add 000)
176	SF 5000 Plus	838,699
177	Yasmin 28	837,743
178	Bactroban	824,689
179	Ranexa	816,279
180	Metadate CD	810,541
181	Lamictal	801,627
182	Atrovent HFA	800,659
183	Simcor	800,564
184	Opana ER	794,188
185	Rhinocort Aqua	774,768
186	Humalog Mix 75/25 Pen	769,785
187	Carafate	764,966
188	Norvir	762,060
189	Aspir-Low	760,731
190	BenzaClin	759,929
191	Skelaxin	759,046
192	Duac Care System	755,382
193	Wellbutrin XL	753,516
194	Arthrotec	752,560
195	Epiduo	742,395
196	Pulmicort Flexhaler	735,413
197	Omnaris	734,773
198	Ortho Tri-Cyclen	732,714
199	Prandin	726,766
200	Nevanac	725,667

Source: Drug Topics, June 2011

INDEX

A

Abortive treatment options, 164
Absence seizures, 149
Absorption, 452
Absorption barriers, 440–441
Accreditation, 540
ACE (angiotensin-converting enzyme) inhibitors
  heart failure, 21, 23, 46
  hypertension, 8
  ischemic heart disease, 39, 41
  MI prevention, 42
  patient education, 13, 28
Acetic acids
  osteoarthritis, 262
  pain management, 289
Acetylation, 449
Acne
  definitions, 323
  diagnosis, 323
  drug storage/administration, 327
  guidelines, 324
  learning points, 331, 344
  medication charts, 325–326
  patient education, 327
  signs/symptoms, 323
ACS (acute coronary syndrome), 37
Activated charcoal, 337
Active transport, 438–439
Acute coronary syndrome (ACS), 37
Acute lymphocytic leukemia (ALL), 196–197
Acute mania, 240, 241
Acute myeloid leukemia (AML), 196–197
Acute pain management, 285
Acute poisoning, 336–338
Addison's disease, 128
Adjunctive therapy, 265
Adverse drug reaction
  chemotherapy agents, 211
  decongestants, 389
  hormonal imbalance, 349
  resources, 525
AEDs. *See* Anti-epileptic drugs
Aldosterone receptor antagonists (ARAs)
  heart failure, 21, 42
  medication charts, 25

  MI prevention, 42
  patient education, 28
ALL (acute lymphocytic leukemia), 196–197
Allergic rhinitis, 392, 393
Allergy tuberculosis testing, 432
Alligation, 479–480
Allogenic HSCT, 197
Alpha agonists, 368
Alpha antagonists, 367, 369
α_2-agonists
  medication chart, 302
  POAG, 300, 302
α_2-receptor agonists
  medication chart, 11
  patient education, 13
α_1-receptor antagonists
  medication chart, 11
  patient education, 13
Alzheimer's disease
  definition, 252
  diagnosis, 252
  drug storage/administration, 256
  guidelines, 252–253
  patient education, 256
  signs/symptoms, 252
Ambulatory pneumonia, 56
Amenorrhea, 135
American College of Cardiology, staging system, 21
American College of Physicians, asthma
  guidelines, 110
American Diabetes Association (ADA),
  guidelines, 120
American Heart Association, staging system, 21
Aminoglycosides, 80
Aminosalicylates, 184, 190
AML (acute myeloid leukemia), 196–197
Amorphous solids, 417
Amphotericin B, 92
Anaerobes, 98
Analgesic therapy
  STEMI, 41
  UA/NSTEMI, 38–39
Analgesics
  adjuncts medication chart, 295
  migraine headaches, 164
Anemia. *See* Hematologic disorders

Total parenteral nutrition (TPN), 487
Traditional release oral products, 420–422
Transdermal contraceptives, 354
Transdermal delivery, 433
Transfusion, 310
Trapezoidal rule, 460
Treatment naive patients, 61, 62
Triglycerides (TG), 13
   classification, 14
Tuberculosis
   allergy tuberculosis testing, 432
   definitions, 69
   diagnosis, 69
   drug storage/administration, 74
   guidelines, 70–71
   learning points, 74
   medication charts, 71–73
   patient education, 74
   signs/symptoms, 70
Tubular reabsorption, 450, 452
Tubular secretion, 450
Two-compartment model, 456
Typical antipsychotics, 245–247
Tyrosine kinase inhibitors, 197, 213–214

U

Ulcerative colitis (UC)
   clinical findings, 181
   definitions, 181
   non-pharmacologic therapy, 182
   pharmacologic therapy, 183
   severity, 182
   symptoms, 181
Ultrafiltration/hemofiltration, 313
Ultrasound, 433
Unstable angina (UA)
   definition, 37
   pharmacologic management, 38–40
Urea breath test, 173
Urethral suppositories, 428
Urge incontinence, 367. *See also* Urinary incontinence
Urinary incontinence
   definition, 366
   diagnosis, 366
   drug storage/administration, 370
   guidelines, 367
   medication charts, 368–369

   patient education, 370
   signs/symptoms, 366–367
   treatment recommendations, 367
Urinary tract infection (UTI)
   common organisms, 52
   diagnosis, 52
   guidelines, 53–54
   signs/symptoms, 53
Urologic disorders
   erectile dysfunction, 362–366
   learning points, 370
   urinary incontinence, 366–370

V

Vaginal dosing, 428
Vancomycin, 88
Varicella-zoster virus, 95
Vasodilators
   heart failure, 27
   storage/administration, 28
VEGF inhibitors, 213–214
Viscosity, 418
Volume (of distribution), 460
Vomiting, 214

W

Wagner-Nelson method, 462
Warfarin (Coumadin), 35
Water-soluble ointment base, 427
Weak acids/bases, 415
White clot, 37
Whole-bowel irrigation, 338
Women's Health Initiative (WHI), 358

X

Xarelto (rivarozaban), 36